Osteosarcopenia

Osteosarcopenia

Edited by

Gustavo Duque
Chair of Medicine and Director, Australian Institute for Musculoskeletal Science (AIMSS), The University of Melbourne and Western Health, St Albans, VIC, Australia

Bruce R. Troen
Professor and Chief, Division of Geriatrics and Palliative Medicine; Director, Center for Successful Aging; Director, Center of Excellence for Alzheimer's Disease; Jacobs School of Medicine and Biomedical Sciences, University at Buffalo;
Physician-Investigator, Geriatrics and Extended Care and Research Service, Veterans Affairs Western New York Healthcare System, Buffalo, NY, United States

ELSEVIER

Elsevier
Radarweg 29, PO Box 211, 1000 AE Amsterdam, Netherlands
The Boulevard, Langford Lane, Kidlington, Oxford OX5 1GB, United Kingdom
50 Hampshire Street, 5th Floor, Cambridge, MA 02139, United States

Notices
Knowledge and best practice in this field are constantly changing. As new research and experience broaden our understanding, changes in research methods, professional practices, or medical treatment may become necessary.

Practitioners and researchers must always rely on their own experience and knowledge in evaluating and using any information, methods, compounds, or experiments described herein. In using such information or methods they should be mindful of their own safety and the safety of others, including parties for whom they have a professional responsibility.

To the fullest extent of the law, neither the Publisher nor the authors, contributors, or editors, assume any liability for any injury and/or damage to persons or property as a matter of products liability, negligence or otherwise, or from any use or operation of any methods, products, instructions, or ideas contained in the material herein.

ISBN: 978-0-12-820088-9

Publisher: Stacy Masucci
Acquisitions Editor: Ana Claudia A. Garcia
Editorial Project Manager: Timothy Bennett
Production Project Manager: Niranjan Bhaskaran
Cover Designer: Miles Hitchen

Typeset by STRAIVE, India

Dedication

To the most wonderful women in my life—my mother Rubiela and my aunts Olga, Alba, and Fabiola—for providing me with the strength and support during the most challenging and also during the happiest times, and to God—the Great Architect of everything that is described in this book.

—Gustavo Duque

To my wife Suzanne and my sons Ben and Eli, for your unerring and continued support in my professional and personal endeavors.

—Bruce R. Troen

Contents

Contributors

Numbers in parentheses indicate the pages on which the authors' contributions begin.

Kate Anderson (287), Deakin University, School of Health and Social Development; Institute for Health Transformation, Deakin University, Geelong, VIC, Australia

Rahul D. Barmanray (117), Department of Medicine, The University of Melbourne; Department of Diabetes & Endocrinology, The Royal Melbourne Hospital, Parkville, VIC, Australia

Alison Beauchamp (287), Department of Medicine-Western Health, University of Melbourne; Australian Institute for Musculoskeletal Science (AIMSS), University of Melbourne and Western Health, St Albans; School of Rural Health, Monash University, Warragul, VIC, Australia

Dario Boschiero (161), Biotekna®, Marcon-Venice, Venice, Italy

Sharon L. Brennan-Olsen (287), Deakin University, School of Health and Social Development, Geelong; Department of Medicine-Western Health, University of Melbourne; Australian Institute for Musculoskeletal Science (AIMSS), University of Melbourne and Western Health, St Albans; Institute for Health Transformation, Deakin University, Geelong, VIC, Australia

Cathleen Colón-Emeric (147), Geriatrics Division, Department of Medicine, Duke University; Durham VA Geriatric Research Education and Clinical Center, Durham, NC, United States

Natanael Perez Cordero (51), School of Medicine, Universidad Central del Caribe, Bayamon, PR, United States

Selma Cvijetic (161), Institute for Medical Research and Occupational Health, Zagreb, Croatia

Andrea L. Darling (133), Department of Nutrition, Food and Exercise Sciences, School of Biosciences and Medicine, Faculty of Health and Medical Sciences, University of Surrey, Guildford, United Kingdom

Larry Dian (307), Division of Geriatrics; Center for Hip Health and Mobility, Faculty of Medicine, University of British Columbia, Vancouver, BC, Canada

Rachel L. Duckham (287), Department of Medicine-Western Health, University of Melbourne; Australian Institute for Musculoskeletal Science (AIMSS), University of Melbourne and Western Health, St Albans; Institute for Physical Activity and Nutrition (IPAN), Deakin University, Geelong, VIC, Australia

Gustavo Duque (275), Australian Institute for Musculoskeletal Science (AIMSS), The University of Melbourne and Western Health; Department of Medicine-Western Health, The University of Melbourne, St. Albans, VIC, Australia

Joshua N. Farr (19), Division of Endocrinology; Robert and Arlene Kogod Center on Aging; Division of Physiology and Biomedical Engineering, Mayo Clinic College of Medicine, Mayo Clinic, Rochester, MN, United States

Jack Feehan (275), Australian Institute for Musculoskeletal Science (AIMSS), The University of Melbourne and Western Health; Department of Medicine-Western Health, The University of Melbourne, St. Albans, VIC, Australia

Sadanand Fulzele (51), Department of Cell Biology and Anatomy; Department of Orthopedics; Departments of Medicine; Center for Healthy Aging, Augusta University, Augusta, GA, United States

Ali Ghasem-Zadeh (205), Endocrinology and Medicine, Austin Health, The University of Melbourne, Heidelberg, VIC, Australia

Jennifer C. Gilman (161), Independent Writer, Conroe, TX, United States

Ebrahim Bani Hassan (205), Department of Medicine, Western Health and Australian Institute for Musculoskeletal Science (AIMSS), The University of Melbourne, Melbourne, VIC, Australia

William D. Hill (51), Center for Healthy Aging, Augusta University, Augusta, GA; Department of Pathology and Laboratory Medicine, Medical University of South Carolina, Charleston, SC; Ralph H. Johnson Veterans Affairs Medical Center, Charleston, SC, United States

Eisuke Hiruma (1), Department of Sport and Medical Science, Teikyo University, Tokyo, Japan

Yushu Huang (91), Brandeis University, Waltham, MA, United States

Jasminka Z. Ilich (161), Florida State University, Tallahassee, FL, United States

Mahdi Imani (205), Department of Medicine, Western Health and Australian Institute for Musculoskeletal Science (AIMSS); Faculty of Medicine, Dentistry and Health Sciences, The University of Melbourne, Melbourne, VIC, Australia

David Karasik (217), The Azrieli Faculty of Medicine, Bar-Ilan University, Safed, Israel; Marcus Institute for Aging Research, Hebrew SeniorLife, Boston, MA, United States

Japneet Kaur (19), Division of Endocrinology; Robert and Arlene Kogod Center on Aging, Mayo Clinic College of Medicine, Mayo Clinic, Rochester, MN, United States

Owen J. Kelly (161), Sam Houston State University College of Osteopathic Medicine, Conroe, TX, United States

Iryna Khrystoforova (217), The Azrieli Faculty of Medicine, Bar-Ilan University, Safed, Israel

Peter Lee (39), Department of Biomedical Engineering, Faculty of Engineering and Information Technology, The University of Melbourne, Melbourne, VIC, Australia

Sean X. Leng (91), Division of Geriatric Medicine & Gerontology, Department of Medicine, Johns Hopkins University School of Medicine, Baltimore, MD, United States

Yukang Li (91), Division of Geriatric Medicine & Gerontology, Department of Medicine, Johns Hopkins University School of Medicine, Baltimore, MD, United States

Ching-Ti Liu (217), Department of Biostatistics, Boston University School of Public Health, Boston, MA, United States

Brian Alexander MacDonald (239), Division of Geriatrics and Palliative Medicine, Jacobs School of Medicine and Biomedical Sciences, University at Buffalo and Research Service, Veterans Affairs Western New York Healthcare System, Buffalo, NY, United States

Fatemeh Malekipour (39), Department of Biomedical Engineering, Faculty of Engineering and Information Technology, The University of Melbourne, Melbourne, VIC, Australia

Hossein Mokhtarzadeh (39), Department of Biomedical Engineering, Faculty of Engineering and Information Technology, The University of Melbourne, Melbourne, VIC, Australia

Ahmed M. Negm (181), GERAS Centre for Aging Research, St Peter's Hospital, Hamilton, ON; Department of Surgery, University of Calgary, Calgary, AB, Canada

Jordan O'Connor (287), Federation University, School of Health and Life Science, Ballarat, VIC, Australia

Alexandra Papaioannou (181), GERAS Centre for Aging Research, St Peter's Hospital; Division of Geriatric Medicine, McMaster University, Hamilton, ON, Canada

Naaz Parmar (307), Division of Geriatrics, Faculty of Medicine, University of British Columbia; Pacific Geriatricians Group, Vancouver, BC, Canada

Patricia V. Schoenlein (51), Department of Cell Biology and Anatomy, Augusta University, Augusta, GA, United States

Kenneth Ladd Seldeen (239), Division of Geriatrics and Palliative Medicine, Jacobs School of Medicine and Biomedical Sciences, University at Buffalo and Research Service, Veterans Affairs Western New York Healthcare System, Buffalo, NY, United States

Neema Sharda (147), Geriatrics Division, Department of Medicine, Duke University, Durham, NC, United States

Charikleia Stefanaki (77), University Research Institute of Maternal and Child Health & Precision Medicine; UNESCO Chair on Adolescent Health Care, National and Kapodistrian University of Athens, "Aghia Sophia" Children's Hospital; Unit of Endocrinology, Diabetes mellitus, and Metabolism, School of Medicine, National and Kapodistrian University of Athens, Aretaieion Hospital, Athens, Greece

Bruce Robert Troen (239), Division of Geriatrics and Palliative Medicine, Jacobs School of Medicine and Biomedical Sciences, University at Buffalo and Research Service, Veterans Affairs Western New York Healthcare System, Buffalo, NY, United States

Debra L. Waters (255), Department of Medicine and School of Physiotherapy, University of Otago, Dunedin, New Zealand

Christopher J. Yates (117), Department of Medicine, The University of Melbourne; Department of Diabetes & Endocrinology, The Royal Melbourne Hospital, Parkville, VIC, Australia

Foreword

Over the last 5years, osteosarcopenia has included itself among the giants of geriatrics. In 1965, Professor Bernard Isaacs described the major syndromes in older persons, which he designated the "geriatric giants." The syndromes that he considered made up these giants were immobility, instability, falls, incontinence, and cognitive dysfunction. He believed in the importance of defining these syndromes because although geriatricians know they are specialists they are uncertain of what they specialize in.

In 2016/2017, at Saint Louis University, we suggested that a new set of syndromes would be more appropriate as "geriatric giants" in the 21st century. We suggested that these modern giants should be frailty, sarcopenia, anorexia of aging, and cognitive dysfunction. We developed simple screening tests, i.e., FRAIL, SARC-F, SNAQ, and RCS (rapid cognitive screen) to make it simple for primary healthcare professionals to screen for these syndromes. We stressed that early recognition of these syndromes would allow primary and secondary prevention, thus reducing the likelihood of the development of disability.

In 2017, the John A. Hartford Foundation stated that the competencies of geriatric medicine were changing and suggested replacing the "geriatric giants" with the five Ms. of geriatrics. They suggested that the core competencies of geriatrics should be mind, mobility, medications, multicomplexity, and what matters most to the older person. They believed that these should be screened for regularly to adopt an age-friendly approach to older persons.

Osteoporosis, which occurs in more than 200 million persons worldwide, has always been a giant of endocrinology alongside diabetes mellitus. Roubenoff suggested that sarcopenia increases the risk of fractures in those with osteoporosis. In 2015, Binkley and Buehring suggested that the term "sarco-osteopenia" should be introduced to recognize the increased risk of fractures in persons who have both osteoporosis and sarcopenia. Duque and his group, among others, have utilized the term "osteosarcopenia" and demonstrated that it is a major risk factor for multiple adverse outcomes.

This book provides a compilation of the pathophysiology, clinical features, and management of osteosarcopenia. There is recognition that many of the factors that cause osteoporosis also play a role in muscle loss. It is also recognized that bone-muscle communication and vice versa is a key component of physiology. The book highlights the role of inflammation, sex steroids, vitamin D, and parathyroid hormones in the development of osteosarcopenia.

Clinically, the approaches to the diagnosis of osteosarcopenia and the non-pharmacological and pharmacological management are covered in detail. One chapter focuses on the models of care for falls and fracture prevention and another on the relationship of osteosarcopenia with the development of physical frailty.

Overall, the book provides a comprehensive overview of the pathophysiology, diagnosis, and management of osteosarcopenia. It is central to establishing osteosarcopenia as an important geriatric giant.

John Morley
Saint Louis University School of Medicine, St. Louis, MO, United States

Preface

Bone and muscle represent more than 55% of the body composition of a healthy human adult. The close connection between bone and muscle tissues is striking, and the multiple pathological conditions that affect them result in numerous adverse outcomes, including reduced quality of life, disability, institutionalization, and premature mortality. However, the biological and clinical approaches to muscle and bone have very much been conducted via clinical and research silos and fragmented models of care. Therefore, bone loss (osteopenia/osteoporosis) and muscle loss (sarcopenia) have been approached separately as unlinked conditions. Unfortunately, this has hindered awareness and the ability to improve care to these highly prevalent conditions in our older population. Therefore, we propose that osteosarcopenia is the unifying concept that can increase the understanding of these conditions within a newly designated geriatric syndrome. Thus, the main aim of this book is to summarize novel evidence on the concept of osteosarcopenia and provide practical tips to clinicians and investigators on how to approach this syndrome, optimize care, and reduce costs to our health systems.

Biologically, the usual paradigm is that bone and muscle tissues connect mechanically and regulate each other only when they are in a close connection. This narrow perspective was questioned a while ago, when pioneers in the field demonstrated that this relationship goes beyond mechanical forces and that there is a complex communication system between muscle and bone that involves factors secreted by each one of them, usually reaching the circulation and affecting their growth, function, and survival. In addition, an important new player has been identified more recently when the role of fat was better discerned as not just a generalized phenomenon but also a localized one where adipose infiltration plays an important role in the biology and cell-cell interactions within the local bone and muscle microenvironment.

This purely translational book is divided into three main sections. Chapter 1 summarizes current evidence on the biology of muscle and bone, including their similarities and differences. Initially, the authors describe how alike muscle and bone are, including their common origin from mesenchymal stem cells (MSCs), followed by the multiple shared pathways regulating their growth and function. This is followed by Chapter 2 that provides a comprehensive review of the effect that the aging process has on all those cells, pathways, and growth factors. Aging seems to be the most critical risk factor for muscle and bone deterioration, which, when reaching pathological stages, are identified as sarcopenia and osteopenia/osteoporosis, respectively. The chapter describes the significant joint changes that happen during the aging process and approaches the recently described concept of geroscience to explain those biological changes frequently observed in osteosarcopenia.

Although there is a prevailing concept of a purely mechanical connection between muscle and bone, there is no doubt that these tissues have a set of critical interactions that regulate their growth and function. Several types of cells within muscle, bone, and fat respond to changes in mechanical stress and are strongly associated with the pathogenesis of osteosarcopenia, which provides potentially innovative therapeutic approaches. Chapter 3 on mechanobiology summarizes the mechanical components of those interactions and delineates how such connections go beyond physical forces and are transformed into biological stimuli in the musculoskeletal system.

A particular novelty of this book is the understanding of osteosarcopenia as a lifespan and healthspan syndrome that starts from childhood during muscle and bone growth that is regulated by multiple factors such as genetics, diet, physical activity, ethnicity, etc. Chapter 4 summarizes those changes and risk factors that, when present in early life, will predispose individuals to further deterioration of their muscle and bone mass and function during their adulthood or older age.

Chapter 5 is dedicated to osteosarcopenia and inflammation, which in older persons is often identified as inflammaging. Multiple inflammatory factors affect bone and muscle either positively or negatively and subsequently impact cellular and biological components that can increase or reduce bone and muscle mass and function. In addition, therapeutic approaches to reduce inflammation in osteosarcopenia are also summarized.

To close with chapters focused on biology and start the transition into more clinical aspects of osteosarcopenia, we dedicate Chapters 6 and 7 to summarize the roles of sex steroids and calcitropic hormones on the biology of muscle and bone and in the pathogenesis and potential therapeutic approaches to osteosarcopenia. We focused the scope due to their crucial role in the regulation of muscle and bone from their role in stem cells to their impact on metabolism and the well-described associations between their deficiency or, in the case of parathyroid hormone, high levels, with osteosarcopenia, falls, and fractures.

After presenting highly comprehensive evidence on the biological basis of osteosarcopenia, Chapters 9–16 cover multiple clinical aspects of this syndrome: epidemiology and identification in clinical practice, association with obesity (known as osteosarcopenic obesity), association with adverse outcomes, and the prediction of those outcomes via innovative imaging and biochemical markers that are focused on bone and muscle tissues with solid potential to become valid and robust biomarkers for musculoskeletal diseases.

A fundamental question that we seek to address in this book is whether osteosarcopenia could increase the risk not only for adverse outcomes but also, more specifically, for frailty. Since frailty syndrome is increasingly being recognized as a core element in geriatric practice, identifying the similarities and differences between osteosarcopenia and frailty while also describing their common biological pathways is an important component of the book. Overall, the authors propose that early identification and treatment of osteosarcopenia in clinical practice could lead to the prevention of frailty and its catastrophic consequences in our older population.

When considering treatments for osteosarcopenia, Chapter 15 is dedicated to nonpharmacological interventions with dual impacts on muscle and bone. This is particularly relevant since most of the clinical trials testing novel drugs for sarcopenia have been unsuccessful. The authors propose that interventions such as nutrition and exercise effectively increase muscle and bone mass and function and provide practical guidelines for their implementation. However, their benefit for preventing fractures is significantly lower than current pharmacological approaches for osteoporosis. Therefore, the current pharmacological treatments and treatment pathways for osteosarcopenia that include pharmacological approaches are described in Chapter 16. Importantly, there is growing evidence that some of those osteoporosis treatments could have a dual effect on muscle and bone, which deserves further exploration.

Last but not least, Chapters 17 and 18 are dedicated to translating evidence into practice. Chapter 17 brings an excellent and highly comprehensive description of osteosarcopenia from its social, demographic, and economic risk factors to the broad impact that this condition has on our societies and health systems, thus highlighting the importance of designing appropriate unified interventions to prevent and treat osteosarcopenia in multiple settings. This concept is exemplified by the innovative care model of Falls and Fractures Clinics. Using their personal experience combined with current evidence in the field, Chapter 18 (our last chapter) summarizes the rationale for implementing Falls and Fractures Clinics to target our most vulnerable populations at high risk of osteosarcopenia and its associated adverse outcomes.

In summary, medicine is constantly evolving, and our field is not immune to change. With time, we have realized that osteopenia/osteoporosis and sarcopenia are two closely interconnected elements of a more complex syndrome that requires a specific understanding and a combination of interventions that we are just starting to identify. This book is an initial step that we hope will significantly impact clinical and research practice, facilitating the understanding of this particular geriatric syndrome and generating multiple novel interventions and research hypotheses in the future.

Gustavo Duque
Bruce R. Troen

Acknowledgments

The editors thank Timothy Bennett from Elsevier for his outstanding support of this project. Special thanks goes to all the chapter authors who share the same interest in osteosarcopenia and muscle and bone health. Without their collaboration, this project would have never been successful.

Chapter 1

Muscles and bones

Eisuke Hiruma
Department of Sport and Medical Science, Teikyo University, Tokyo, Japan

Introduction

Organisms undergo growth and development. They give birth to new individuals and multiply. They respond to internal and external stimuli to adapt to their environment and sustain life. They metabolize substances captured from outside of the body and excrete unnecessary ones. They continually use the energy generated by this metabolism to carry out life processes. Each cell and tissue is connected to each other through a network to perform these processes. The organism eventually undergoes senescence and death.

Bone and muscle are the two largest tissues in the musculoskeletal system. The main function of musculoskeletal system is locomotion, in which the mechanical interaction between bones and muscles work together. Both bone and muscle tissues act as a system of pulleys and levers whereby bones provide an attachment and muscles provide a load. There is a very close relationship between bones and muscles from embryogenesis to growth and development to aging. Bone and muscle develops synchronously during embryogenesis, which is regulated by multiple signaling pathways and stimulatory phenomena. Aging results in progressive bones loss known as osteopenia and osteoporosis and in progressive muscle loss known as sarcopenia. A healthy musculoskeletal system is essential for healthy people to regularly maintain physical activity, although aging results in decreases in physical performance and in nonmusculoskeletal systems. In the last two decades, the multiple findings have expanded our knowledge regarding the molecular and biomechanical interaction between bones and muscles.

In this chapter, we will focus on the structure and function of muscle and bone, changes in both tissues associated with growth and senescence, biochemical networks of muscle and bone tissue (cross-talk), and cytokines secreted by muscle and bone tissue that regulate muscle and bone health.

Osteosarcopenia. https://doi.org/10.1016/B978-0-12-820088-9.00021-4

Structure and function of bones

Human bones undergo continuous renewal throughout life (Fig. 1). This phenomenon is called modeling. The functions of bones include shaping the human body (body support), protecting the brain and internal organs (organ protection), maintaining static stability and performing dynamic activity together with muscles (body movement), storing calcium (99% of the calcium in the body), phosphorus (85% of the phosphorus in the body), and other minerals (mineral storage), and producing blood cells (blood cell production).

Bones are formed by calcification of the bone matrix secreted by osteoblasts, and there are two types of formation: intermembranous ossification and endochondral ossification. In both cases, undifferentiated mesenchymal cells differentiate into osteoblast progenitor cells and receive commitment to osteoblastic cells. Mature osteoblasts become osteocytes and are buried in the substrate secreted by the osteoblasts themselves, calcifying the bone matrix. These cells need to undergo the state of the germ layer from which they were originally derived, that is, the ectoderm, mesoderm, and endoderm, and then differentiate into specific cells of each tissue. Bones are classified according to their shape, and each bone is connected to each other by ligaments to form a skeleton that serves as a support for the body. Blood vessels and nerves in bone tissue are distributed in various parts of bone and are involved in the control of various functions. The bones also constitute the locomotorium by attaching tendons that connect the muscles. Bone tissue consists of a tight, dense cortical bone on the outside and a cancellous bone on the inside, with bone marrow filling the space between the trabeculae within the surface bone. The hematopoietic red bone marrow in childhood is present in bones throughout the body. With aging, the

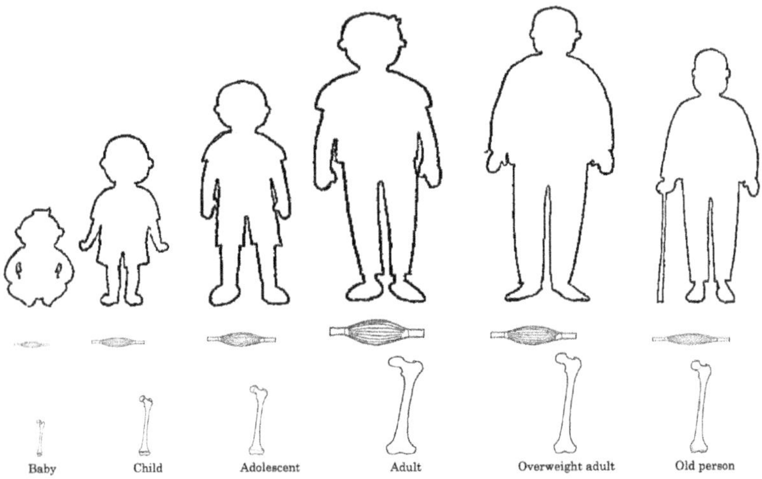

FIG. 1 The changes during growth and development, and effects of aging on bones and muscles in humans.

hematopoietic function of the long bones of the extremities is lost and replaced by fatty yellow bone marrow. However, in the bones of the trunk near the central axis of the body, such as the sternum and rib vertebrae, red bone marrow is present even in old age and is responsible for hematopoiesis.

During growth, the growing cartilage plates at both ends of the bone contribute to the longitudinal growth of long bones, but the cartilage endplates close in adulthood. The ends of the bone are covered with hyaline cartilage, which has no blood vessels or nerves, and constitutes a joint together with the synovium, which is rich in ligaments and vascular network. The outer surface of the bone other than the articular surface is covered with the periosteum, which is a strong fibrous connective tissue existing outside the dense bone. The outer side of the periosteum, which is rich in thick type I collagen fibers, provides tendon and ligament attachments, while the inner side, which is rich in cell fibers and rich in blood vessels, is involved in bone formation and maintenance.

Bones change with age, and aging affects the quality and quantity of the bone matrix. Remodeling involves removal of old bone tissue and replacement with new bone tissue after bone shaping is complete. Remodeling affects bone strength whereby osteoclasts resorb bone, preosteoblasts that migrate and colonize, and osteoblasts and osteocytes that form bone. In addition to coupling factors that maintain communication between osteoclasts and osteoblasts, this remodeling required for maintaining bone strength has also been suggested to occur outside the bones due to mechanical stresses such as locomotion and the nervous and immune systems. Bone strength is dictated by hydroxyapatite, a crystal of calcium phosphate, as the main component of bones, and bone mineral density is dictated by the bone matrix, with type I collagen (collagen fiber) as the main component (for flexibility and binding of collagen molecules) [1]. This chapter introduces the aforementioned coupling factors and the effects of aging; the external effects of locomotion are introduced in later chapters (Fig. 2).

Differentiation and function of osteoclasts

Osteoclasts are multinucleated cells that control the resorption of mineralization and are modulated by osteocytes and osteoblasts that are involved in bone formation. Osteoclast activity is regulated by vitamin D, parathyroid hormone, calcitonin, and leptin. Osteoclast progenitor cells differentiating from the mononuclear phagocyte system possess the receptor activator of nuclear factor-κB (RANK) receptor, which binds RANK ligand secreted by osteoblasts. Osteoclasts maintain serum calcium homeostasis and bone resorption by promoting and suppressing bone resorption. In addition to the release and activation of the transforming growth factor-β (TGF-β) family, bone marrow mesenchymal stem cell recruitment and osteoblast differentiation promote bone regeneration. Leptin suppresses the proliferation of osteoblasts via the sympathetic nervous system and suppresses bone formation. This promotes the secretion of nuclear factor-κB ligand (RANKL) from osteoblasts and promotes bone

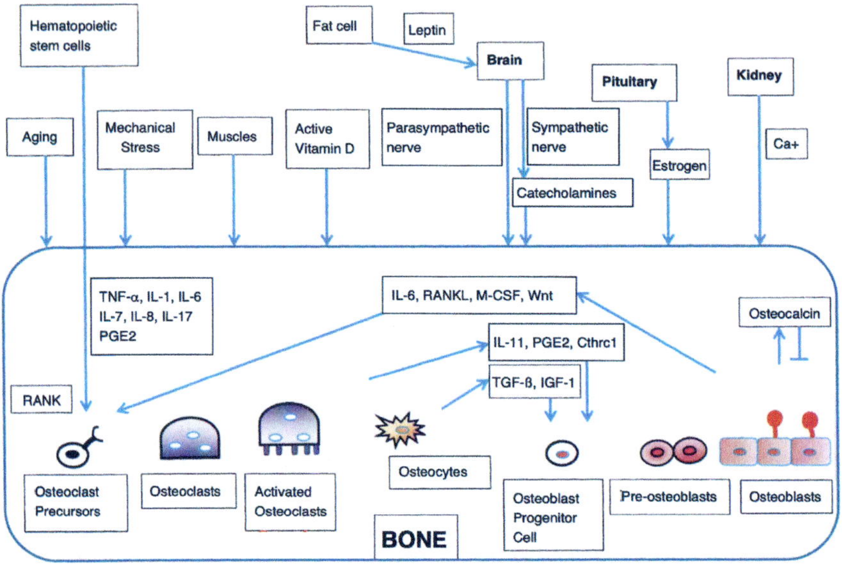

FIG. 2 Intrabone cell dynamics of humoral factors and their effects on osteoclasts and osteoblasts, and their cross-talk. Bones that have completed growth and development activate osteoclasts and promote bone resorption by stimulating osteoblasts and osteocytes. This induces bone remodeling via the proliferation of osteocytes and osteoblasts. Osteoblasts that have not become bone tissue are calcified in the bones and prepare for the next remodeling. *RANK*, receptor activator of nuclear factor-kappa B; *TNF-α*, tumor necrosis factor-α; *IL-1*, interleukin-1; *IL-6*, interleukin-6; *IL-7*, interleukin-7; *IL-8*, interleukin-8; *IL-17*, interleukin-17; *PGE2*, prostaglandin E2; *RANKL*, receptor activator of nuclear factor-kappa B ligand; *M-CSF*, macrophage colony-stimulating factor; *IL-11*, interleukin-11; *Cthre1*, collagen triple helix repeat containing protein 1; *TGF-β*, transforming growth factor-β; *FGF-2*, fibroblast growth factor-2; *HGF*, hepatocyte growth factor; *LIF*, leukemia inhibitory factor; *IGF-1*, insulin-like growth factor-1.

resorption of osteoclasts. Osteoclast differentiation is regulated by RANK and M-CSF (macrophage colony-stimulating factor 1). Osteoclast progenitor cells express RANK receptors and M-CSF receptors, which recognize RANKL and M-CSF produced by osteoblasts, leading to differentiation and bone resorption. A decrease in blood calcium stimulates the secretion of parathyroid hormone (PTH) and promotes bone resorption by osteoclasts. In contrast, an increase in blood calcium promotes the secretion of calcitonin and suppresses bone resorption by osteoclasts. Regulation by cytokines and vitamins is explained below with effects of aging on bones and age-related osteoporosis.

Differentiation and function of osteoblasts

Osteoblasts derived from differentiation of mesenchymal stem cells activate intracellular factors via diverse signaling pathways and induce or suppress the expression of various mRNAs. Furthermore, the differentiation of bone cells is modulated by various transcription factors and humoral factors. The regulation of transcription involves Runx2 (Runt-related transcription factor-2) which belongs to the Runx family and Osterix which is a transcription factor induced by BMP2 (bone morphogenetic protein-2). Runx2 differentiates pluripotent undifferentiated mesenchymal cells into preosteoblasts, and Runx2 and Osterix are essential for subsequent mature osteoblast differentiation. Runx2 and Ostrix are also involved in chondrocyte proliferation and hypertrophy. The transcription factors Runx2 and Osterix are induced by type I collagen, noncollagen proteins such as osteocalcin and osteopontin, and cytokines that also modulate osteoblast differentiation and activation. Humoral factors, including the TGF-β family, regulate the migration and differentiation of bone-forming mesenchymal stem cells, which are involved in bone formation, into bone-resorption sites. Wnt, which promotes bone formation, and sclerostin, which suppresses bone formation, are involved in the regulation by humoral factors. Wnt binds to Wnt co-receptor LRP5, suppresses GSK-β (glycogen synthase kinase-β), and inhibits the degradation of β-catenin. The activated β-catenin translocates to the nucleus and promotes differentiation from pluripotent undifferentiated mesenchymal cells into osteoblasts. Sclerostin suppresses the action of Wnt, suppresses the differentiation and calcification of osteoblasts, and induces apoptosis. Osteocalcin, a hormone that acts on β cells of the pancreas to increase insulin secretory capacity, suppresses bone formation. Recent studies have reported that leptin, which is secreted by adipocytes with a contact-suppressing action, suppresses osteoblast proliferation and bone formation via sympathetic nerves. Thus, various transcription and humoral factors are involved in promotion and suppression of osteoblasts. Most osteoblasts die by apoptosis, but some are buried in the bone matrix produced by themselves and differentiate into mature osteocytes in the process of mineralization. Mechanical stimulation suppresses the action of sclerostin and promotes osteoblast differentiation.

Differentiation and function of osteocytes

Osteocytes are buried in the calcified osteoid as mature osteoblasts are incorporated into the bone matrix. Osteocytes produced by the differentiation of osteoblasts have projections that form a cellular network. Mechanical stress applied to the bones stimulates osteocytes to transmit a signal among themselves. Via the osteocyte projections, these signals modulate bone metabolism and the functions of both osteoclasts and osteoblasts on the bone surface. Furthermore, since most phosphorus is stored in bones, bone cells modulate phosphorus metabolism. Phosphorus in the blood is absorbed from the intestinal tract, and excreted and reabsorbed from the kidneys to control the phosphorus level in blood. Therefore, when blood phosphorus concentration increases, bone cells suppress resorption in the kidneys.

Thus, bone remodeling causes bone formation, and in a healthy adult, bone resorption and bone formation are in equilibrium to maintain bone strength and fragility.

Effects of aging on bones and age-related osteoporosis

The progressively older adult population in developed countries is increasing at risk for osteoporosis, which constitutes a major public health threat. With aging, bone resorption exceeds bone formation, and bone strength decreases due to a decrease in bone mass and deterioration of bone quality. This is called age-related osteoporosis. This chapter describes the morphological changes in age-related osteoporosis, endocrine and hormonal effects, and vitamin D effects.

Bone strength can be evaluated by changes in the bone mass of the cancellous (trabecular or spongy bones) and cortical bones (compact or substantia bones). Although there are various methods to measure bone strength, the current standard methods for bone density measurement include quantitative computed tomography and dual energy X-ray absorptiometry. In females, the age at puberty between 10.5 and 12.5 years overlaps with peak height development due to the burst in bone growth. Similarly, in males, the age at puberty (between 13 and 14 years) coincides with the peak in height development. At this peak, 26% of adult bone mass is acquired [2]. Subsequently, the bone mineral density reaches the average value for young adults at 29 years of ages in the proximal femur and the lumbar spine. It is almost constant until 40 years old. Recent study presented reductions in cortical and tubercular in hydroxyapatite. At the distal radius of postmenopausal females, the decrease in hydroxyapatite at aged 50–64 years and at older than 80 years was −17.1 mg and −16.3 mg, respectively. However, the significant decrease in hydroxyapatite between aged 65 and 79 years was −73.1 mg, of which cortical bone was −50.2 mg and trabecular bone was −22.9 mg. The bone mass in human body composes 80% of trabecular and 20% of cortical compartment. Therefore, the cortical compartment, which is originally small volume in the bone compartment, is significantly reduced with aging. This quality of bone, is deteriorated, may result in the developing osteoporosis and stress fracture. [3].

In age-related osteoporosis, structural bone quality (bone microstructure) breaks down due to increased bone resorption and deterioration of material quality due to increased oxidative stress associated with menopause and aging [4]. It has been reported that this oxidative stress is further exacerbated by lifestyle-related diseases [5]. Further, advanced glycation end products (AGEs), which accumulate with age, affect bone fragility [6].

Sclerostin and Wnt family

Sclerostin, secreted by osteocytes, acts to suppress bone formation. Sclerostin, which is a product of the SOST gene, binds directly to the Wnt co-receptors LRP4 and LRP5. This inhibition induces osteoblast differentiation, proliferation, and activity resulting in bone formation. The Wnt/β-catenin signaling pathway promotes bone formation and osteocyte transmission of mechanical loading by binding Wnt/β-catenin to its receptors Frizzled and co-receptors LRP4 and LRP5. The pathway is triggered by cross-talk with the prostaglandin pathway in response to loading, thereby decreasing negative regulators of bone formation such as sclerostin. Sclerostin suppresses the differentiation and calcification of osteoblasts responsible for bone formation and induces apoptosis of bone cells. Mechanical stress and parathyroid hormone (PTH) suppress TGF-β-mediated SOST expression, suppress sclerostin production, and promote bone formation. Vitamin D, also, increases bone formation in a manner inversely related to sclerostin. The marker of osteocyte mechano-sensing is sclerostin, which suppresses stimulation of bone formation by differentiated osteocytes.

Estrogen

Estrogen enhances the function of osteoblasts and suppresses the function of osteoclasts. It also increases vitamin D synthesis in the kidneys. Therefore, when estrogen secretion decreases due to menopause, osteoblastic bone formation is reduced and osteoclast bone resorption is enhanced, resulting in osteoporosis.

Vitamin D

When calcium metabolism is normal, active vitamin D promotes calcium absorption in the small intestine and reabsorption of calcium in the kidneys to maintain the calcium concentration in the blood, resulting in bone formation. Active vitamin D promotes the deposition of calcium and contributes to bone formation. On the other hand, when the calcium concentration in the blood decreases, the synthesis of active vitamin D in the kidneys increases, and in collaboration with PTH, calcium is removed from the bones and the homeostasis of the calcium concentration in the blood is maintained. A recent study demonstrated that vitamin D increases bone formation in an animal model for osteoporosis [7].

Vitamin D is abundant in blood and control two different receptors for sphingosine-1-phosphate (S1P), a lysophospholipid mediator enriched in blood. These receptors play a vital role in regulating the migration and positioning the osteoclast precursors on the bone surface [8]. One receptor is S1PR1 perform positive chemotaxis to S1P and is involved in the migration of osteoclast precursor cells from the bone surface to blood vessels. Another receptor is S1PR2 play negative chemotaxis to S1P. Osteoclast precursors control the activity and inhibition of bone resorption via these two receptors. Therefore, the active vitamin D promotes bone formation and control bone remodeling. [8].

Structure and function of muscle

Muscles are involved in various physical activities. Different shapes of muscles have different functuion and role. The function of muscle includes body movement, posture retention, breathing, oxygen and energy consumption, heat production, organ and blood vessel construction, heart contraction and relaxation, glycogen storage, external shock buffering, and blood circulation support (milking action). Muscles are classified into three types according to their function: skeletal muscles, smooth muscles, and myocardium. Skeletal muscles and myocardium have a striated structure whereas smooth muscles and myocardium are involuntary muscles. Thus, the myocardium is a muscle with structural features of skeletal muscle and neurological features of smooth muscle. This section introduces the physiological characteristics and functions of skeletal muscles and the endocrine organs of skeletal muscles.

Skeletal muscles contract spontaneously and account for approximately 40% of body weight. Skeletal muscles are generally attached to the bone by tendons, which are connective tissues that attach the muscle to the periosteum of the bone. The muscle fiber structure of skeletal muscles has a parallel or pennate arrangement. Muscle spindles have bundles that are organized parallel to the semimajor axis of the muscle. Muscle spindles are also greatly shortened because the fasciculation lines up directly with the tendons. The lesser the number of total bundles attached to the tendon, the lesser force required to contract the muscle spindle. Therefore, spindle-shaped muscles can generate a large force quickly. For this reason, they are involved in the function of elbow and shoulder joints, which move quickly and with great mobility. Pennate muscles have a bundle associated with the tendon and can span the length of the entire muscle. The long tendons of skeletal muscles may extend to some distance between the origin and insertion of the muscle. Due to its pennate shape, many bundles are attached to a single tendon. Examples of pennate muscles are quadriceps femoris and calf muscles, which can generate as well as withstand large outside forces. Skeletal muscle is composed of skeletal muscle, nervous, connective, and adipose tissues.

Skeletal muscles are surrounded by several connective tissue layers that support the muscle during contraction. Skeletal muscles are composed of three layers of connective tissue: epimysium, perimysium, and endomysium. In addition, there are two types of skeletal muscle cells: slow-twitch (type I) and fast-twitch fibers (FT or type II), depending on their contractile characteristics. The composition ratio of these fibers are different in each muscle and do not have the same functional capacity. These muscle fiber types are controlled by myosin heavy chains and molecules, blood supply, motor neurons, and mitochondria for exertion and endurance. Type I muscle fibers have high oxidase activity due to their volume density and large number of mitochondria. They are reddish due to their high myoglobin content and capillary density. Therefore, type I muscle fibers contract slowly, have a large blood supply, and are more resistant to fatigue. Type II muscle fibers exert great force and contract at a high rate because of high sarcoplasmic reticulum content. Their glycolytic enzyme activity is high due to the large amount of glycogen stored in cells. The composition of type I and II muscle fibers is affected by genetics regardless of gender. Type II muscle fibers have high contractile resistance and oxidase activity, and can be divided into subtypes: type IIa (FT oxidative glycolytic fiber) and low type IIb (FT glycolytic fiber).

For skeletal muscle, isometric contraction (static contraction) is involved in posture maintenance, isotonic contraction (concentric and eccentric contraction) is involved in physical activity accompanied by muscle shortening and stretching, and isokinetic contraction is involved in exerting tension with constant velocity. Isometric contraction occurs when a muscle that develops tension is unable to move the load and does not change length. When a muscle maintains a constant length, it produces increasing tension. Muscle strength is measured when isometric contraction action is performed with maximum effort; this is referred to as maximum muscle strength. The effort exerted by the muscle is insufficient to move when the load is too heavy or when dealing muscles contract in opposition to each other, thus preventing movement. This is called engaged isometric contraction. The effort during the contracted isometric contraction is higher the isometric contraction by 10%.

There are two types of isotonic contraction: concentric and eccentric contraction. Concentric contraction means that the muscle develops sufficient tension to overcome resistance and shortens. Eccentric contraction means that the muscle produces tension as it resists lengthening. Eccentric contraction may occur when muscle is used to oppose a movement, but not to stop it. When an equal load is applied, the tension created in a muscle during an eccentric contraction is higher than that created during a concentric contraction. Eccentric contraction can induce delayed-onset muscle soreness (DOMS) which leads to an increase in inflammation, pain, and muscle damage along with a decrease in strength and range of motion. When DOMS occurs, interleukin-6 (IL-6), cortisol, and creatine kinase significantly increase for the few days after the first eccentric contraction training. The combination of eccentric and concentric contraction is referred to as a stretch-shortening cycle (counter-movement). Putting a muscle under stretch in the eccentric contraction phase enables the muscle to store potential (elastic) energy.

Thus, a mixture of isotonic and eccentric contractions, and complex elongation-shortening cycles are used in everyday life. The effects on the muscle tissue are different since the muscles are loaded differently. Subsequently, the quality and quantity of muscle damage and various secreted substances differ. Eccentric contraction affects the secretion of a large number of humoral factors for muscle regeneration such as IL-6, IL-15, and cortisol.

Growth and development of muscles and effects of aging on muscles

Skeletal muscle cells, similar to central nerve cells, are mitotic cells that do not undergo cell division or regeneration after birth. The increase in skeletal muscle weight from infancy to adolescence is due to cell hypertrophy and vertical growth due to increased cell and sarcomere numbers.

A positive correlation has been found between the growth and development of muscle fibers between the ages of 7 and 18 and voluntary muscle strength.

Voluntary muscle exertion in humans is dictated by the level of excitement of the cerebral cortex, rate of motor nerve participation, and cross-section of a unit muscle. Muscle fiber development during this period involves hypertrophy of myofibrils and extension of muscle length, but in children up to 10 years old, muscle strength per unit area tends to be low. This is thought to be due to the underdeveloped nervous system function. In addition, gender differences are observed after the age of 13; in girls, there is a difference in muscle cross-sectional area and strength due to an increase in blood estrogen concentration, which suppresses long bone growth and white muscle fiber hypertrophy [9].

Age-related loss of muscle strength and mass increases the likelihood of bed-rest or long-term care due to decreased activity in the elderly, injuries due to falls, and the onset of sarcopenia. The rate of decrease in muscle mass, number of muscle fibers, and muscle strength with aging is consistent. The loss of muscle mass results from changes in the balance between protein synthesis and protein degradation. The decrease in secreted IGF-1 and physical activity, bed rest, lack of nutrition and chronic diseases (including noncommunicable diseases) have been related to enhanced protein degradation and depletion of muscle mass. The decrease in hormones also appears to impact the pathogenesis of muscle loss. The reduced levels of estrogen and testosterone may indirectly affect muscle mass due to their inhibitory effects on the regulation of IL-1 and IL-6, which are pro-inflammatory and pro-catabolic cytokine. These changes are related to maximum muscle strength (isometric muscle strength), which depends on muscle mass and the maximum tension generated by motor units during concentric contraction; thus, muscle power is not significantly affected by aging. Various physiological mechanisms are involved in the power reduction of lower limb muscle strength in elderly people with healthy muscle strength per unit cross-section of muscle and mobility-limited older adults [10,11]. Thus, age-related muscle weakness is due to decreased neuromuscular facilitation rather than decreased muscle mass in FT muscle fibers. The single surviving muscle fasciculation function acts as a compensatory action to maintain the required strength and function in the event of age-related loss of major muscle groups throughout the body (Fig. 3).

Development of skeletal muscles

Skeletal muscles can undergo a range of injuries from asymptomatic injuries due to overload and trauma to severe injuries with significant pain and muscle rupture. However, these muscles have excellent regenerative capabilities, and inactive satellite cells in skeletal muscle play a central role in muscle regeneration. Satellite cells, which are systemic stem cells, receive and activate stimuli associated with damage to surrounding muscle fibers. Subsequently, they form muscle progenitor cells and proliferate by repetitive division. The proliferated cells fuse with each other and contribute to the formation, repair, and hypertrophy of muscle fibers. In this process, some muscle progenitor cells return to the

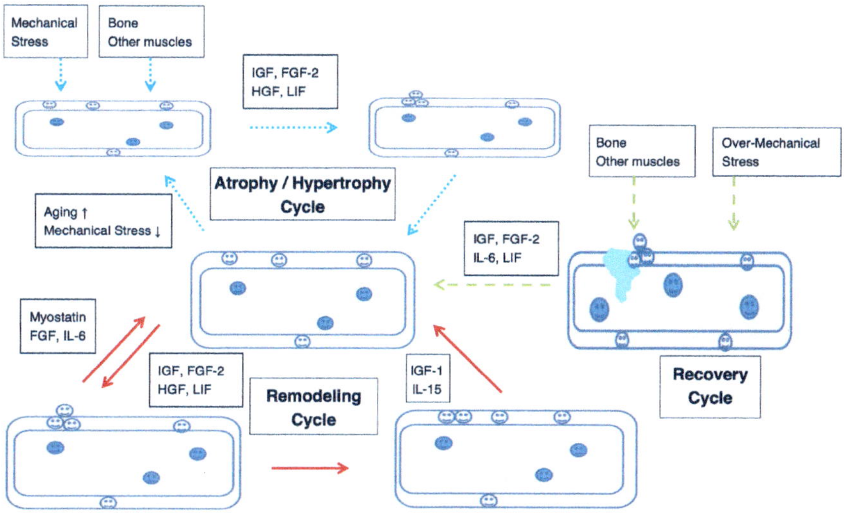

FIG. 3 Intramuscular dynamics of myokines on satellite cells. Atrophy/hypertrophy cycle shows that the decreased muscle fibers due to aging or lack of exercise and various stimuli such as mechanical stress and nutrition, indicating recovery of muscle fibers activate myoblast activity [2]. Recovery cycle shows that cells damaged by excessive mechanical stress accumulate due to the proliferation of myoblasts, indicating the proliferation of myocytes [3]. Remodeling cycle shows how the muscle fibers that mature are remodeled with cytokines. *IGF*, insulin-like growth factor; *FGF-2*, fibroblast growth factor-2; *HGF*, hepatocyte growth factor; *LIF*, leukemia inhibitory factor; *FGF*, fibroblast growth factor; *IL-6*, interleukin-6.

resting phase and become undifferentiated satellite cells. The function of satellite cells during skeletal muscle regeneration is modulated by physical factors such as locomotion and heat, mechanical stresses, and humoral factors such as growth hormone and cytokines.

In recent years, hormone-like humoral factors named myokines secreted by skeletal muscles have garnered interest. It was previously thought that myokines are synthesized in skeletal muscles by shear stress stimulation and secreted extracellularly when physical exercise and locomotion are performed. However, recent studies have shown that in addition to muscle contraction, myokine secretion is constant and is modulated by mechanical, drug, and thermal stimulation. Moreover, some of the identified myokines have physiological actions such as systemic metabolic function and antioxidant and antiinflammatory actions. I summarize and introduce the effects and mechanism of action of satellite cell activation, functional regulation, skeletal muscle regeneration, and hypertrophy.

Skeletal muscles are plastic tissues modulated by various physiological and physical stimuli. This regulation involves muscle proteins, organelles, and tissue turnover or remodeling. Nonhypertrophic remodeling of skeletal muscle fibers involves removal of "old" or damaged cellular components and replacement with new muscle proteins. Therefore, muscle remodeling is essential for the maintenance and composition of genes and cells involved in skeletal muscle health and physical fitness throughout adult life. Muscle fiber remodeling is modulated at various levels, including (1) myogenic stem cells (satellite cells), (2) nonmyogenic cells, (3) gene transcription, and (4) protein synthesis and degradation [12].

Recent studies have shown that satellite cells in the healthy tissue may control skeletal muscle remodeling for the accumulation of skeletal muscle fibrous and adipose tissues due to aging, obesity, and inactivity. In addition, it has been reported that satellite cell in the disease tissue content and regenerative ability of skeletal muscle are reduced [13].

Bone-muscle interaction

It is well known that bone mass and strength are highly correlated with body weight, and lean body mass may have a particularly strong relationship with bone mineral content and area moment of inertia, which affect bone strength and vulnerability [14]. Muscles are a major source of mechanical stimulation of bones, and are involved in bone formation at high frequency and low intensity in addition to high bone strain at peak load [15]. Bone growth and development involves modeling whereas bone renewal involves remodeling achieved by the cooperation of osteoclasts and osteoblasts; osteoporosis occurs due to aging and lack of exercise. Similarly, growth and development in muscles involve modeling whereas muscle renewal involves remodeling due to satellite cell differentiation; muscle fiber loss occurs due to aging and lack of exercise, and they continue to have the same function throughout life. Physical factors such as locomotion and humoral factors such as cytokines are involved in such bone and muscle neoplasia and deterioration. Regenerating bone with Ilizarov external fixator, it has bought about a treatment of orthopedic problems which are fracture fixation, limb lengthening, deformity correction, joint mobilization, and reconstruction of bone. Ilizarov treatment to regenerate bone revealed that the optimum rate of distraction is 0.25 mm, four times per day [16]. Osgood-Schlatter in young athletes results from the unequal of growth speed between bone and muscle. Thus, muscles and bones may act in the same way, but they may act differently in terms of development, remodeling, and regeneration.

In recent years, studies have focused on muscle-bone interaction, cross-talk, and/or communication. Hamrick [17] first submitted a paper on muscle-bone interactions. Recent studies on muscle-bone interactions have reported that muscle-covered fractures heal faster than uncovered or damaged muscles. Moreover, if a porous barrier is placed between muscle and bone, pores large enough for growth factors and other peptides to pass through facilitate healing [18]. Moreover, IGF-1, is abundant in wound exudates of skeletal muscle flap, not only important myokine for muscle hypertrophy, but also osteogenic myokine for the healing development of new blood vessel and bone formation from

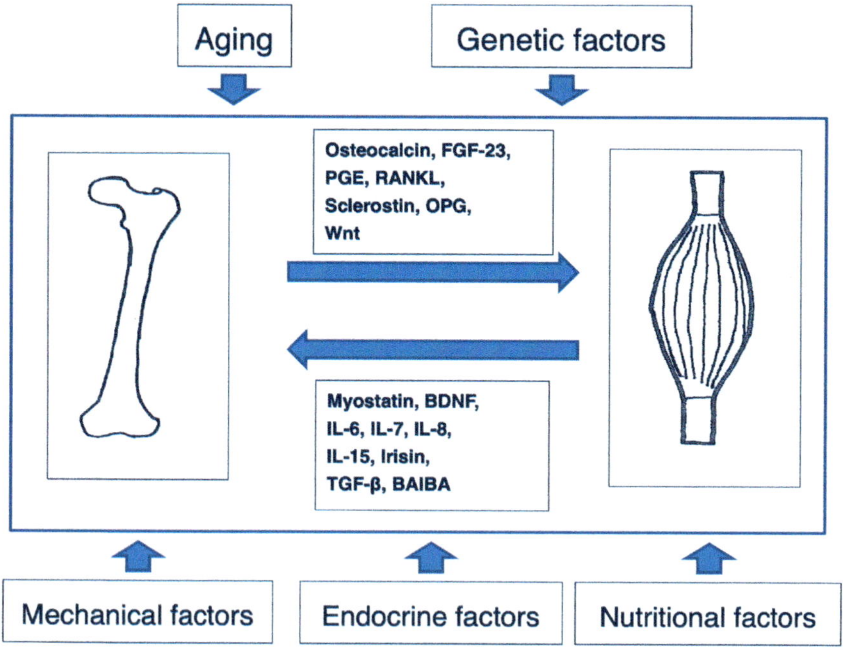

FIG. 4 Cross-talk between bone and muscle. *FGF-23*, fibroblast growth factor-23; *PGE*, prostaglandin E; *RANKL*, receptor activator of NF-κB ligand; *OPG*, osteoprotegerin; *BNDF*, brain-derived neurotrophic factor; *IL-6*, interleukin-6; *IL-7*, interleukin-7; *IL-8*, interleukin-8; *IL-15*, interleukin-15; *TGF*-β, transforming growth factor-β; *BAIBA*, β-aminoisobutyric acid.

the adjacent muscle bed. These findings suggest that muscle-derived factors are directly related to the bone repair process. In this manner, bones and muscles work together without stimulating each other. This section introduces the humoral factors that bridge the relationship between bones and muscles, and the effects of physical factors such as exercise are introduced in another chapter (Fig. 4).

Osteocalcin (bone-to-muscle interaction)

Osteocalcin is a calcium-binding protein that acts as an inhibitor of bone formation by mature osteoblasts. It has been reported that osteocalcin-deficient mice have increased bone mass and strength. Osteocalcin has been recognized as a factor that modulates glycolipid metabolism [19,20]. Osteocalcin also acts on pancreatic β-cells to enhance insulin and glucagon-like peptide-1 secretion. Therefore, it improves insulin sensitivity and glucose tolerance, and enhances lipid metabolism [21], and is a regulator of bone formation and glycolipid metabolism via endocrine action.

Myostatin (muscle-to-bone interaction)

Myostatin, a cytokine that belongs to the TGF-β family, suppresses skeletal muscle regeneration and hypertrophy. It is produced, secreted, and acts in skeletal muscles [22]. Myostatin is a major regulator of proliferation and differentiation of mesenchymal stem cells such as satellite cells. Myostatin secretion suppresses the differentiation of satellite cells, causing a decrease in its self-renewal ability [23]. It has also been shown that myostatin-null mice have reduced body fat and increased bone mineral density, bone marrow-derived stem cells, bone formation, differentiation, and repair, and muscle strength. It was also found that myostatin inhibitors, which affect the inhibition of myostatin receptor (ActRIIB) in osteoblasts, lead to increased bone formation in mice. Myostatin directly affects the proliferation and differentiation of osteoprogenitor cells, suggesting that myostatin suppression is likely to enhance both muscle mass and bone strength [24].

Insulin-like growth factor (muscle-to-bone interaction)

There are two types of insulin-like growth factors (IGF): IGF-1 and IGF-2. IGF-1 is involved in bone formation and muscle regeneration and hypertrophy. In addition to being secreted from the liver stimulated by the growth hormone, IGF-1 is secreted from skeletal muscles near the periosteum [25]. In bone tissue, IGF-1 plays an important role as a bone metabolism regulator. It is involved in both facilitation and inhibition of IGF-1 binding to the receptor in osteoblast, thereby regulating bone formation. Furthermore, IGF-1 accumulates in large quantities in the bone matrix and is involved in the promotion of chondrocyte and osteoblast proliferation and differentiation, and substrate synthesis [26].

IGF-1 and IGF-2 present in skeletal muscles and periosteum enhance satellite cell differentiation and muscle protein synthesis, and are involved in muscle regeneration and hypertrophy. IGF-1 is a potent anabolic factor, and IGF-1 secreted from muscle fibers binds to IGF-1 receptors on satellite cells, promoting muscle growth and hypertrophy. In addition to being secreted from the liver stimulated by growth hormone, IGF-1 is also secreted from skeletal muscle near the periosteum [25]. The increase in IGF-1 expression associated with muscle hypertrophy occurs due to a local increase in IGF-1 secretion and muscle-bone action. Thus, paracrine interactions on the surface of muscle and periosteum may directly support biochemical communication between muscle and bone.

Since 2011, many studies on muscle-bone interactions have been performed. In this chapter, we introduced osteocalcin, which mediates bone-to-muscle interactions and myostatin and IGF-β, which mediate muscle-to-bone interactions, and their effects on each organ. Humoral factors related to muscle-bone interaction that could not be presented here are shown in Fig. 4 and Tables 1 and 2.

TABLE 1 Bone to muscle interactions.

Factor	Impact	Reference
FGF-23 (fibroblast growth factor)	Regulate mineral homeostasis and cardiac muscle function	Shimada et al. [27]
PGE (prostaglandin E)	Enhance myoblast differentiation	Mo et al. [28]
RANKL (nuclear factor kappa-B ligand)	Reduces muscle strength, whereas inhibition of RANKL improves muscle strength	Bonnet et al. [29]
Sclerostin	Enhance myoblast differentiation	Huang et al. [30]
OPG (osteoprotegerin)	Inhibit differentiation and function of osteoclasts	Udagawa et al. [31]
Wnt (wingless-related MMTV integration site)	Enhance differentiation and function of osteogenesis	Basoli et al. [32]

TABLE 2 Muscle to bone interactions.

Factor	Impact	Reference
BDNF (brain-derived neurotrophic factor)	Regulate neuronal development and increase satellite cell activation and skeletal muscle regulation	Zhang et al. [33]
IL-6 (interleukin-6)	Enhance osteoblast and osteoclasts differentiation	Jeffer et al. [34]
IL-7 (interleukin-7)	Promote osteoclast differentiation	Weizmann et al. [35]
IL-8 (interleukin-8)	Stimulate angiogenesis	Pedersen et al. [36]
IL-15 (interleukin-15)	Increase bone mineral content	Quinn et al. [37]
Irisin	Supports osteocytes and inhibits bone formation	Kim et al. [38]
TGF-β (transforming growth factor)	Generate osteogenic growth and release osteoclast	McPherron et al. [22]
BAIBA (β-aminoisobutyric acid)	Prevent bone loss and osteocytes death	Kitase et al. [39]

Future research on humoral factors of bone and muscle in aging

Bones and muscles play a structural role in supporting our body and storing various substances. Recent studies have shown that humoral factors secreted by bone tissues and muscles modulate interactions between bone tissue and muscle and those between other organs and tissues.

In the 1950s, an animal study was conducted in which different individuals were sutured at the subcutaneous level, a technique known as parabiosis, and the circulating body fluids of both individuals were mixed and shared. Heterochronic parabiosis was studied in old and young rats [40]. As a result, it was found that humoral factors are involved in rejuvenation of the circulating blood due and extended lifespan of aged rats. In 2000, various parabiosis studies were conducted, and the rejuvenation of the living body of aged mice was reported. In particular, it was found that satellite cells of aged mice were activated without a decrease in their number and an inhibitory effect on aged cells was observed; thus, it was clarified that there are factors that modulate satellite cells [41]. Furthermore, it was reported that administration of growth differentiation factor 11 (GDF11), which is a regulator of satellite cells, to aged mice improves satellite cell function, muscle strength, and exercise tolerance [42]. However, other studies refuting the results of this study have been published. It was reported that administration of GDF11 to aged rats inhibits the function of satellite cells, and its administration to young mice suppressed satellite cell differentiation and muscle regeneration. It also activates osteoclasts in bone tissue and reduces bone mass to suppress the action of osteoblasts [43]. Recent animal studies have reported that certain humoral factors in blood may enhance or suppress certain aspects of aging. These studies aid understanding methods to maintain and improve our health. Further research is needed to determine whether the network of homeostatic systems that are double or triple barriers in humans can produce results similar to those in animal experiments.

References

[1] Schwartz AV, Vittinghoff E, Bauer DC, et al. Association of BMD and FRAX score with risk of fracture in older adults with type 2 diabetes. JAMA 2011;305:2184–92.

[2] Bailey DA, McKay HA, Mirwald RL, et al. A six-year longitudinal study of the relationship of physical activity to bone mineral accrual in growing children: the University of Saskatchewan Bone Mineral Accrual Study. J Bone Miner Res 1999;14:1672–9.

[3] Zebaze RMD, Ghasem-Zadeh A, Bohte A, et al. Intercortical remodeling and porosity in the distal radius and post-mortem femurs of women: a cross-sectional study. Lancet 2010;375:1729–36.

[4] Saito M, Marumo K. Collagen cross-links as a determinant of bone quality: a possible explanation for bone fragility in aging, osteoporosis, and diabetes mellitus. Osteoporos Int 2010;21:195–214.

[5] Yamamoto M, Sugimoto T. Advanced glycation end products, diabetes, and bone strength. Curr Osteoporos Rep 2016;14:320–6.

[6] Goh SY, Cooper ME. Clinical review: the role of advanced glycation end products in progression and complications of diabetes. J Clin Endocrinol Metab 2008;93:1143–52.
[7] Kikuta J, Kawamura S, Okiji F, et al. Sphingosine-1-phosphate-mediated osteoclast precursor monocyte migration is a critical point of control in antibone-resorptive action of active vitamin D. Proc Natl Acad Sci U S A 2013;110:7009–13.
[8] Ishii M, Egen JG, Klauschen F, et al. Sphingosine-1-phosphate mobilizes osteoclast precursors and modulates bone homeostasis. Nature 2009;458:524–8.
[9] Kanehisa H. Growth and development in muscular training. In: Muscle training science. Tokyo: Kobundo Publishing; 1989. p. 72–80.
[10] Frontera WR, Reid KF, Phillips EM, et al. Muscle fiber size and function in elderly humans: a longitudinal study. J Appl Physiol 1985;105:637–42.
[11] Reid KF, Pasha E, Doros G, et al. Longitudinal decline of lower extremity muscle power in healthy and mobility-limited older adults: influence of muscle mass, strength, composition, neuromuscular activation and single fiber contractile properties. Eur J Appl Physiol 2014;114:29–39.
[12] Burd NA, Lisio MD. Skeletal muscle remodeling: interconnections between stem cells and protein turnover. Exerc Sport Sci Rev 2017;45:187–91.
[13] Judson RN, Zhang RH, Rossi FMA. Tissue-resident mesenchymal stem/progeneitor cells in skeletal muscle: collaborators or saboteurs? FEBS J 2013;280:4100–8.
[14] Reid IR. Relationships between fat and bone. Ostroporos Int 2008;19:595–606.
[15] Judex S, Rubin CT. Is bone formation induced by high-frequency mechanical signals modulated by muscle activity? J Musculoskelet Neuronal Interact 2010;10:3–11.
[16] Littlewood R, Lynch R. Cosmos, gods and madmen frameworks in the anthropologies of medicine. New York, Oxford: Berghahn; 2011. p. 1–14.
[17] Hamrick MW. A role for myokines in muscle-bone interactions. Exerc Sport Sci Rev 2011;39:43–7.
[18] Stein H, Perren SM, Cordey J, et al. The muscle bed—a crucial factor in fracture healing: a physiological concept. Orthopedics 2002;25:1379–83.
[19] Fulzele K, Riddle RC, DiGirolamo DJ, et al. Insulin receptor signaling in osteoblasts modulates postnatal bone acquisition and body composition. Cell 2010;142:309–19.
[20] Lee NK, Sowa H, Hinoi E, et al. Endocrine regulation of energy metabolism by the skeleton. Cell 2010;130:309–19.
[21] Kanazawa I. Osteocalcin as a hormone regulating glucose metabolism. World J Diabetes 2015;6:1345–54.
[22] McPherron AC, Lawler AM, Lee SJ. Regulation of skeletal muscle mass in mice by a new TGF-beta superfamily member. Nature 1997;387:83–90.
[23] McCroskery S, Thomas M, Maxwell L, et al. Myostatin negatively modulates satellite cell activation and self-renewal. J Cell Biol 2003;162:1135–47.
[24] Elasrawy M, Hamrick MW. Myostatin (GFD-8) as a key factor linking muscle mass and bone structure. J Musculoskelet Neuronal Interact 2010;10:25–34.
[25] Turner JD, Rotwein P, Novakofski J, BEtchel, P. J. Induction of mRNA for IGF-1 and IGF-II during growth-hormone stimulated muscle hypertrophy. Am J Physiol 1988;255:E513–7.
[26] Hamrick MW, McNeil PL, Patterson SL. Role of muscle-derived growth factors in bone formation. J Musculoskelet Neuronal Interact 2010;2010:64–70.
[27] Shimada T, et al. Targeted ablation of FGF-23 demonstrates an essential physiological role of FGF-23 in phosphate and vitamin D metabolism. J Clin Invest 2004;113(4):561–8.
[28] Mo C, et al. Prostaglandin E2 promotes proliferation of skeletal muscle myoblasts via EP4 receptor activation. Cell Cycle 2015;14(10):1507–16.

[29] Bonnet N, et al. RANKL inhibition improves muscle strength and insulin sensitivity and restores bone mass. J Clin Invest 2019;129(8):3214–23.

[30] Huang J, et al. Cross-talk between MLO-Y4 osteocytes and C2C12 muscle cells is mediated by the Wnt/β-catenin pagthway. JBMR Plus 2017;1:86–100.

[31] Udagawa N, et al. Osteoprotegerin produced by osteoblasts is an important regulator in osteoclast development and function. Endocrinology 2000;141(9):3478–84.

[32] Basoli V, et al. Physical stimulation by REAC and BMP4/WNT-1 inhibitor synergistically enhance cardiogenic commitment in iPSCs. PLoS One 2019;14(1), e0211188.

[33] Zhang Z, et al. BDNF regulates the expression and secretion of VEGF from osteoblasts via the TrkB/ERK1/2 signaling pathway during fracture healing. Mol Med Rep 2017;15(3):1362–7.

[34] Jeffer P, et al. Mechanically loads myotubes affect osteoclast formation. Calcif Tissue Int 2014;94(3):319–26.

[35] Weizmann MN, et al. Increased production of Il-7 uncouples bone formation from bone resorption during estrogen deficiency. J Clin Invest 2002;110(10):1643–50.

[36] Pedersen BK, et al. Muscle as a secretory organ. Compr Physiol 2013;3(3):1337–62.

[37] Quinn LS, et al. Oversecretion of interleukin-15 from skeletal muscle switch. Am J Endocrinol Metab 2009;296(1):E191–202.

[38] Kim H, et al. Irisin mediates effects on bone and fat via aV integrin receptors. Cell 2018;175(7):1756–68.

[39] Kitase Y, et al. β-Aminoisobutyric acid, l-BAIBA, is a muscle-derived osteocyte survival factor. Cell Rep 2018;22(6):1531–44.

[40] McCay CM, Pope F, Lunsford W. Parabiosis between old and young rats. Geron 1963;7:7–17.

[41] Conboy IM, Conboy MJ, Wagers AJ, et al. Rejuvenation of aged progenitor cells by exposure to a young systemic environment. Nature 2005;317:760–4.

[42] Sinha M, Jang YC, Oh J, et al. Restoring systemic GDF11 levels reverses age-related dysfunction in mouse skeletal muscle. Science 2014;344:649–52.

[43] Lie W, Zhou L, Zhou C, et al. GDF11 decreases bone mass by stimulating osteoclastogenesis and inhibiting osteoblast differentiation. Nat Commun 2016;7:12794.

Chapter 2

Cellular senescence and other aging mechanisms in bone and muscle

Japneet Kaur[a,b] and Joshua N. Farr[a,b,c]

[a]*Division of Endocrinology, Mayo Clinic College of Medicine, Mayo Clinic, Rochester, MN, United States,* [b]*Robert and Arlene Kogod Center on Aging, Mayo Clinic College of Medicine, Mayo Clinic, Rochester, MN, United States,* [c]*Division of Physiology and Biomedical Engineering, Mayo Clinic College of Medicine, Mayo Clinic, Rochester, MN, United States*

Introduction

Aging is associated with universal cellular damage and the simultaneous decline of several crucial biological processes. Lopez-Otin et al. [1] grouped these fundamental mechanisms or "*hallmarks of aging*" into nine categories as follows: telomere attrition, genomic instability, loss of proteostasis, epigenetic alterations, mitochondrial dysfunction, deregulated nutrient signaling, stem cell exhaustion, altered intercellular communication, and cellular senescence. Each of these hallmarks of aging meets the following criteria: (i) it manifests during normal chronological aging; (ii) its experimental induction accelerates aging; and (iii) its experimental amelioration slows or delays the natural aging process and hence extends healthspan (i.e., the period of life free of chronic disease).

There is now mounting evidence that each of these hallmarks of aging apply to essentially every tissue and system throughout the body, including bone and skeletal muscle (as previously reviewed [2,3]). Thus, there is direct experimental data in several preclinical models and some evidence in humans for each of the nine fundamental aging mechanisms to have causal roles in mediating multiple diseases and co-morbidities of aging, including osteoporosis and sarcopenia. The extent to which individual aging hallmarks drive aging is important because these mechanisms are linked and overlap, and thus each contribute to the overall aging process [1]. Indeed, based on their interconnections and overlap, interventions that therapeutically target one hallmark should in theory prevent or delay age-related co-morbidities across tissues and systems. Therefore, interfering with one hallmark has the potential to simultaneously ameliorate a majority of age-associated chronic diseases as a group. This approach is

Osteosarcopenia. https://doi.org/10.1016/B978-0-12-820088-9.00008-1

fundamentally different that the current paradigm of one drug to treat each disease of aging, which ultimately leads to polypharmacy and potential adverse drug interactions in the older population. One such hallmark of aging that fits the above criteria and appears to be particularly amendable to therapeutic targeting to prevent multiple age-related co-morbidities, at least in mice, is cellular senescence. Here we review the evidence for reducing the cellular senescence burden to alleviate musculoskeletal aging.

Cellular senescence

Cellular senescence is a cell-intrinsic phenomenon that has been observed both in vitro and in vivo. The senescence pathways are triggered by various forms of cellular stress or metabolic insults that cause the accumulation of cellular damage. Specific examples of intrinsic and extrinsic stressors that converge to cause a cell to enter the senescence program include DNA damage, telomere shortening, oxidative and proteotoxic stress, activation of oncoproteins such as Ras and its sequelae, as well as prolonged shifts in nutrient homeostasis in the forms of both deprivation and excess. Over time, these cumulative insults can eventually cause a cell to enter an essentially irreversible proliferative arrest, making the cell resistant to apoptosis yet metabolically active and immune to mitogenic stimuli. Senescent cells undergo dramatic changes in gene expression, chromatin organization, and morphological changes resulting in cell enlargement and flattening [4–7]. Although not always the case, senescent cells frequently produce a pro-inflammatory secretome that contributes to the spread of senescence and is responsible for driving damage across tissues [8–10].

First described by Dr. Leonard Hayflick in the early 1960s [11], cellular senescence was demonstrated in a series of elegant cell culture experiments establishing that normal embryonic human fibroblasts grown in culture cease to divide after numerous cell divisions, even under favorable conditions. These experiments revealed that cells initially start dividing gradually (Phase I), which is followed by a period of profuse cell growth (Phase II). After phase II cells gradually lose their ability to divide and enter phase III, termed "cellular senescence" [11]. The number of cell divisions or population doublings that a cell undergoes before reaching the senescence phase (which differs among cell types and species) is referred to as the Hayflick Limit [11]. For example, human fibroblasts undergo ~50 population doublings (or cell divisions propagated in a 1:2 ratio) before they enter the senescence phase [11]. It was later established that the reason there is an inherent limit to cell division is because with each mitosis, telemetric DNA shortens, which after many population doublings makes cell division impossible [12].

Telomeres are functional chromosomal ends that protect the genome. They are rich in 5′-TTAGGG-3′ nucleotide sequence repeats; however, with each ensuing DNA replication the terminal segment of the telomere in the lagging strand is lost, leading to telomere attrition over time. On average, human telomeres shorten at a rate of 24.8 to 27.7 base pairs per year with the rate of shortening directly related to the biological age of the individual and the risk for age-related diseases [13]. This loss of sequence from the ends of the chromosomes can be reversed by telomerase, an enzyme responsible for synthesizing chromosomal ends by elongating telomeres. Nonetheless, most human somatic cells have minimal or no telomerase activity and thus their telomeres shorten with each replication until their length reaches a critical threshold which triggers cellular senescence—termed "replicative senescence." Telomere shortening is thus considered a "*mitotic clock*" that can be used to estimate the history of replication for a given cell. It has been hypothesized that the amount of telomere shortening occurring with each division remains constant in a particular cell population; however, the rate of shortening can increase in response to various types of cellular stress resulting in premature telomere shortening and senescence of the cell at an earlier age [14]. Poor lifestyle habits and other risk factors such as cigarette smoking, obesity, anxiety, and stress have been linked to accelerating the pace of telomere shortening in human cells [13].

The shortening of telomeres leads to their "uncapping"—i.e., loss of the terminal t-loop configuration, which can activate a DNA damage response (DDR) [4–7]. This genomic damage caused by telomere shortening or due to other insults such as ionizing radiation as well as chemotherapeutic agents mimics DNA double-stranded breaks (DSBs) that trigger the DDR through the activity of sensory kinases (ATM/ATR, DNA-PK), resulting in the formation of DNA damage foci, and phosphorylated histone H2A.X (γH2A.X). This in turn can trigger the tumor suppressor protein, p53, to activate its downstream transcriptional target, $p21^{Cip1}$ (a cyclin-dependent kinase inhibitor [CDKi], also known as *Cdkn1a*), thus halting the cell-cycle. If, however, the nature of the damage is severe and irreparable, $p53/p21^{Cip1}$ signaling will persist and thereby activate other signaling pathways such as p38 MAPK and protein kinase C, upregulating the expression of $p16^{Ink4a}$ (a CDKi encoded by the Ink4a/Arf locus, also known as *Cdkn2a*) which activates Rb, another tumor suppressor protein, thereby causing a more persistent and pronounced cell-cycle arrest [4–7]. Cellular senescence triggered via the DDR can also occur through direct activation of the $p16^{Ink4a}$/Rb pathway, although in most cases $p16^{Ink4a}$ is activated secondary to the $p53/p21^{Cip1}$ pathway [15]. Some stressors, such as elevated reactive oxygen species (ROS) can induce senescence through direct activation of $p16^{Ink4a}$/Rb resulting in a persistent cell-cycle arrest [4]. Thus, cellular senescence is activated and maintained by chronic signaling of either the $p53/p21^{Cip1}$ or $p16^{Ink4a}$/Rb tumor-suppressor pathways, or by both [4–7].

Senescence-associated secretory phenotype (SASP)

Persistent DDR signaling and the enhanced metabolic activity of senescent cells can result in revved-up intracellular machinery that permits the secretion of a complex *S̲enescence-A̲ssociated S̲ecretory P̲henotype* (termed, the "*SASP*") typically comprised of cytokines, chemokines, matrix-degrading remodeling proteins (e.g., MMPs), and growth factors [8–10]. Important SASP regulators in senescent cells can include IL-1α, IL-6, NFκB, C/EBPβ, or GATA4 [7]. Although the exact composition of the SASP is dependent on the cell type and the type of the senescence inducing stimuli, SASP components are generally pro-inflammatory in nature, including factors such as interleukins, various monocyte chemoattractant proteins and macrophage inflammatory proteins, as well as granulocyte/macrophage colony-stimulating factors, and MMPs [8–10]. Elevated SASP factors have been shown to mediate the spread of senescence to neighboring, nonsenescent cells (at least in vitro) via the senescence-induced bystander effect, resulting in a greater accumulation of senescent cells and further amplification of the SASP [16]. Likewise, through this spreading mechanism an elevated in vivo senescent cell and SASP burden may, at least in part, propel the chronic, sterile low-grade inflammation associated with aging (termed "*inflammaging*") that has been hypothesized to contribute substantially to morbidity and mortality [17]. Therefore, senescent cells represent promising therapeutic targets to prevent or delay age-related diseases. Indeed, mounting evidence, predominantly from mice and more recently from studies in humans, has shown that senescent cells and their accompanying SASP increase with aging and in the context of several age-associated co-morbidities such as metabolic dysfunction, hepatic steatosis, neurodegenerative diseases, renal disease, pulmonary fibrosis, cardiovascular disease, osteoarthritis, frailty, sarcopenia, and osteoporosis [18–46].

Senescent cells have the ability to protect themselves from their own pro-apoptotic SASP via a pro-survival mechanism that involves the upregulation of multiple *Senescent Cell Anti-apoptotic Pathways*, termed "*SCAPs*" [34,47,48]. Among those SCAPs that have been discovered to date, include the B-cell lymphoma (BCL) family inhibitors (BCL-2, BCL-xL, BCL-W), PI3K/AKT pathways, p53/p21^{Cip1}/serpine pathways, HSP-90 pathway, serpine (PAI-1, PAI-2), HIF-1α, ephrins, and dependence receptors/tyrosine kinases [34,47,48]. Originally coined as the "*Achilles' Heel*" of the senescent cells, SCAPs are the targets of drugs referred to in the field as "*senolytics*" that selectively kill senescent cells by inducing their apoptosis without having detrimental effects on nonsenescent cells [34]. Among the first-generation senolytic compounds identified were Dasatinib (D; an FDA-approved tyrosine kinase inhibitor) and Quercetin (Q; a flavonoid present in many fruits and vegetables) that, when administered intermittently have both in vitro and in vivo senolytic activity [34].

Given that senescent cells are present at the time and location of aging and diseases in both animals and humans alike, there has been heightened recent interest in the therapeutic potential of senolytics to delay aging and extend healthspan [47]. In addition to using senolytics, in order to examine the mechanisms and consequences of senescent cell removal in preclinical animal models of aging and various diseases, several groups have developed transgenic mouse models that harbor "suicide" transgenes driven by senescence gene promoters. For example, the "*INK-ATTAC*" (i.e., *p16Ink4a-linked apoptosis through targeted activation of caspase*) mouse model permits inducible removal of cells positive for $p16^{Ink4a}$ (a marker expressed at high levels in many types of senescent cells) by activation of an FKBP-caspase 8 fusion protein that dimerizes upon administration of a synthetic drug, AP20187, which in turn activates an apoptosis cascade within $p16^{Ink4a}$-positive senescent cells to permit their inducible killing or "clearance" [18]. In addition, $p16^{Ink4a}$ trimodality reporter (p16-3MR) transgenic mice have been developed to harbor a different senescent cell killing system which utilizes ganciclovir as an activator molecule that triggers a mitochondrial DNA damage cascade in an inducible manner to specifically eliminate $p16^{Ink4a}$-positive senescent cells [19]. Several studies, some of which are described below, have used either genetic or senolytic approaches (or the combination of both strategies) in old mice and models of accelerated age-associated diseases to study the biological functions of senescent cells in vivo as well as the consequences of their selective removal [18–44].

Biomarkers of cellular senescence

Although a single universal marker to unequivocally identify a senescent cell has yet to be discovered, *p16Ink4a* appears to be expressed at higher levels in many types of senescent cells in both human and rodent tissues and thus far has been regarded by many as a critical senescent cell-specific marker [6]. Nevertheless, because not all senescent cells express high levels of $p16^{Ink4a}$, the field has recommended the application of multiple criteria to identify and characterize senescent cells both in vitro and in vivo [49]. For example, additional effectors and regulators of the $p53/p21^{Cip1}$, $p16^{Ink4a}$/Rb as well as other potential pathways that induce senescence such as p15 and p27 have been implicated as potential markers to identify senescent cells [7,50]. In addition, among the first assay biomarkers of cellular senescence was senescence-associated β-galactosidase (SA-β-Gal) [51], which at pH 6.0 measures endogenous lysosomal β-galactosidase staining that tends to be higher in senescent cells. However, SA-β-Gal activity as a senescence biomarker can be problematic in some tissues, such as bone, due to high background staining and potential false-positive staining in macrophages and osteoclasts [52]. Therefore, as noted above, the combination of more specific markers is recommended. Perhaps the most robust senescent cell biomarker identified to date is referred to as telomere-associated foci (or "*TAF*" [53]), which are sites of DNA damage co-localized with telomeres.

In addition to TAF-positive nuclei, the cellular senescence phenotype is associated with profound changes in chromatin organization. Altered heterochromatin can result in the formation of senescence-associated heterochromatin foci (SAHFs) that have been shown to accumulate in senescent cells [54].

For example, the presence of SAHFs has been shown by distinct bright DNA foci on DAPI-stained senescent human cells compared to normal human cells [55]. However, the inability to trace SAHFs in models of normal and accelerated aging may render this approach as a less consistent marker of cellular senescence [50,56]. Another perhaps more reliable marker of senescence based on altered heterochromatin organization that has been more widely reported in both human and preclinical animal models is senescence-associated distension of satellites (or "*SADS*"), which is a measure of the nuclear decondensation of peri-centromeric satellite heterochromatin found in senescent cells [56]. Although these approaches highlight some of the well-established methods to detect senescence, biomarker expression can vary among senescent cell populations, across species and based on the senescence inducing stimuli, which underscores the need to characterize senescence based on a combination of biomarkers.

Identification of senescent cells in old bone

In order to identify the cell type(s) within the bone microenvironment that become senescent in old age, our group [57] studied female and male young (6-month-old) and old (24-month-old) C57BL/6 wild-type (WT) mice from which we isolated highly enriched populations of osteoblast progenitors, osteoblasts, osteocytes, myeloid cells, as well as B- and T-cells. These populations were isolated from either bone itself (using liberase to digest the sample to release osteoblasts and enrich the remaining sample for osteocytes) or from bone marrow using magnetic-activated cell sorting (MACS) based on novel approaches described in our publication [57]. Our data revealed a significant increase in mRNA expression of senescence effector genes, most notably *p16Ink4a*, but also in some cases *p21Cip1* and *p53*, in the various cell populations of old as compared to young mice. More specifically, *p16Ink4a* mRNA expression increased ~5–10-fold with aging in each of the cell types isolated in both female and male mice, whereas *p21Cip1* and *p53* levels increased to varying degrees in osteocytes and myeloid cells [57]. Our finding of increased senescence with aging in osteocytes was supported by the presence of a significantly higher percentage of in vivo SADS in osteocytes of bone cortices from old relative to young mice [57]. In addition, we found that the percentage of TAF-positive cells and the number of TAFs per osteocyte were both significantly higher in primary osteocytes isolated from older as compared to young mice [57]. Corresponding with these age-related increase in senescence biomarkers, was upregulation of the SASP with aging that was assessed based on an a priori panel of 36 SASP genes identified from the literature [8–10]. Most notably was the significant upregulation of SASP factors with old age in osteocytes (23 out of 36 SASP genes queried) and myeloid cells (26 out of 36 SASP genes queried) [57]. We also determined that these findings of an increased senescence burden with aging in old mice were also applicable to humans as demonstrated by increased mRNA levels of *p16Ink4a* and *p21Cip1* and SASP components (12 out of 36 genes queried) in posterior iliac crest needle bone biopsies isolated from older postmenopausal women relative to younger women [57]. Therefore, senescent cells are present at the time and location of age-related bone loss in both mice and humans.

Consistent with findings from our young versus old mouse study [57], Piemontese and colleagues [58] found an increase in osteocyte senescence, including higher *p16Ink4a* mRNA levels and γH2A.X in osteocyte-enriched bone samples isolated from old as compared to young mice. In addition, they identified a potential link between increased osteocyte senescence and higher levels of receptor activator of nuclear factor kappa-B ligand (RANKL—an essential osteoclast differentiation factor) that both correlated with greater endocortical bone resorption and increased cortical porosity with aging [58]. Thus, based on the collective data in mice, it appears that at least a subset of senescent osteocytes accumulate in old bone where potentially through their detrimental pro-inflammatory SASP they accelerate bone resorption in the setting of aging.

Accelerated cellular senescence and skeletal fragility in mice with type 2 diabetes (T2D)

An increased senescent cell burden has also been shown to be found in conditions of accelerated aging attributed to obesity and metabolic dysfunction, including preclinical models of type 2 diabetes (T2D). For example, in response to high-fat diet (HFD) feeding, senescent cells have been shown to accumulate prematurely in obese young adult mice in several tissues, such as adipose [32], brain [30], liver [26], and pancreatic β cells [33], thus contributing to metabolic dysfunction in these animals [59]. Moreover, Aguayo-Mazzucato et al. [33] recently showed that increased insulin resistance in mice with T2D is associated with pancreatic β-cell senescence and acquisition of the SASP in β-cells, while removal of these senescent cells using either genic *INK-ATTAC* or senolytic (D + Q) approaches in these mice with metabolic dysfunction improved glucose metabolism as well as insulin secretion, and reduced expression of senescence and SASP markers in pancreatic β-cells.

Evidence from several studies in humans has established higher fracture risk in individuals with T2D despite a normal to higher bone mineral density (BMD) [60,61]. Therefore, we hypothesized that senescent cells may represent an underlying mechanism at the nexus of skeletal fragility and T2D [62]. Thus, in order to begin to investigate whether bone-resident senescent cells accumulate prematurely in the setting of T2D, our group [62] subjected young adult mice to HFD and a single relatively low dose of streptozotocin (STZ) to induce obesity and adult-onset T2D—i.e., the HFD/STZ mouse model that is commonly used throughout the diabetes field [63,64]. Consistent with previous studies, we showed that these mice display several key features of T2D such as increased body weight, fat mass, consistently higher glucose (≥ 250 mg/dL) and HbA1c levels, insulin resistance, and decreased pancreatic β-cell area [62]. T2D mice also displayed deteriorated bone quality (assessed by longitudinal micro-CT scanning), including decreased trabecular bone volume fraction (BV/TV), cortical vBMD and thickness as well as micro-finite element analysis (μFEA)-derived bone strength in comparison to control mice [62]. Along with these detrimental changes in bone microarchitecture, directly measured biomechanical bone strength and material properties such as failure load, ultimate stress, and stiffness were significantly diminished in T2D as compared to control mice [62]. Skeletal histomorphometric and serum bone turnover analyses revealed higher bone resorption (osteoclast numbers and cross-linked C-telopeptide of type I collagen [CTx] levels) and lower bone formation rates in T2D mice relative to controls [62]. Additional analyses of osteocyte-enriched bone samples from these mice demonstrated increased mRNA expression of the cellular senescence markers, *p16Ink4a* and *p21Cip1*, as well as SASP factors—most notably Mmp's (*Mmp3*, *Mmp9*, *Mmp12*, and *Mmp13*) and NFκB [62]. In addition, mice with T2D displayed a significantly higher proportion of senescent osteocytes in vivo in bone cortices as characterized by increased SADS- and TAF-positive staining [62]. These data thus provide compelling evidence for accelerated osteocyte senescence and skeletal fragility in young adult obese mice with T2D.

Effects of reducing the senescent cell burden on bone

Our group has demonstrated that elimination of senescent cells in old *INK-ATTAC* mice using AP20187 (a synthetic drug that activates the *ATTAC* suicide transgene and thus apoptosis of $p16^{Ink4a}$-positive senescent cells) effectively eliminates senescent osteocytes as well as senescent preadipocytes in old AP20187-treated as compared to age-matched vehicle-treated control mice [28]. Furthermore, the older mice treated with AP20187 displayed better cortical and trabecular bone microarchitecture and improved biomechanical bone strength properties compared to their age-matched vehicle-treated counterparts [28]. Elimination of senescent cells caused a reduction in osteoclast numbers and decreased levels of bone resorption marker—CTX; whereas, senescent cell elimination increased osteoblast numbers and improved bone formation rates on endocortical surfaces assessed by histomorphometry [28].

As an alternative to the transgenetic *INK-ATTAC* approach and one potentially more adaptable to human translation, we randomized old WT mice to either intermittent senolytic (D+Q) therapy or vehicle treatments over the course of 4 months. Similar to the old *INKA-TTAC* mice treated with AP20187, old mice treated with the combination of D+Q displayed better bone microarchitecture and strength and had lower levels of bone resorption along with improved bone formation rates on endocortical surfaces [28].

It should be noted, however, that removal of senescent osteoclast progenitors using ganciclovir in aged p16-3MR mice was not sufficient to alleviate age-related bone loss, perhaps because senescent osteocytes were not eliminated in this model [65].

As mentioned earlier, senescence-related DDR activation can also occur following high doses of ionizing radiation and chemotherapy, limiting the capacity of the immune system to clear senescent cells from the body, even earlier in life at younger ages. However, both radiation and chemotherapy are used clinically to treat patients with cancer. Although both strategies are effective in limiting the spread of malignant cells, a byproduct is the premature, accelerated accumulation of senescent cells. To examine the bystander effects of senescent cell accumulation on bone loss in the setting of radiation, Chandra et al. [43] performed single-limb (at the femoral metaphysis) focal radiation therapy (FRT) on young adult mice. They found a 4.4-fold increase in SA-β-Gal-positive osteoblasts in the radiated femur versus the contralateral nonradiated femur of these mice [43]. This was accompanied by a 4.7-fold increase in TAF-positive osteocytes and a 3.7-fold increase in TAF-positive osteoblasts in the radiated femur as compared to the contralateral femur [43]. Increased mRNA expression of senescent markers, *p16Ink4a*, *p21Cip1*, *p15*, and *p27*, and SASP components (18 out of 46 genes queried) were also found in the radiated femur compared to the nonradiated contralateral limb [43]. This increased senescence burden in radiated bone was accompanied by deterioration of trabecular bone microarchitecture, and treatment of radiated mice with senolytics (D + Q) decreased bone mRNA expression of *p16Ink4a*, *p21Cip1*, and SASP genes (e.g., *Ccl-2*, *Ccl-4*, *Cxcl-9*, *Cxcl-13*, *IL-10*, *IL-18*, and *Mmp2*) as compared to vehicle-treated mice [43]. Removal of senescent cells restored trabecular bone parameters, increased osteoblast numbers and levels of the bone formation marker, P1NP, and decreased the numbers of bone marrow adipocytes, compared to the vehicle-treated mice also receiving FRT [43]. Therefore, targeting senescent cells with senolytics may represent an effective strategy to preserve bone in cancer patients receiving radiotherapy.

In addition to radiotherapy, chemotherapy-induced bone loss has also been hypothesized to be at least partially a consequence of increased senescent cell accumulation. To test this hypothesis, Yao et al. [44] recently examined the effects of doxorubicin (DOXO), a chemotherapeutic agent used for the treatment of early and advanced-stage breast cancer, on bone parameters and cellular senescence in the bone microenvironment of young adult mice. As anticipated, mice given DOXO developed a lower bone mass phenotype affecting both trabecular and cortical bone parameters as compared to vehicle-treated mice [44]. Female DOXO-treated mice also had a greater reduction in bone parameters compared to ovariectomized (OVX) mice thus establishing that chemotherapy induces bone loss independent of estrogen deficiency [44]. Similar results were found with another chemotherapeutic agent, paclitaxel

[44]. Mice treated with DOXO also displayed higher bone mRNA expression of *p16Ink4a* and lower levels of HMGB1 as compared to the vehicle-treated mice [44], which are both indicative of a higher senescent cell burden in bone. Additionally, DOXO-treated mice displayed upregulated SASP components in bone samples such as *IL-6*, *Ccl3*, *MCSF*, and *MMP12* relative to vehicle-treated mice [44]. By contrast, similar senescence- and SASP-associated changes were not observed in OVX mice implying that lack of estrogen by itself is not sufficient to cause cellular senescence [44]. Treatment of DOXO-induced *INK-ATTAC* mice using AP20187 resulted in decreased *p16Ink4a* and *IL-6* and increased HMGB1 levels, and a concomitant increase in cortical and trabecular bone parameters, bone formation rates, and decreased osteoclast numbers as compared to the vehicle group [44]. Therefore, consist with clearance of senescent cells in old mice to prevent age-related bone loss [28], genetic clearance of $p16^{Ink4a}$-positive cells may represent a novel strategy to alleviate cancer-induced bone loss.

Cellular senescence and aged skeletal muscle

Although heterogeneous in nature, mammalian skeletal muscle is predominantly a mitotically stable tissue with limited turnover yet there is a small population of quiescent muscle stem cells (i.e., satellite cells) that have important biological roles and have been implicated in cellular senescence. Traumatic muscle injury or genetic defects, such as muscular dystrophies, can activate quiescent satellite cells that then undergo dynamic interactions to repair damaged myofibers. Proliferation and differentiation of activated satellite cells can result in their fusion with the damaged myofibers and with other satellite cells to initiate a repair response of the damaged skeletal muscle fibers or can give rise to new fibers.

Satellite cells can self-renew to maintain the skeletal muscle stem cell pool by dividing into daughter stem cells and returning to quiescence following muscle repair thereby maintaining skeletal muscle regenerative capacity [66,67]. However, satellite cell regenerative capabilities have been shown to decline with aging, and the molecular mechanisms regulating quiescence in satellite cells have been linked to the regulation of senescence-associated genes [68]. In particular, quiescent satellite cells in sarcopenic myofibers of geriatric mice display hallmarks of sarcopenia, including impaired activation in response to injury and reduced regenerative capacity [68]. In old age, these cells tend to break away from their state of quiescence and enter into a presenescence state under homoeostatic conditions which is evidenced by their increased *p16Ink4a* mRNA expression compared to younger mice [68]. This quiescence to senescence shift of satellite cells has been attributed to the accumulation of genomic damage with advancing age, which can be reversed by repression of *p16Ink4a* using short-hairpin RNA (shRNA) to thereby decreasing *p16Ink4a* levels and increase the activation rate and self-renewal capacity of satellite cells following muscle injury [68]. Similar to the findings in mice, assessment of human satellite cells isolated from older individuals with sarcopenia (aged ~75 years) showed significantly increased *p16Ink4a* mRNA levels, SA-β-Gal staining, and a dysregulated p16-Rb pathway as compared to satellite cells isolated from younger human subjects [68]. Collectively, these data provide evidence that in response to age-related stress, quiescent muscle satellite cells can enter a state of cellular senescence that limits their resilience and regenerative capacity, thus contributing to aging, frailty, and sarcopenia.

Causal roles of senescent cells in physical dysfunction and frailty

The link between natural aging and declining physical function and increased frailty is clear. In addition to maintaining skeletal muscle regeneration, several studies have shown reduced physical function and lifespan, most notably in mouse models of cancer therapy or accelerated aging, characterized with an increased senescent cell burden. For example, Zhu and colleagues [34] reported that clearance of senescent cells using senolytics, D + Q, improved physical function in mice by alleviating impairment induced by radiation exposure. Indeed, months after radiation, mice that were treated with senolytics had the ability to exercise longer on a treadmill (i.e., more time, distance, as well as total work) and maintained their greater endurance capacity for at least 7 months following senolytic therapy as compared to the vehicle-treated mice [34]. Furthermore, senolytic therapy resulted in decreased expression of *p16Ink4a* in skeletal muscle and a reduced proportion of SA-β-Gal-positive cells in inguinal fat [34], suggesting that the benefits on physical function where potentially mediated through senescent cell clearance in skeletal muscle and adipose tissue depots.

As an extension to this study, Xu and colleagues [41] more recently investigated the causal roles of cellular senescence in mediating physical dysfunction and frailty using multiple approaches. In the first of a series of elegant experiments, they transplanted a small number of senescent preadipocytes intraperitoneally into young adult WT mice, which after only 1 month caused persistent physical dysfunction, including decreased maximal walking speed, shorter hanging endurance, and reduced grip strength as compared to control mice transplanted with control, nonsenescent preadipocytes [41]. Furthermore, an increased senescence burden (e.g., higher *p16Ink4a* expression, increased TAF-positive cells, and SA-β-Gal-positive cells) was observed locally in visceral adipose tissue (near the injection site) in mice transplanted with senescent cells even after the transplanted cells (which were traced in vivo using a luciferase reporter) were cleared from the body of these animals [41]. In addition, the spread of senescence was noted in tissues distant from the site of injection (e.g., skeletal muscle) as evidenced by increased expression of *p16Ink4a* and proinflammatory SASP cytokines such as TNFα and IL-6, thus demonstrating the systemic spread of cellular senescence to the host's tissues [41]. Transplantation of even fewer senescent cells into older mice was sufficient to accelerate physical dysfunction and frailty in these animals and significantly increased their mortality [41]. In complementary experiments, clearance of senescent cells in normal, chronologically aged WT mice by periodically administering senolytics, D+Q, to these animals alleviated physical dysfunction and aspects of frailty by reducing senescent cell abundance; importantly, senescent cell clearance in these animals also extended posttreatment survival (by 36%) while simultaneously compressing morbidity [41]. Interestingly, senescent cell clearance was also observed following administration of D+Q to surgically excised ex vivo adipose tissue explants from obese humans [41], pointing to the translational relevance of this strategy to target cellular senescence to potentially improve physical function and alleviate aspects of frailty with aging and in the setting of metabolic dysfunction. Whether these or similar approaches are effective in ameliorating sarcopenia remains to be established.

Further potential translational evidence for the roles of cellular senescence in driving physical dysfunction with aging comes from studies performed in humans that have reported an accumulation of *p16Ink4a*-positive cells in thigh adipose tissue biopsies obtained from older as compared to younger subjects [69]. Furthermore, the elevated proportion of *p16Ink4a*-positive cells in thigh adipose tissue correlated negatively with measures of physical performance such as grip strength, gait speed on 4-m course and self-perceived mobility, even after controlling for potentially confounding factors including age and measures of body composition [69]. Although these studies provide initial evidence for the association between a greater senescent cell burden and physical dysfunction in humans, additional larger prospective studies are warranted.

Senolytics in clinical trials

Clinical trials investigating the safety and efficacy of senolytics in humans are currently underway, and results from the first studies were recently reported. For example, in the first-in-human pilot study of D+Q conducted on 14 patients with idiopathic pulmonary fibrosis (IPF), a chronic, rapidly progressing fibrotic lung disease linked to cellular senescence [70], Justice and colleagues [45] administered D+Q intermittently in the form of 9 doses over the course of 3 weeks to 14 IPF patients. Although this study lacked a placebo-controlled group, a significant improvement was observed in these patients in 6-min walk distance, 4-m gait speed, chair stand time, and short physical performance battery scores in response to intermittent senolytic therapy [45]. There was also a trend for a decrease in SASP factors within the circulation, although changes did not reach statistical significance potentially due to the relatively small sample size [45]. Nevertheless, given the modest improvements in physical function and that D+Q was found to be well-tolerated and safe, this study supports the need for additional senolytic trials. One such ongoing phase 1, open-label, trial in patients with diabetic kidney disease has reported interim results [46]. Indeed, Hickson and colleagues [46] administered the combination of D+Q to patients with diabetic kidney disease for three consecutive days and then examined the in vivo senescent cell burden in these subjects 11 days following the final dose. Consistent with data form preclinical studies, a significant reduction in *p16Ink4a*- and *p21Cip1*-positive cells as well as significantly reduced SA-β-Gal staining was observed in subcutaneous abdominal tissue samples of D+Q-treated subjects with similar findings observed in skin biopsies [46]. In addition, several SASP factors including IL-1α, -2, -6, and -9, and MMP-2, -9, and -12 were significant reduced in the circulation of subjects treated with D+Q [46]. Although again not placebo-controlled and preliminary, this study provides initial "*proof-of-concept*" evidence that senolytic therapy can reduce the in vivo cellular senescence burden in humans, as observed in mice. It should be noted that multiple other placebo-controlled, randomized controlled clinical trials involving senolytics are currently underway as more data on safety, tolerability, side effects, and efficacy are needed in humans. Furthermore, additional carefully monitored trials in humans with other conditions, such as elderly subjects with age-related bone loss, will be initiating soon.

Conclusion

In summary, there is hope that the enormous burden of age-related comorbidities, including osteosarcopenia, can be mitigated by therapeutically targeting fundamental mechanisms of aging, such as cellular senescence. Indeed, mounting evidence, predominantly in mice (as summarized in Table 1), points to reducing the senescent cell burden to prevent or delay age-related bone loss and physical dysfunction as well as aspects of frailty in old age. Additional clinical studies and trials are needed to establish whether these exciting preclinical findings can be translated to humans.

Funding

This work was supported by National Institutes of Health (NIH) grants P01 AG062413 (J.N.F.), R21 AG065868 (J.N.F), K01 AR070241 (J.N.F.), as well as a High-Risk Pilot Award (J.N.F.) and Career Development Award (J.N.F.) from the Mayo Clinic Robert and Arlene Kogod Center on Aging, and the Richard F. Emslander Career Development Award in Endocrinology (J.N.F.).

Conflict of interest

Japneet Kaur and Joshua Farr have nothing to disclose.

TABLE 1 Summary of the senescence markers and the effects of senolytic therapy for the major studies included in the review.

Reference	Animal or human characteristics	Senescence markers	Effects of senolytics on senescence/SASP markers	Functional implications of senolytic therapy
Farr et al. [57]	Mice: **Old** vs young	↑p16^{Ink4a} (OP, OB, OCY, B, T, Myeloid) ↑p21 (OCY); ↑p53 (OCY, Myeloid) ↑SASP, senescent OCY, TIF$^+$ OCY	NA	NA
	Human: **Old** vs young	↑p16^{Ink4a}, p21, SASP	NA	NA
Farr et al. [28]	Mice: **Old** vs young	↑p16^{Ink4a}	↓p16^{Ink4a}, EGFP, ↓Senescent OCY	↑Spine BV/TV, Tb.N, Tb.Th ↓Spine Tb.Sp, SMI ↑Femur Ct.Th, failure load ↑Femur Ec. N.Ob/B.Pm, MAR, BFR/BS ↓Femur Ec. N.Oc/B.Pm
Chandra et al. [43]	Mice: **R** vs NR	↑p16^{Ink4a}, p21, SASP ↑SA-β-Gal+ and TAF$^+$ bone lining cells ↑TAF$^+$ OCY	↓p^{16Ink4a}, p21, SASP ↓TAF$^+$ OCY and bone lining cells	↑Femur BV/TV, Conn. D. ↑Femur N.Ob/B.Pm ↓Femur N.Ad/T.Ar
Eckhardt et al. [62]	Mice: **HFD/STZ** vs control	↑p16^{Ink4a}, p21, SASP, senescent OCY	NA	NA
Yao et al. [44]	Mice: **R** vs NR	↑p16^{Ink4a}, SASP ↓HMGB1	NA	NA
	Mice: **DOXO** vs VEH	↑p16^{Ink4a}, SASP, SA-β-Gal+ cells ↓HMGB1	↓p16^{Ink4a}, SASP ↑HMGB1	↑Femur Tb BV/TV ↓Oc.S/BS, N.Oc/BS ↑Femur BFR/BS

Kim et al. [65]			↓p16^{Ink4a} ↓Senescent OC progenitors	No effect on age related loss of bone mass
Sousa-Victor et al. [68]	Mice: **Geriatric**, old, adult and young	↑p16^{Ink4a} in satellite cells	↓p16^{Ink4a}	Restoration of muscle regenerative functions
	Human: **Geriatric** vs young	↑p16^{Ink4a} in satellite cells	NA	NA
Zhu et al. [34]			↓p16^{Ink4a} in quadriceps muscle ↓SA-β-Gal in inguinal fat	↑Treadmill exercise time, distance, total work
Xu et al. [41]	Mice: Senescent cell transplantation	↑p16^{Ink4a} ↑SA-β-Gal ↑TAF+ cells ↑TNFα, IL-6	↓p16^{Ink4a} ↓IL-6, Cxcl1	↑Maximal walking speed, hanging and treadmill endurance, grip strength, daily activity
Justice et al. [69]	Human: Overweight/obese old	↑p16Ink4a^{INK4a}+cells	NA	NA

Key: *B*, B-cells; *BFR/BS*, bone formation rate per bone surface; *BV/TV*, bone volume fraction; *Ct*, cortical; *DOXO*, doxorubicin; *Ec*, endocortical; *HFD*, high-fat diet; *STZ*, streptozotocin; *MAR*, mineral apposition rate; *N*, number; *N.Ad/T.Ar*, adipocyte numbers per total area; *N.Ob/B.Pm*, osteoblast numbers per bone perimeter; *N.Oc/B.Pm*, osteoclast numbers per bone perimeter; *OB*, osteoblast; *OCY*, osteocytes; *OP*, osteoprogenitor; *R*, radiated; *NR*, nonradiated; *SASP*, senescence-associated secretory phenotype; *SA-β-Gal*, senescence-associated beta-galactosidase; *Sp*, separation; *T*, T-cells; *TAF*, telomere associated foci; *Tb.*, trabecular; *Th*, thickness. The upward (↑) and downward (↓) arrows represent the results for the study group in **bold** versus the contralateral group.

References

[1] Lopez-Otin C, Blasco MA, Partridge L, Serrano M, Kroemer G. The hallmarks of aging. Cell 2013;153(6):1194–217.

[2] Farr JN, Almeida M. The spectrum of fundamental basic science discoveries contributing to organismal aging. J Bone Miner Res 2018;33(9):1568–84.

[3] Aversa Z, Zhang X, Fielding RA, Lanza I, LeBrasseur NK. The clinical impact and biological mechanisms of skeletal muscle aging. Bone 2019;127:26–36.

[4] Campisi J. Aging, cellular senescence, and cancer. Annu Rev Physiol 2013;75:685–705.

[5] Ben-Porath I, Weinberg RA. The signals and pathways activating cellular senescence. Int J Biochem Cell Biol 2005;37(5):961–76.

[6] van Deursen JM. The role of senescent cells in ageing. Nature 2014;509(7501):439–46.

[7] Khosla S, Farr JN, Tchkonia T, Kirkland JL. The role of cellular senescence in ageing and endocrine disease. Nat Rev Endocrinol 2020;16(5):263–75.

[8] Coppe JP, Patil CK, Rodier F, Sun Y, Munoz DP, Goldstein J, et al. Senescence-associated secretory phenotypes reveal cell-nonautonomous functions of oncogenic RAS and the p53 tumor suppressor. PLoS Biol 2008;6(12):2853–68.

[9] Acosta JC, Banito A, Wuestefeld T, Georgilis A, Janich P, Morton JP, et al. A complex secretory program orchestrated by the inflammasome controls paracrine senescence. Nat Cell Biol 2013;15(8):978–90.

[10] Coppe JP, Desprez PY, Krtolica A, Campisi J. The senescence-associated secretory phenotype: the dark side of tumor suppression. Annu Rev Pathol 2010;5:99–118.

[11] Hayflick L, Moorhead PS. The serial cultivation of human diploid cell strains. Exp Cell Res 1961;25:585–621.

[12] Shay JW, Wright WE. Hayflick, his limit, and cellular ageing. Nat Rev Mol Cell Biol 2000;1(1):72–6.

[13] Shammas MA. Telomeres, lifestyle, cancer, and aging. Curr Opin Clin Nutr Metab Care 2011;14(1):28–34.

[14] von Zglinicki T. Oxidative stress shortens telomeres. Trends Biochem Sci 2002;27(7):339–44.

[15] Campisi J, d'Adda di Fagagna F. Cellular senescence: when bad things happen to good cells. Nat Rev Mol Cell Biol 2007;8:729–40.

[16] Nelson G, Wordsworth J, Wang C, Jurk D, Lawless C, Martin-Ruiz C, et al. A senescent cell bystander effect: senescence-induced senescence. Aging Cell 2012;11(2):345–9.

[17] Tchkonia T, Zhu Y, van Deursen J, Campisi J, Kirkland JL. Cellular senescence and the senescent secretory phenotype: therapeutic opportunities. J Clin Invest 2013;123(3):966–72.

[18] Baker DJ, Wijshake T, Tchkonia T, LeBrasseur NK, Childs BG, van de Sluis B, et al. Clearance of p16Ink4a-positive senescent cells delay aging-associated disorders. Nature 2011;479(7372):232–6.

[19] Laberge RM, Adler D, DeMaria M, Mechtouf N, Teachenor R, Cardin GB, et al. Mitochondrial DNA damage induces apoptosis in senescent cells. Cell Death Dis 2013;4, e727.

[20] Demaria M, Ohtani N, Youssef SA, Rodier F, Toussaint W, Mitchell JR, et al. An essential role for senescent cells in optimal wound healing through secretion of PDGF-AA. Dev Cell 2014;31(6):722–33.

[21] Xu M, Palmer AK, Ding H, Weivoda MM, Pirtskhalava T, White TA, et al. Targeting senescent cells enhances adipogenesis and metabolic function in old age. Elife 2015;4, e12997.

[22] Roos CM, Zhang B, Palmer AK, Ogrodnik MB, Pirtskhalava T, Thalji NM, et al. Chronic senolytic treatment alleviates established vasomotor dysfunction in aged or atherosclerotic mice. Aging Cell 2016;15(5):973–7.

[23] Baker DJ, Childs BG, Durik M, Wijers ME, Sieben CJ, Zhong J, et al. Naturally occurring p16(Ink4a)-positive cells shorten healthy lifespan. Nature 2016;530(7589):184–9.

[24] Childs BG, Baker DJ, Wijshake T, Conover CA, Campisi J, van Deursen JM. Senescent intimal foam cells are deleterious at all stages of atherosclerosis. Science 2016;354(6311):472–7.

[25] Jeon OH, Kim C, Laberge RM, Demaria M, Rathod S, Vasserot AP, et al. Local clearance of senescent cells attenuates the development of post-traumatic osteoarthritis and creates a pro-regenerative environment. Nat Med 2017;23(6):775–81.

[26] Ogrodnik M, Miwa S, Tchkonia T, Tiniakos D, Wilson CL, Lahat A, et al. Cellular senescence drives age-dependent hepatic steatosis. Nat Commun 2017;8:15691.

[27] Schafer MJ, White TA, Iijima K, Haak AJ, Ligresti G, Atkinson EJ, et al. Cellular senescence mediates fibrotic pulmonary disease. Nat Commun 2017;8:14532.

[28] Farr JN, Xu M, Weivoda MM, Monroe DG, Fraser DG, Onken JL, et al. Targeting cellular senescence prevents age-related bone loss in mice. Nat Med 2017;23(9):1072–9.

[29] Bussian TJ, Aziz A, Meyer CF, Swenson BL, van Deursen JM, Baker DJ. Clearance of senescent glial cells prevents tau-dependent pathology and cognitive decline. Nature 2018;562(7728):578–82.

[30] Ogrodnik M, Zhu Y, Langhi LGP, Tchkonia T, Kruger P, Fielder E, et al. Obesity-induced cellular senescence drives anxiety and impairs neurogenesis. Cell Metab 2019;29(5):1061–77 e8.

[31] Anderson R, Lagnado A, Maggiorani D, Walaszczyk A, Dookun E, Chapman J, et al. Length-independent telomere damage drives post-mitotic cardiomyocyte senescence. EMBO J 2019;38(5).

[32] Palmer AK, Xu M, Zhu Y, Pirtskhalava T, Weivoda MM, Hachfeld CM, et al. Targeting senescent cells alleviates obesity-induced metabolic dysfunction. Aging Cell 2019;18(3), e12950.

[33] Aguayo-Mazzucato C, Andle J, Lee Jr TB, Midha A, Talemal L, Chipashvili V, et al. Acceleration of beta cell aging determines diabetes and senolysis improves disease outcomes. Cell Metab 2019;30(1):129–42.

[34] Zhu Y, Tchkonia T, Pirtskhalava T, Gower AC, Ding H, Giorgadze N, et al. The Achilles' heel of senescent cells: from transcriptome to senolytic drugs. Aging Cell 2015;14(4):644–58.

[35] Yosef R, Pilpel N, Tokarsky-Amiel R, Biran A, Ovadya Y, Cohen S, et al. Directed elimination of senescent cells by inhibition of BCL-W and BCL-XL. Nat Commun 2016;7:11190.

[36] Chang J, Wang Y, Shao L, Laberge RM, Demaria M, Campisi J, et al. Clearance of senescent cells by ABT263 rejuvenates aged hematopoietic stem cells in mice. Nat Med 2016;22(1):78–83.

[37] Zhu Y, Doornebal EJ, Pirtskhalava T, Giorgadze N, Wentworth M, Fuhrmann-Stroissnigg H, et al. New agents that target senescent cells: the flavone, fisetin, and the BCL-XL inhibitors, A1331852 and A1155463. Aging (Albany NY) 2017;9(3):955–63.

[38] Fuhrmann-Stroissnigg H, Ling YY, Zhao J, McGowan SJ, Zhu Y, Brooks RW, et al. Identification of HSP90 inhibitors as a novel class of senolytics. Nat Commun 2017;8(1):422.

[39] Baar MP, Brandt RMC, Putavet DA, Klein JDD, Derks KWJ, Bourgeois BRM, et al. Targeted apoptosis of senescent cells restores tissue homeostasis in response to chemotoxicity and aging. Cell 2017;169(1):132–47 e16.

[40] Yousefzadeh MJ, Zhu Y, McGowan SJ, Angelini L, Fuhrmann-Stroissnigg H, Xu M, et al. Fisetin is a senotherapeutic that extends health and lifespan. EBioMedicine 2018;36:18–28.

[41] Xu M, Pirtskhalava T, Farr JN, Weigand BM, Palmer AK, Weivoda MM, et al. Senolytics improve physical function and increase lifespan in old age. Nat Med 2018;24(8):1246–56.

[42] Musi N, Valentine JM, Sickora KR, Baeuerle E, Thompson CS, Shen Q, et al. Tau protein aggregation is associated with cellular senescence in the brain. Aging Cell 2018, e12840.

[43] Chandra A, Lagnado AB, Farr JN, Monroe DG, Park S, Hachfeld C, et al. Targeted reduction of senescent cell burden alleviates focal radiotherapy-related bone loss. J Bone Miner Res 2020.

[44] Yao Z, Murali B, Ren Q, Luo X, Faget DV, Cole T, et al. Therapy-induced senescence drives bone loss. Cancer Res 2020;80(5):1171–82.
[45] Justice JN, Nambiar AM, Tchkonia T, LeBrasseur NK, Pascual R, Hashmi SK, et al. Senolytics in idiopathic pulmonary fibrosis: results from a first-in-human, open-label, pilot study. EBioMedicine 2019;40:554–63.
[46] Hickson LJ, Langhi Prata LGP, Bobart SA, Evans TK, Giorgadze N, Hashmi SK, et al. Senolytics decrease senescent cells in humans: preliminary report from a clinical trial of dasatinib plus quercetin in individuals with diabetic kidney disease. EBioMedicine 2019;47:446–56.
[47] Kirkland JL, Tchkonia T, Zhu Y, Niedernhofer LJ, Robbins PD. The clinical potential of senolytic drugs. J Am Geriatr Soc 2017;65(10):2297–301.
[48] Wissler Gerdes EO, Zhu Y, Tchkonia T, Kirkland JL. Discovery, development, and future application of senolytics: theories and predictions. FEBS J 2020;287(12):2418–27.
[49] Gorgoulis V, Adams PD, Alimonti A, Bennett DC, Bischof O, Bishop C, et al. Cellular senescence: defining a path forward. Cell 2019;179(4):813–27.
[50] Munoz-Espin D, Serrano M. Cellular senescence: from physiology to pathology. Nat Rev Mol Cell Biol 2014;15(7):482–96.
[51] Dimri GP, Lee X, Basile G, Acosta M, Scott G, Roskelley C, et al. A biomarker that identifies senescent human cells in culture and in aging skin in vivo. Proc Natl Acad Sci U S A 1995;92(20):9363–7.
[52] Odgren PR, MacKay CA, Mason-Savas A, Yang M, Mailhot G, Birnbaum MJ. False-positive beta-galactosidase staining in osteoclasts by endogenous enzyme: studies in neonatal and month-old wild-type mice. Connect Tissue Res 2006;47(4):229–34.
[53] Hewitt G, Jurk D, Marques FD, Correia-Melo C, Hardy T, Gackowska A, et al. Telomeres are favoured targets of a persistent DNA damage response in ageing and stress-induced senescence. Nat Commun 2012;3:708.
[54] Criscione SW, De Cecco M, Siranosian B, Zhang Y, Kreiling JA, Sedivy JM, et al. Reorganization of chromosome architecture in replicative cellular senescence. Sci Adv 2016;2(2), e1500882.
[55] Zhang R, Adams PD. Heterochromatin and its relationship to cell senescence and cancer therapy. Cell Cycle 2007;6(7):784–9.
[56] Swanson EC, Manning B, Zhang H, Lawrence JB. Higher-order unfolding of satellite heterochromatin is a consistent and early event in cell senescence. J Cell Biol 2013;203(6):929–42.
[57] Farr JN, Fraser DG, Wang H, Jaehn K, Ogrodnik MB, Weivoda MM, et al. Identification of senescent cells in the bone microenvironment. J Bone Miner Res 2016;31(11):1920–9.
[58] Piemontese M, Almeida M, Robling AG, Kim HN, Xiong J, Thostenson JD, et al. Old age causes de novo intracortical bone remodeling and porosity in mice. JCI Insight 2017;2(17).
[59] Palmer AK, Gustafson B, Kirkland JL, Smith U. Cellular senescence: at the nexus between ageing and diabetes. Diabetologia 2019;62(10):1835–41.
[60] Ma L, Oei L, Jiang L, Estrada K, Chen H, Wang Z, et al. Association between bone mineral density and type 2 diabetes mellitus: a meta-analysis of observational studies. Eur J Epidemiol 2012;27(5):319–32.
[61] Bonds DE, Larson JC, Schwartz AV, Strotmeyer ES, Robbins J, Rodriguez BL, et al. Risk of fracture in women with type 2 diabetes: the Women's Health Initiative observational study. J Clin Endocrinol Metab 2006;91(9):3404–10.
[62] Eckhardt BA, Rowsey JL, Thicke BS, Fraser DG, O'Grady KL, Bondar OP, et al. Accelerated osteocyte senescence and skeletal fragility in mice with type 2 diabetes. JCI Insight 2020;5(9).
[63] Luo J, Quan J, Tsai J, Hobensack CK, Sullivan C, Hector R, et al. Nongenetic mouse models of non-insulin-dependent diabetes mellitus. Metabolism 1998;47(6):663–8.

[64] Mu J, Woods J, Zhou YP, Roy RS, Li Z, Zycband E, et al. Chronic inhibition of dipeptidyl peptidase-4 with a sitagliptin analog preserves pancreatic beta-cell mass and function in a rodent model of type 2 diabetes. Diabetes 2006;55(6):1695–704.

[65] Kim HN, Chang J, Iyer S, Han L, Campisi J, Manolagas SC, et al. Elimination of senescent osteoclast progenitors has no effect on the age-associated loss of bone mass in mice. Aging Cell 2019;18(3), e12923.

[66] Yin H, Price F, Rudnicki MA. Satellite cells and the muscle stem cell niche. Physiol Rev 2013;93(1):23–67.

[67] Sampath SC, Sampath SC, Ho ATV, Corbel SY, Millstone JD, Lamb J, et al. Induction of muscle stem cell quiescence by the secreted niche factor Oncostatin M. Nat Commun 2018;9(1):1531.

[68] Sousa-Victor P, Gutarra S, Garcia-Prat L, Rodriguez-Ubreva J, Ortet L, Ruiz-Bonilla V, et al. Geriatric muscle stem cells switch reversible quiescence into senescence. Nature 2014;506(7488):316–21.

[69] Justice JN, Gregory H, Tchkonia T, LeBrasseur NK, Kirkland JL, Kritchevsky SB, et al. Cellular senescence biomarker p16INK4a+ cell burden in thigh adipose is associated with poor physical function in older women. J Gerontol A Biol Sci Med Sci 2018;73(7):939–45.

[70] Schafer MJ, Haak AJ, Tschumperlin DJ, LeBrasseur NK. Targeting senescent cells in fibrosis: pathology, paradox, and practical considerations. Curr Rheumatol Rep 2018;20(1):3.

Chapter 3

Biomechanics and mechanobiology of bone and muscle: Current and future musculoskeletal modeling research directions in osteosarcopenia

Hossein Mokhtarzadeh, Fatemeh Malekipour, and Peter Lee
Department of Biomedical Engineering, Faculty of Engineering and Information Technology, The University of Melbourne, Melbourne, VIC, Australia

Background

Osteosarcopenia is the concurrent occurrence of osteoporosis and sarcopenia which may be worsen with advancing age [1]. Several clinical or research tools have been developed to identify these two conditions including measurements of bone mineral density (BMD) and muscle strength [2–6]. These techniques are used to avoid devastating sequelae of these conditions including but not limited to bone fracture and falls [7]. The current clinical bone and muscle biomarkers can detect those at risk but may still fail to provide information regarding high-risk activities [8,9]. This lack of predictability in the clinical setting may be the reason why the number of falls and fractures are significantly on the rise particularly among older adults [10,11].

In addition to the consequences of age-related deterioration in bone and muscle, these conditions are costly both for individuals and the society [12,13]. For instance, on average, the direct cost of osteoporotic fractures was reported between $5000 and $6500 billion in United States, Canada, and Europe per year. This estimate excludes indirect costs [14]. Moreover, recent estimate of hospitalization cost for those with sarcopenia has been $40.4 billion (average $260/person) which was shown to be race-, gender-, and age-specific in the United States [12]. Apart from the cost, unfortunately, patients with osteosarcopenia [15] may be at greater risk of fall, fracture, hospitalization [16] and

Osteosarcopenia. https://doi.org/10.1016/B978-0-12-820088-9.00005-6

significantly greater mortality rate compared with the patients with osteoporosis or sarcopenia alone [17,18]. The significance of age-related conditions is further pronounced by the WHO initiative to call this the decade of healthy aging [19].

Another challenge that investigators may face with these patients is their limited ability to perform high-risk diagnostic experiments due to fragile bone and muscles. Thus, development of noninvasive techniques and clinical tools complementing imaging techniques are required to avoid any unintended falls or fractures during diagnoses of those with either osteoporosis and sarcopenia or both [9,20,21]. Imaging techniques such as DXA scans are routinely used as a clinical and noninvasive tool for osteoporosis patients. However, current imaging techniques do not provide information about more dynamic scenarios such as walking or lifting. More importantly, they do not provide any information about bone and muscle function and their interactions during various activities. To address these shortcomings, numerous musculoskeletal (MSK) and computer models have been developed [9,22]. These noninvasive methods can provide powerful tools that can potentially and safely predict the consequences of osteosarcopenia [22,23].

This chapter reviews the role of personalized MSK models for predicting the risk of falls and fracture in patients with osteosarcopenia toward addressing the following questions: (1) can we predict high-risk activities that lead to falls and fractures during daily activities?, (2) In a given high-risk activity, which bone is more susceptible to fracture, and finally (3) can we identify the role of individual muscles and bone during high-risk activities to eventually develop preventive and protective methods against fall and fracture? In summary, this book chapter focuses on state-of-the-art biomechanical models to develop novel and complementary therapeutic approaches toward predictive tools to screen those with sarcopenia, osteoporosis or osteosarcopenia and their associations with fractures and falls.

Why personalized musculoskeletal modeling?

Clinical assessment of osteosarcopenia considers personalized measurements of patients including previous falls, timed up and go (TUG), handgrip strength, walking speed or BMD level [7]. However, to predict risk of structural failure of bone, fracture and falls, measurements of each individual are compared with population-based studies, which may not precisely identify the consequences of those at risk of osteosarcopenia. However, there may be a strong association between these parameters such as fall and handgrip strength or BMD level and osteoporotic fractures [24]. For instance, bone fracture assessment using the FRAX score has been developed as a useful and simple tool based on statistical analyses of a population using several risk factors such as BMD, smoking, and BMI [25]. Nonetheless, such scores may not fully represent the ability of the bone to maintain structure and function for an individual during different daily activities [25].

Bone fracture depends not only on the bone quality, but the magnitude and its rate (time to peak) of the applied load during various activities. Fracture occurs when the applied load exceeds the bone strength at a particular location (i.e., Load Strength Ratio > 1). Bone strength varies under different loading conditions (quasistatic, cyclic loading or impact loads such as those during a fall) [26]. Moreover, different individuals exert different loads on their bones in each activity, which can affect the Load Strength Ratio in a certain scenario. Thus, the risk of fracture is subject-specific in any given activity [9]. Consequently, bone fracture analyses require a well-defined loading conditions (i.e., loading profile versus time) and bone strength [27]. Loading conditions in turn require an accurate measure of the muscle contribution, as major load generating actuators. Overall, there is a complex interdependence between bone and muscle strength and the generated loads in them during various activities. An accurate calculation of this interdependence can help identify the high-risk activities and anatomical locations in each individual.

During daily activities, muscles, and bone work in concert. Smooth performance of a daily activity occurs because of proper activation of several muscles that can move the joints and bones in a right direction. This process applies mechanical loads via muscles and ligaments to the bones and joints while the whole body keeps its balance during a dynamic situation. However, at any given time, any internal (e.g., muscle weakness or lack of synergy) or external (e.g., trip or slip scenarios) perturbations could affect the balance thus leading to a likely fall or fracture. Moreover, following mechanical perturbation, the strategy in recovering from perturbations is subject-specific [28] though some overall approaches have been identified involving the ankle or hip strategies [29–31]. Thus, understanding underlying causes of fall and fracture in bone and muscle quality and their anatomical variations (both function and forms) should be considered in implementing personalized methodologies.

Personalized MSK models are powerful tools that have shown a promising pathway toward such an individualized prediction of muscle and bone loading due to internal (e.g., intraabdominal pressure) or external loading (e.g., ground reaction forces) to the body [9,20,22,23,32,33]. In these modeling approaches, muscle and bone morphology and their quality are computationally quantified for each individual and a set of mathematical and physical equations are used to quantify the interaction between bone-muscle and how their function/form could lead to fall and fractures [27,34]. Next, we will discuss how a personalized MSK modeling (a.k.a., computer-based, or biomechanical modeling) can be created and eventually help clinicians to better screen osteosarcopenia and predict consequences of such age-related conditions.

Personalized musculoskeletal modeling as a predictive tool

Prediction of high-risk activities leading to osteoporotic fractures

MSK models use physics-based models of human movement and can be used to predict the forces that cause the motion or vice versa. Let us consider Newton's second law where $F=m\times a$. F is the force on a mass (m) such as a body segment where it causes the mass to accelerate (i.e., a). If we can assess forces on the human body (e.g., muscles, external forces, etc.), one can predict how the joints move (a) given the mass. Similarly, if we can measure joint motions (a), one can predict forces (F) that cause the joint motions. This simple explanation is the basis of MSK modeling using engineering principles.

Bone fracture occurs when mechanical load (L) exceeds its strength (S) or load/strength ratio (LSR) is greater than 1, i.e., LSR > 1. To better understand the risk of fracture, LSR needs to be quantified during daily activities for an individual. Several experimental and computational methods have been developed to measure these variables to identify those at risk of fracture [9,20,35]. Mechanical crush testing of cadaveric specimens using material testing machines has been extensively used to quantify strength of bone for a variety of loading rates [36] and can eventually help predict bone strength of others using correlation and regression analyses [9,37]. Moreover, sensors placed on the intervertebral joint to measure disc pressure can be related to intervertebral loading [38,39]. However, these methods are extremely invasive and are not practical for those with osteosarcopenia at risk of fracture and fall. On the other hand, image-based methods have been developed to predict bone strength and the risk of fracture, such as Quantitative computed tomography (QCT) and Dual-energy X-ray absorptiometry (DEXA) [9,21,40]. These imaging techniques have also been combined with Finite Element Analysis (FEA), a stress analysis method to predict bone strength (FEA) [21]. Though such methods are noninvasive, they are not free of side effects including high dose of X-rays and costs due to high computational and labor efforts to develop these complex models [17].

These imaging methods are still the best way to measure (or predict) bone strength in a noninvasive manner. Though, biomechanical loading experienced by bone cannot be predicted by only imaging techniques. It is because such a loading strongly depends on the type of a movement, joint motions, and external forces. In addition, most imaging techniques are conducted in stationary situation while most of daily activities are dynamic. MSK models enable us to obtain internal loading given joint motions and external loading, e.g., ground reaction forces (GRFs).

One of the most comprehensive biomechanical modeling studies was performed using the Framingham Heart Study (FHS) database, where MSK models were used to predict spinal loading and the risk of vertebral fracture at every intervertebral joint. A total of 250 individuals from the FHS database were recruited in the study [20,41,42]. Subject-specific MSK models were developed by scaling a generic MSK model, and each model was adjusted for the major muscles in terms of their respective cross-sectional area, moment arms where QCT data was available, as well as the position of each vertebrae from X-ray images [20]. Inverse dynamic and joint reaction analyses were performed in OpenSim [22] to predict individuals' muscle forces (for over 500 muscle fascicles) and all 17 interverbal joint across the spine for 126 different

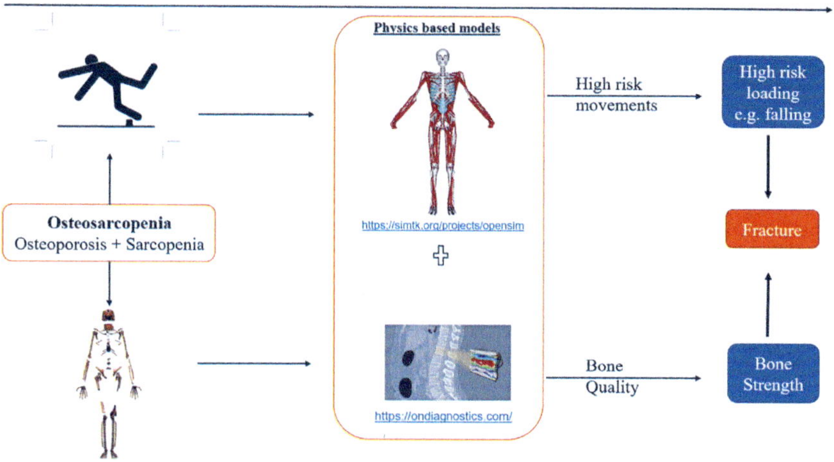

FIG. 1 Prediction of consequences of osteosarcopenia using combined musculoskeletal modeling and finite element analyses. Each step to develop models can benefit from AI algorithms given relevant information such as large muscle and skeletal imaging or motion data. These computer base models not only predict fall and fractures but also can reveal the function of the MSK system during high-risk activities. *(The image is copyright of O.N. Diagnostics, and the permission to reproduce was provided by O.N. Diagnostics (https://ondiagnostics.com/).)*

activities [9,20]. In the meantime, the vertebral strengths were predicted based on Quantitative Computed Tomography-based Finite Element Analysis (QCT-FEA) models and then a regression analyses provided the strength of each vertebra (Fig. 1) [9,20]. QCT data provide 3D geometry models and BMD levels (associated with bone strength) then using a mathematical model, i.e., FEA, one can predict the stress/strain level of bone including its strength. Having both intervertebral joint loading (L) and their respective vertebral strength (S), the risk of fracture (load/strength or LSR) was predicted for every spinal level for each person performing all 126 activities. The results revealed high-risk activities due to maximum LSRs along the spine including: "*lateral bending with a weight in one hand (upper thoracic), holding weights with elbows flexed (lower thoracic) and forward flexion with weight (lumbar).*" The findings indicated that a wide range of asymmetric activities of weightlifting, carrying nonsymmetric postures should be evaluated in the future studies of vertebral fracture. Such outcomes from biomechanical modeling could eventually be used for clinical practice when proven in a longitudinal human study. Finally, these findings provide evidence on variety of high-risk activities and static postures that need to be scrutinized in more dynamic scenarios in the future to study osteoporotic vertebral fracture biomechanics. We envision that future studies of MSK modeling approaches can improve their usability so that they become a part of clinical practice. It should be noted that the protocols developed in this study can be used for other joints as a novel tool to predict a risk of bone fracture.

Prediction of risk of falls following sarcopenia

Patients with sarcopenia may suffer from future falls [43]. Generally, falls occur when the body is unable to maintain its balance in a given activity. A fall is defined as an incidence in which an individual comes to a resting or lower position while muscles cannot prevent such unintentional movement (WHO definition). The musculoskeletal system is responsible for keeping the balance. Age-related conditions such as sarcopenia adversely affect muscle mass, strength, and possibly neural activities, affecting stability and thereby increasing the risk of falls and bone fractures. The clinical consequences of sarcopenia and its risk factors have been assessed using walking performance (e.g., gait speed), timed up and go (TUG) test, muscle strength and imaging techniques such as DEXA scans. One shortcoming regarding these measures is that they may not consider the role of high-risk activities that can lead to falls [1,7,44]. Having information regarding the quality of muscles including muscle morphology, their activation patterns and strength would be valuable adjunct to predict sarcopenia's adverse effects in addition to the current clinical tools [45].

A physical moment following a fall incidence, large mechanical loading is generated between the human body and environment—usually a hard surface—in which the person is in contact. Prior to or at the time of a fall, muscles and joints may respond differently compared to normal walking [46] or sit to stand [47] experiments which involve slow speed movements. Thus, the following question can be raised: what kind of activities can pose high-risk situations and how do individual muscles and joints respond for individuals during these activities?

To address such challenging questions, a holistic view of neuromusculoskeletal system is required. Bioengineering methods utilizing MSK modeling can provide such a platform to give us insights regarding the high-risk situations—including perturbation-based or dual tasking scenarios [2,48–50]—and muscle and joint contributions during these scenarios.

Currently, there are not many biomechanical studies where age-related conditions such as sarcopenia are considered [51]. For instance, in the recent study on the role of sarcopenia on spinal loading, researchers used a MSK model approach [51]. The authors virtually reduced the strength of certain spinal muscles to simulate age-related muscle parameters such as erector spinae's strength. It was found that severe and very severe (36% and 24%, respectively) sarcopenia levels, led to an increase in spinal compressive load of up to 36% or 318N. These age-related changes in spinal loading increased muscle activities of up to 100% of their muscle strength [51]. The effect of aging on spinal loading was simulated and revealed that spinal loading and even load-to-strength ratio could increase with aging (part of [9] not published yet). These changes in muscle activation with aging could not only lead to increased risk of spinal fracture but also may affect the balance of the trunk and the whole body, which could further lead to subsequent falls.

In another recent perturbation-based study to compare healthy young and older adults, researchers found that there is no difference as a result of age on gait stability measures (i.e., margin of stability) following ipsi- and contralateral sway, belt acceleration/deceleration and even visual/auditory perturbations on medio-lateral direction [52]. Moreover, a recent computational and experimental model of fall scenarios have focused on the role of lower limb muscles contribution to center of mass acceleration [53] and how strategies of older versus younger individuals [54] lead to loss of balance.

Again, such an investigation may have found no significant difference between muscle contributions to the overall center of mass acceleration due to advancing age. However, older people needed to take several steps (shorter and faster initial step in recovery) and then adjust their upper body flexion across the recovery stage versus those elders with single step recovery strategy [54]. These insignificant outcomes for muscle contributions to the overall movements could be partially explained by the fact that participants were healthy in these two young and old groups. Though such MSK models are in their infancy, they may still suggest targeting possible interventions on neuromuscular control of certain muscles such as Gastrocnemius, Soleus, Vasti and Hip Abductors that can enhance the balance recovery performance [53]. However, more detailed MSK models of those with osteosarcopenia are needed to better understand how muscles and joints will undertake recovery maneuvers following simulated fall risk as we age [53]. Individualized MSK model can quantify the interaction between bone and muscle and adjust for individual changes with aging. Such a modeling approach could help better identity high-risk activities and develop personalized recovery strategies particularly for those with sarcopenia.

Prediction of consequences of osteosarcopenia

The modeling approaches discussed in previous sections for either osteoporosis or sarcopenia can be applied to study the consequences of osteosarcopenia given the relevant information on bone and muscle quality during human movement. The current literature provides enough evidence that using MSK modeling to predict the consequences of osteoporosis or sarcopenia are promising [9,37,51]. For instance, epidemiological observation of spinal fracture is being explained by MSK modeling [9,20], while the same modeling approaches could provide bone fracture risk assessment [55] including hip fracture risk assessment during exercises recommend for enhancing bone health [56].

Risk of falls were investigated by MSK models [57] using wearables, lab-based motion analyses, or Artificial Intelligence (AI) or Machine Learning (ML) based models [58,59]. As a result, using MSK modeling for diagnosis of MSK conditions seems to be plausible for those at risk of osteosarcopenia. As shown in Fig. 1, regardless of type of MSK conditions (sarcopenia, osteoporosis), MSK models can consider quality of bone and muscles thus provide useful information on fall and fractures.

MSK models use several input variables including external loads, joint motions, and anatomical variations, to predict internal biomechanical variables including joint loadings, muscle activations [9,20,22,23,37,60]. If one could adjust the MSK models to predict osteoporosis and age-related sarcopenia separately [51], the same MSK could provide insights as to whether the patient might suffer from both. Moreover, MSK models do not require an assumption of the underlying conditions while their consequences (fall or fracture) can be quantified. Later on, having access to a large database of MSK models and their outcomes as we have shown recently [9], other researchers can potentially develop novel thresholds for possible falls or fractures or categories by investigating muscle and bone interactions in a wholistic view of both conditions.

Again, MSK models are powerful tools that can be used for prediction of fall and fractures; however, more needs to be done in terms of changes over time in both bone and muscle quality and their interactions. One can develop a model of human at a given time, but MSK models (Fig. 1) with longitudinal data can better evaluate people with osteosarcopenia. Mechanobiological models combined with MSK models are being developed to consider such changes over time, but still in their infancy [61,62].

Future directions

Development of advanced MSK models combined with imaging data and cutting-edge machine learning techniques will be a promising pathway to detect, screen and evaluate those at risk of osteosarcopenia. We envisage that current imaging scans routinely taken in the clinics can be repurposed and be input into MSK models such that the existing preventive measures can be improved. Such improvements could eventually reduce devastating consequences of those with osteosarcopenia and improve quality of life of older adults.

References

[1] Zanker J, Duque G. Osteosarcopenia: the path beyond controversy. Curr Osteoporos Rep 2020;18(2):81–4. Springer.

[2] Sepúlveda-Loyola W, Phu S, Hassan EB, Brennan-Olsen SL, Zanker J, Vogrin S, Conzade R, Kirk B, Al Saedi A, Probst V. The joint occurrence of osteoporosis and sarcopenia (osteosarcopenia): definitions and characteristics. J Am Med Dir Assoc 2020;21(2):220–5. Elsevier.

[3] Laurent MR, Dubois V, Claessens F, Verschueren SMP, Vanderschueren D, Gielen E, Jardí F. Muscle-bone interactions: from experimental models to the clinic? A critical update. Mol Cell Endocrinol 2016;432:14–36. Elsevier.

[4] Yang M, Lu J, Jiang J, Zeng Y, Tang H. Comparison of four sarcopenia screening tools in nursing home residents. Aging Clin Exp Res 2019;31(10):1481–9. Springer.

[5] Cruz-Jentoft AJ, Bahat G, Bauer J, Boirie Y, Bruyère O, Cederholm T, Cooper C, Landi F, Rolland Y, Sayer AA. Sarcopenia: revised European consensus on definition and diagnosis. Age Ageing 2019;48(1):16–31. Oxford University Press.

[6] Black DM, Cauley JA, Wagman R, Ensrud K, Fink HA, Hillier TA, Lui L-Y, Cummings SR, Schousboe JT, Napoli N. The ability of a single BMD and fracture history assessment to predict fracture over 25 years in postmenopausal women: the study of osteoporotic fractures. J Bone Miner Res 2017;33(3):389–95. [Internet] Available from http://doi.wiley.com/10.1002/jbmr.3194.
[7] Kirk B, Zanker J, Duque G. Osteosarcopenia: epidemiology, diagnosis, and treatment—facts and numbers. J Cachexia Sarcopenia Muscle 2020;609–18. Wiley Online Library.
[8] Cosman F, Krege JH, Looker AC, Schousboe JT, Fan B, Sarafrazi Isfahani N, Shepherd JA, Krohn KD, Steiger P, Wilson KE, Genant HK. Spine fracture prevalence in a nationally representative sample of US women and men aged ≥40 years: results from the National Health and Nutrition Examination Survey (NHANES) 2013–2014. Osteoporos Int 2017;28(6):1857–66. [Internet]. Osteoporosis International; Available from: http://link.springer.com/10.1007/s00198-017-3948-9.
[9] Mokhtarzadeh H, Anderson DE, Allaire BT, Bouxsein ML. Patterns of load-to-strength ratios along the spine in a population-based cohort to evaluate the contribution of spinal loading to vertebral fractures. J Bone Miner Res 2021;36(4):704–11.
[10] Berry SD, Miller RR. Falls: epidemiology, pathophysiology, and relationship to fracture. Curr Osteoporos Rep 2008;6(4):149–54.
[11] Möckel L. Risk of falls in patients with low bone mineral density. Z Gerontol Geriatr 2020;1–6. Springer.
[12] Goates S, Du K, Arensberg MB, Gaillard T, Guralnik J, Pereira SL. Economic impact of hospitalizations in US adults with sarcopenia. J Frailty Aging 2019;8(2):93–9. Springer.
[13] Al Saedi A, Hassan EB, Duque G. The diagnostic role of fat in osteosarcopenia. J Lab Precis Med 2019;4(7):1–8.
[14] Kemmak AR, Rezapour A, Jahangiri R, Nikjoo S, Farabi H, Soleimanpour S. Economic burden of osteoporosis in the world: a systematic review. Med J Islam Repub Iran 2020;34(154):1–23. Iran University of Medical Sciences.
[15] Binkley N, Buehring B. Beyond FRAX: it's time to consider "sarco-osteopenia". J Clin Densitom 2009;12(4):413.
[16] Huo YR, Suriyaarachchi P, Gomez F, Curcio CL, Boersma D, Muir SW, Montero-Odasso M, Gunawardene P, Demontiero O, Duque G. Phenotype of osteosarcopenia in older individuals with a history of falling. J Am Med Dir Assoc 2015;16(4):290–5. Elsevier.
[17] Paintin J, Cooper C, Dennison E. Osteosarcopenia. Br J Hosp Med 2018;79(5):253–8. MA Healthcare London.
[18] Yoo J-I, Kim H, Ha Y-C, Kwon H-B, Koo K-H. Osteosarcopenia in patients with hip fracture is related with high mortality. J Korean Med Sci 2017;33(4).
[19] World Health Organization. Decade of healthy ageing, 2020. [Internet]. Available from https://www.who.int/initiatives/decade-of-healthy-ageing.
[20] Bruno AG, Mokhtarzadeh H, Allaire BT, Velie KR, De Paolis Kaluza MC, Anderson DE, et al. Incorporation of CT-based measurements of trunk anatomy into subject-specific musculoskeletal models of the spine influences vertebral loading predictions. J Orthop Res 2017;35(10):2164–73.
[21] Martelli S, Mokhtarzadeh H, Pivonka P, Ebeling PR. The femoral neck mechanoresponse to hip extensors exercise: a case study. J Osteoporos 2017;2017:1–9. [Internet] Available from https://www.hindawi.com/journals/jos/2017/5219541/.
[22] Delp SL, Anderson FC, Arnold AS, Loan P, Habib A, John CT, Guendelman E, Thelen DG. OpenSim: open-source software to create and analyze dynamic simulations of movement. IEEE Trans Biomed Eng 2007;54(11):1940–50.

[23] Blemker SS, Asakawa DS, Gold GE, Delp SL. Image-based musculoskeletal modeling: applications, advances, and future opportunities. J Magn Reson Imaging 2007;25(2):441–51.
[24] Cheung C-L, Tan KCB, Bow CH, Soong CSS, Loong CHN, Kung AW-C. Low handgrip strength is a predictor of osteoporotic fractures: cross-sectional and prospective evidence from the Hong Kong osteoporosis study. Age (Omaha) 2012;34(5):1239–48. Springer.
[25] Kanis JA, Johnell O, Oden A, Johansson H, McCloskey E. FRAX and the assessment of fracture probability in men and women from the UK. Osteoporos Int 2008;19(4):385–97. [Internet]. Available from http://www.ncbi.nlm.nih.gov/pubmed/18292978.
[26] Hansen U, Zioupos P, Simpson R, Currey JD, Hynd D. The effect of strain rate on the mechanical properties of human cortical bone. J Biomech Eng 2008;130(1). American Society of Mechanical Engineers Digital Collection.
[27] Mokhtarzadeh H, Anderson DE. The role of trunk musculature in osteoporotic vertebral fractures: implications for prediction, prevention, and management. Curr Osteoporos Rep 2016;14(3):67–76. [Internet] Available from http://link.springer.com/10.1007/s11914-016-0305-4.
[28] Shirota C, Simon AM, Kuiken TA. Trip recovery strategies following perturbations of variable duration. J Biomech 2014;47(11):2679–84. Elsevier.
[29] Lynn SG, Sinaki M, Westerlind KC. Balance characteristics of persons with osteoporosis. Arch Phys Med Rehabil 1997;78(3):273–7.
[30] Choi CJ, Lim HW, Park MK, Cho JG, Im GJ, Chae SW. Does the kyphotic change decrease the risk of fall? Clin Exp Otorhinolaryngol 2011;4(3):118–21.
[31] Runge CF, Shupert CL, Horak FB, Zajac FE. Ankle and hip postural strategies defined by joint torques. Gait Posture 1999;10(2):161–70. Elsevier.
[32] Valente G, Pitto L, Testi D, Seth A, Delp SL, Stagni R, Viceconti M, Taddei F. Are subject-specific musculoskeletal models robust to the uncertainties in parameter identification? PLoS One 2014;9(11):e112625. Public Library of Science.
[33] Mokhtarzadeh H, Farahmand F, Shirazi-Adl A, Arjmand N, Malekipour F, Parnianpour M. The effects of intra-abdominal pressure on the stability and unloading of the spine. J Mech Med Biol 2012;12(01):1250014.
[34] Lockhart TE, Smith JL, Woldstad JC. Effects of aging on the biomechanics of slips and falls. Hum Factors 2005;47(4):708–29. SAGE Publications Sage CA: Los Angeles, CA.
[35] Bruno AG. Investigation of spine loading to understand vertebral fractures. Harvard-MIT Program in Health Science; 2015. [Internet]. PhD Thesis. Available from http://hdl.handle.net/1721.1/98727.
[36] Morgan EF, Unnikrisnan GU, Hussein AI. Bone mechanical properties in healthy and diseased states. Annu Rev Biomed Eng 2018;20:119–43. Annual Reviews.
[37] Anderson D, Mokhtarzadeh H, Allaire B, Burkhart K, Bouxsein M. Subject-specific spine models for 250 individuals from the Framingham Heart Study; 2020. p. V1. [Internet]. Available from https://dataverse.harvard.edu/dataverse/SpineModeling.
[38] Guehring T, Unglaub F, Lorenz H, Omlor G, Wilke H-J, Kroeber MW. Intradiscal pressure measurements in normal discs, compressed discs and compressed discs treated with axial posterior disc distraction: an experimental study on the rabbit lumbar spine model. Eur Spine J 2006;15(5):597–604. Springer.
[39] Nachemson A, Morris JM. In vivo measurements of intradiscal pressure. J Bone Joint Surg Am 1964;46(5):1077–92.
[40] Jazinizadeh F, Adachi JD, Quenneville CE. Advanced 2D image processing technique to predict hip fracture risk in an older population based on single DXA scans. Osteoporos Int 2020;31(10):1925–33. Springer.

[41] Meng X, Bruno AG, Cheng B, Wang W, Bouxsein ML, Anderson DE. Incorporating six degree-of-freedom intervertebral joint stiffness in a lumbar spine musculoskeletal model—method and performance in flexed postures. J Biomech Eng 2015;137(10):101008. [Internet] Available from http://biomechanical.asmedigitalcollection.asme.org/article.aspx?doi=10.1115/1.4031417.

[42] Bruno AG, Bouxsein ML, Anderson DE. Development and validation of a musculoskeletal model of the fully articulated thoracolumbar spine and rib cage. J Biomech Eng 2015;137(8):081003. [Internet]. Available from http://biomechanical.asmedigitalcollection.asme.org/article.aspx?doi=10.1115/1.4030408.

[43] Scott D, Daly RM, Sanders KM, Ebeling PR. Fall and fracture risk in sarcopenia and dynapenia with and without obesity: the role of lifestyle interventions. Curr Osteoporos Rep 2015;13(4):235–44. [Internet]. Available from http://link.springer.com/10.1007/s11914-015-0274-z.

[44] Buehring B, Krueger D, Fidler E, Gangnon R, Heiderscheit B, Binkley N. Reproducibility of jumping mechanography and traditional measures of physical and muscle function in older adults. Osteoporos Int 2015;26(2):819–25. [Internet] Available from http://link.springer.com/10.1007/s00198-014-2983-z.

[45] Smith SHL, Coppack RJ, van den Bogert AJ, Bennett AN, Bull AMJ. Review of musculoskeletal modelling in a clinical setting: current use in rehabilitation design, surgical decision making and healthcare interventions. Clin Biomech 2021;83, 105292. Elsevier.

[46] Pandy MG, Andriacchi TP. Muscle and joint function in human locomotion. Annu Rev Biomed Eng 2010;12:401–33.

[47] Caruthers EJ, Thompson JA, Chaudhari AMW, Schmitt LC, Best TM, Saul KR, Siston RA. Muscle forces and their contributions to vertical and horizontal acceleration of the center of mass during sit-to-stand transfer in young, healthy adults. J Appl Biomech 2016;32(5):487–503. Human Kinetics, Inc.

[48] Mokhtarzadeh H, Forte JD, Lee PV-S. Biomechanical and cognitive interactions during visuo motor targeting task. Gait Posture 2021;86:287–91.

[49] Lau LK, Mallya JU, Pang WJB, Chen KK, Bin Abdul Jabbar K, Seah WT, PLK Y, Ng TP, Wee SL. Physiological and cognitive determinants of dual-task costs for gait parameters: the Yishun study. Gerontology 2021;1–10. Karger Publishers.

[50] Silva AS, de Oliveira J, Andrade GS, Nascimento J, Silva JA, Ribeiro AGS, Barbosa CG, et al. Effectiveness of training programs in reducing falls in older adults-systematic review. Biomed J Sci Techn Res 2021;34(3):26816–25.

[51] Ignasiak D, Valenzuela W, Reyes M, Ferguson SJ. The effect of muscle ageing and sarcopenia on spinal segmental loads. Eur Spine J 2018;27(10):2650–9. Springer.

[52] Roeles S, Rowe PJ, Bruijn SM, Childs CR, Tarfali GD, Steenbrink F, Pijnappels M. Gait stability in response to platform, belt, and sensory perturbations in young and older adults. Med Biol Eng Comput 2018;56(12):2325–35. Medical & Biological Engineering & Computing.

[53] Graham DF, Carty CP, Lloyd DG, Barrett RS. Muscle contributions to the acceleration of the whole body centre of mass during recovery from forward loss of balance by stepping in young and older adults. PLoS One 2017;12(10):1–13.

[54] Graham DF, Carty CP, Lloyd DG, Lichtwark G, a, Barrett RS. Muscle contributions to recovery from forward loss of balance by stepping. J Biomech 2014;47(3):667–74. Elsevier.

[55] Geier A, Kebbach M, Soodmand E, Woernle C, Kluess D, Bader R. Neuro-musculoskeletal flexible multibody simulation yields a framework for efficient bone failure risk assessment. Sci Rep 2019;9(1):1–15. Nature Publishing Group.

[56] Martelli S, Kersh ME, Schache AG, Pandy MG. Strain energy in the femoral neck during exercise. J Biomech 2014;47(8):1784–91.

[57] Mortensen J, Merryweather A. Using OpenSim to investigate the effect of active muscles and compliant flooring on head injury risk. Congr Int Ergon Assoc 2018;744–51. Springer.

[58] Collado-Villaverde A, Cobos M, Muñoz P, Barrero F, D. A simulator to support machine learning-based wearable fall detection systems. Electronics 2020;9(11):1831. Multidisciplinary Digital Publishing Institute.

[59] Hossny M, Iskander J. Just don't fall: an AI agent's learning journey towards posture stabilisation. Artif Intell 2020;1(2):286–98. Multidisciplinary Digital Publishing Institute.

[60] Mokhtarzadeh H, Ewing K, Janssen I, Hua Yeow C, Brown N, Vee Sin Lee P. The effect of leg dominance and landing height on ACL loading among female athletes. J Biomech 2017;60:181–7. Elsevier Ltd. 26 July 2017.

[61] Kirby M, Morshed AH, Gomez J, Xiao P, Hu Y, Guo XE, Wang X. Three-dimensional rendering of trabecular bone microarchitecture using a probabilistic approach. Biomech Model Mechanobiol 2020;1–19. Springer.

[62] Pizzolato C, Shim VB, Lloyd DG, Devaprakash D, Obst SJ, Newsham-West R, Graham DF, Besier TF, Zheng MH, Barrett RS. Targeted Achilles tendon training and rehabilitation using personalized and real-time multiscale models of the neuromusculoskeletal system. Front Bioeng Biotechnol 2020;8:878. Frontiers. 12 August 2020.

Chapter 4

A geroscience approach for osteosarcopenia: Autophagy and senescence as therapeutic targets

Natanael Perez Cordero[a], Patricia V. Schoenlein[b], Sadanand Fulzele[b,c,d,e], and William D. Hill[e,f,g]

[a]*School of Medicine, Universidad Central del Caribe, Bayamon, PR, United States,* [b]*Department of Cell Biology and Anatomy, Augusta University, Augusta, GA, United States,* [c]*Department of Orthopedics, Augusta University, Augusta, GA, United States,* [d]*Departments of Medicine, Augusta University, Augusta, GA, United States,* [e]*Center for Healthy Aging, Augusta University, Augusta, GA, United States,* [f]*Department of Pathology and Laboratory Medicine, Medical University of South Carolina, Charleston, SC, United States,* [g]*Ralph H. Johnson Veterans Affairs Medical Center, Charleston, SC, United States*

Introduction

Modern medicine has managed to increase human lifespan by finding better treatments for diseases that at one time were incurable. Diseases like smallpox, carried by the variola virus, killed thousands of people yearly before vaccines were discovered [1]. Not to mention the thousands of lives saved with annual influenza vaccines, or the millions who died worldwide from the Spanish Flu of 1918–19, as well as the current COVID-19 pandemic and the effect of vaccines there [2]. Furthermore, thousands died every year from bacterial infections caused by *Escherichia coli* and *Klebsiella pneumoniae* until Alexander Fleming discovered antibiotics in 1928 [3]. In contrast, the increase in lifespan resulting from medical breakthroughs has not been accompanied by a concomitant rise in health-span, which is the period an individual is generally healthy and free of chronic diseases. The vast majority of diseases worldwide are chronic diseases that have age as a primary, if not the leading underlying cause. Moreover, according to the Center for Disease Control and Prevention (CDC), chronic diseases cost 3.5 trillion dollars to the healthcare system annually [4]. Furthermore, it is estimated that 90% of people aged 65 or older have at least one chronic disease, while 75% have a minimum of two comorbidities [5]. As such, there is imperative to find better treatments against chronic diseases

Osteosarcopenia. https://doi.org/10.1016/B978-0-12-820088-9.00031-7

that affect health and everyday activities, especially those whose underlying mechanisms may be shared; this includes osteoporosis and sarcopenia. Chronic diseases currently limit the human health-span to about 65 years, whereas a healthy human lifespan falls around 72 years. Age is the primary underlying risk for chronic degenerative diseases like osteosarcopenia; hence, novel and more effective ways to target the aging process are necessary [6]. Over the past few years, one of the primary mechanisms integrating and driving aging in cells and tissues has been identified, cellular senescence. Consequently, the development of treatments that can destroy senescent cells, or block their spreading dysfunction to neighboring cells, such as inhibiting their amplification via Senescence Associated Secretory Phenotype (SASP) molecules, is desirable. The SASP involves the expression of multiple molecular processes that result in the secretion of proinflammatory products and extracellular matrix modifiers, including cytokines, growth factors, and proteases [7]. These secreted proteins can ultimately induce nonsenescent cells to undergo senescence, increasing the percentage of senescence cells in a tissue to as high as 20% of the cell population [8].

Thus, the approach of targeting the SASP would also potentially reduce or delay the senescent cell population growth or alleviate some of the senescence's many deleterious effects. For a chronic disease like osteoporosis, senescence would include dysfunctional SASP generating osteoprogenitor cells, osteoblasts, and osteocytes resulting in decreased bone formation, which would be delayed, reduced, or reversed if effective treatments were available, thus increasing patient health-span in the process. In the sections that follow, we will be discussing three major areas of ongoing research that show promise for decreasing the burden of senescent cells on bone and muscle health. We will start by discussing the dual role of autophagy on cellular senescence, highlighting its pro- and antisenescence capabilities. We will discuss senotherapeutic agents, namely senostatics and senolytics. These are novel classes of agents with the potential of treating chronic diseases like osteoporosis and sarcopenia by either inhibiting the SASP produced by senescent cells blocking the spread of senescence, restoring cell function, or inducing senescent cell apoptosis, eliminating senescent populations from tissues broadly. Finally, we will discuss the advantages and disadvantages of each senotherapeutic approach, as well as some of the current limitations on the field, for example, the lack of precise and accurate biomarkers that will be required to successfully implement senotheraputics in the treatment of chronic disease.

Senescence aging effects on bone and osteoporosis

Senescence is a process by which a cell enters growth arrest and stops dividing. This usually happens when the cell is exposed to different types of cellular stress like oxidative, genotoxic, or oncogenic (Fig. 1). Furthermore, "replicative" senescence can also happen when the telomeres become shortened to a

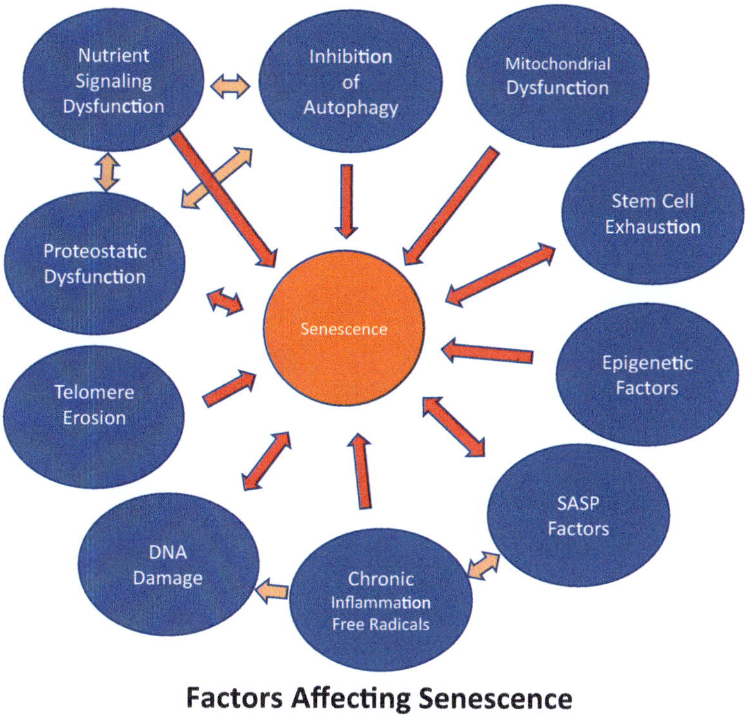

FIG. 1 The pivotal role of aging in disturbing homeostasis and triggering cellular senescence. Aging brings along a myriad of changes at the cellular level, which destabilizes homeostasis at the organism level. These changes increase cellular stress, leading to inflammation and, ultimately, cellular senescence.

point where they are no longer stable [5,9,10]. Evolutionarily senescence is an early process; hence, it must serve a vital positive role in maintaining homeostasis at the cellular and organism levels. Indeed, there is abundant evidence of the beneficial roles of cellular senescence. Among them, research has shown it is essential in suppressing neoplastic growth and in wound healing [11,12]. Nonetheless, cellular senescence can pose detrimental health effects when the senescent cell populations increase to levels that interfere with normal cell and tissue function. The quantity of senescent cells in the body is mainly kept under control by the host's immune system. However, there is growing evidence that the immune system becomes dysfunctional with age. This reduction in immune surveillance/function allows senescent cells to increase and accumulate tying into, and helping to drive, most chronic diseases, including osteoporosis [13–18].

It is now widely accepted that the underlying cause of many chronic diseases like osteoporosis and sarcopenia, which tend to appear with advancing age, is age itself or processes linked to aging (Fig. 2). Furthermore, evidence

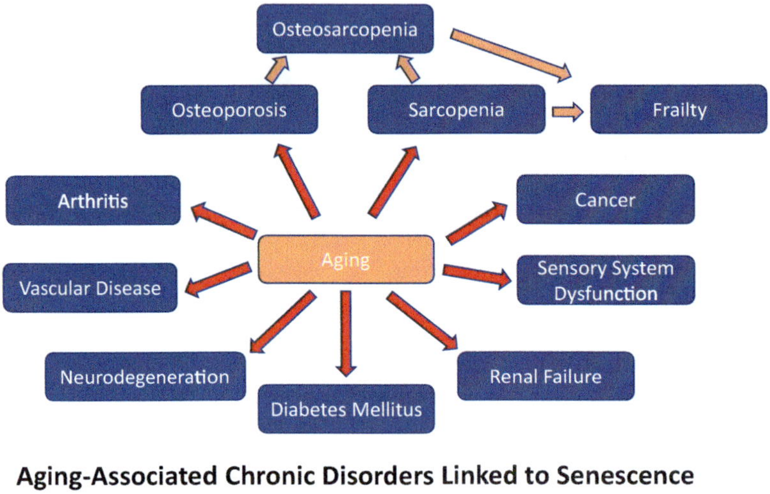

FIG. 2 Multiple chronic diseases have aging as the leading underlying cause. Compiling evidence suggests that age itself may be the culprit of many chronic diseases that tend to appear with advancing age; osteoporosis and sarcopenia being both good examples of them.

suggests that senescent cells tend to increase exponentially with advancing age, suggesting a link between cellular senescence and aging. Senescent cells are characterized by developing a SASP. This phenotype is responsible for chronically producing a myriad of proinflammatory products. Among these, cytokines like IL-15 and IL-1β, growth factors such as Insulin-like Growth Factor Binding Protein-5 (IGFBP-5), and proteases like matrix metalloproteinases (MMP1 and MMP3) [19–21]. The host's immune system usually clears out these SASP products, thereby maintaining homeostasis. The problem arises when the organism undergoes aging. In mice, this happens after 18 months of age, whereas humans typically start entering the senior age after 65 years of age [22,23]. Thus, by 18 months of age, a mouse is similar to a 65+-year-old human. At this point in the aging process, the immune system becomes less functional, making it difficult for the organism to eliminate the SASP proinflammatory products. When these agents are not adequately removed from tissues, they contribute to chronic inflammation, which eventually contributes to multiple diseases, including degenerative diseases, osteosarcopenia being only one of them. Aging, unfortunately, takes its toll in a multiorgan system manner, affecting the immune system, cardiovascular system, metabolome, nervous system, and musculoskeletal system (Fig. 2). In bone, aging eventually compromises osteocytes, with a subset of these bone cells, as well as earlier differentiating and even progenitor populations becoming senescent and developing a SASP releasing proinflammatory products that act in a paracrine or endocrine manner to produce local and systemic inflammation [24–28].

Altogether, in bone, increased osteocyte senescence and SASP products in the local environment and systemic circulation disrupt bone homeostasis by inhibiting osteogenesis and promoting adipogenesis of bone marrow mesenchymal stem cells (BMSCs). This change in the lineage commitment of MSCs toward adipogenesis instead of osteogenesis and inhibition of osteogenesis results in net bone loss by disrupting the balance between bone formation and bone resorption. Ultimately, these age-related, senescence-based alterations in bone homeostasis can advance to the degree of degenerative bone diseases such as osteoporosis and osteosarcopenia.

Unfortunately, osteoporosis is becoming rampant with increased lifespans, with menopause for women and aging for both men and women being primary factors. Over 200 million people currently have osteoporosis. In addition, it is estimated that 1 in every 3 women over the age of 50, and 1 in every 5 men over the age of 50 will suffer from osteoporotic fractures in their lifetime [29]. Furthermore, it is estimated that 25% of patients who suffer an osteoporotic hip fracture will die within a year of the event [30]. Osteoporotic fractures are also associated with sarcopenia and falls. Considering the health costs and morbidities resulting from inadequate bone and muscle health with the newer understanding of the role of senescence driving this process, it highlights the need for research to understand the role of senescence in aging for bone loss as well as more broadly in chronic age-associated disorders. Research studies to date emphasize the need to develop treatments that can either kill senescent cells or inhibit their production of SASP proinflammatory and prosenescent products. More importantly, the development of more accurate and precise biomarkers for detecting senescent cells is imperative. Currently, it requires a number of biomarkers employed together in order to identify senescent cells, since individually they lack precision and accuracy in demonstrating senescence. Furthermore, different cells and tissues have different profiles of SASP factors and other biomarkers. Common biomarkers currently used to identify senescent cells in vitro and in vivo include: increased cell size, intracellular protein content, increased expression of p16, p21 and different combinations of SASP factors (like IL-6, IL-1α, IL-8) depending on cell or tissue type, increased cellular senescence-associated β-galactosidase (SA-βgal) activity, cytoplasmic HMGB1, and the presence of senescence-associated distension satellites (SASDS) [31–35]. These biomarkers can identify various parameters which tend to be present in senescent cells. For example, the overexpression of the tumor suppression genes p16 and p21, give senescent cells the ability to bypass apoptosis. The β-galactosidase activity is increased in senescent cells, originates from the lysosome, and can be selectively detected at a suboptimal pH of 6.0 in senescent cells [36]. Although β-gal activity is primarily in senescent cells, its activity is not required for senescence. Its elevation may be simply due to increased lysosomal populations in senescent cells.

A role for autophagy in antiaging

Autophagy is best known as a survival mechanism employed by a cell under multiple stressors, classically in low nutrient or oxygen conditions (for useful autophagy reviews, see Kirkin, 2020; Klionsky et al., 2016) [37,38]. In response to nutrient deprivation, i.e., amino acid starvation, the cell induces autophagy which is a catabolic process during which the autodegeneration of specific organelles and macromolecules occurs in order to generate needed nutrients and building blocks for essential macromolecules via cellular recycling. Importantly, autophagic catabolism serves to eliminate unwanted and harmful elements such as misfolded proteins and damaged organelles; critically, this includes aged or damaged mitochondria (mitophagy) [39]. The elimination of mitochondria by autophagic catabolism is a type of selective autophagy termed mitophagy. There are many examples of selective autophagy during which specific organelles, proteins, and intracellular pathogens are degraded, with a recent review of the multiple selective autophagy pathways and the key roles of the selective autophagy receptors like ATG19 and p62/SQSTM1, which are used to move targeted molecules or organelles into autophagosomes [37]. Mitophagy, in particular, has been linked to cellular senescence by elegant studies utilizing pharmacological and genetic approaches that have been recently reviewed [40]. They show Senescence-Associated Mitochondrial Dysfunction (SAMD) appears to be necessary for at least part of the specific SASP and may be responsible for tissue-level metabolic dysfunction associated with aging. In these studies, impaired mitophagy promotes senescence, which is consistent with the fact that mitochondrial dysfunction is an independent hallmark of aging [41].

As with other types of selective autophagy, mitophagy utilizes the core autophagy machinery [37,38]. The core machinery of autophagy is dependent on many genes, some of which are designated as autophagy-related genes or *Atg*. To date, there are at least 30 *Atg* genes, and many of these genes encode products (ATG proteins) required for the formation of the autophagosome, the functional unit of autophagy. The autophagosome is a cytoplasmic organelle enclosed by a double membrane that must fuse with the lysosome for the contents within the autophagosome to be degraded. The fusion of the autophagosome with the lysosome generates an organelle referred to as the autolysosome, within which hydrolytic enzymes degrade the macromolecules that were initially sequestered by the autophagosome. There are at least nine genes involved in autophagy initiation, many of which regulate phagophore nucleation. The phagophore is the initial membrane structure that ultimately elongates and develops into the autophagosome, which is enclosed by two membranes, with the outer membrane eventually fusing with the lysosome membrane to form the autolysosome. A minimum of seven genes is involved in phagophore expansion. These genes and their specific functions have been recently reviewed, along with genes involved in the complex process of cargo sequestration within the autophagosome [42]. Induction of autophagy often consists of inhibiting the mammalian target of Rapamycin or mTOR, a master cell growth regulator, a serine/threonine kinase. The regulation of mTOR action is quite complex and involves at least two distinct protein complexes that dictate mTOR action, with blockade of the mTOR complex 1 (mTORC1) able to induce autophagy. The complex mTORC1 includes ATG13, which is released from the complex in response to amino acid starvation such that it can function in autophagy initiation. The targeting (or downregulating) of specific Atg genes or the inhibition of mTOR have been common approaches to establish a role for autophagy in senescence.

A dual role for autophagy in mesenchymal stem cells: Antisenescence versus prosenescence

Although many of the early studies addressing a role for autophagy in senescence have been conducted in fibroblasts, recent studies suggest a role of autophagy in regulating cellular senescence of mesenchymal stem cells (MSCs). The functional roles of autophagy in MSCs, however, are not entirely clear. Evidence supports autophagy as a prosenescence process, albeit evidence also exists that derogates a prosenescence role for autophagy and further suggests that autophagy prevents cellular senescence [43]. Concerning the antisenescence role of autophagy, recent studies showed that inducing elevations in autophagy in aged mice increased health-span by restoring stem cell activity [44,45]. Other studies showed that autophagy is not only essential for sustaining the differentiation of stem cells, but that without autophagic activity, MSCs senescence is almost certain [46]. For example, research done on primary human fibroblasts demonstrated that inhibiting autophagy, by either knocking down (via shRNA targeting) the Atg7 or Atg5 genes, prompted the fibroblasts to enter a senescent state, due to the accumulation of reactive oxygen species (ROS) and mitochondrial impairment [47]. Indeed, depending on the cell/tissue and context, autophagy can inhibit or induce senescence with selective autophagy inhibiting senescence via depletion of key transcription factors and general autophagy, allowing the recycling of amino acids in stressed cells to form SASP molecules [48]. These types of genetic studies provided strong support for an earlier study that established a key role for autophagy as an antiaging process in aged mice [44,45]. This in vivo study showed increased lifespan if mice were treated with Rapamycin, a drug that blocks mTOR activity and induces autophagy. In addition, treating MSCs with Rapamycin resulted in increased autophagy and reduced senescence, whereas reducing Rapamycin resulted in decreased autophagy and increased senescence [49]. We have recently confirmed this inverse relationship between autophagy inhibition and senescence induction in MSCs treated with kynurenine, an age related tryptophan metabolite, signaling via the aryl hydrocarbon receptor system leading to osteogenic inhibition [50]. Moreover, investigations also have found that with aging, MSCs autophagic activity diminishes relative to MSCs from younger sources [51]. This purported antisenescence role of autophagy on MSCs is intriguing and establishes a link between aging in bone, autophagy, and cellular senescence. This suggests that autophagy, at least partly, may be essential in maintaining homeostasis between bone deposition and bone resorption [25].

In human MSCs, one of the most used and reliable biomarkers to detect cells undergoing autophagy is LC3-II, specifically the PE lipidation of LC3-I to LC3-II. LC3 is the product of Atg 8, is typically upregulated during autophagy induction, and is required to form the autophagosomal membrane. Surprisingly, this biomarker has been found in cells entering replicative senescence, suggesting that autophagy plays a role in either promoting or maintaining replicative senescence [52]. A more focused investigation conducted in MSCs showed that cellular senescence was dependent on autophagy induction. In this study, the data showed that when insulin-like growth factor 1 (IGF1) was diminished, the senescent cells were protected by autophagic activity even under hypoxic conditions [53]. A similar prosurvival role for autophagy was reported in an earlier study that showed high glucose concentrations could trigger MSC cellular senescence by promoting the formation of reactive oxygen species (ROS), which then upregulates autophagic activity [54]. MSCs cultivated at high glucose concentrations exhibited telomere attrition and genomic instability, and a higher rate of autophagic activity was required for their survival. This was assessed by measuring the quantity of various biomarkers, including Beclin-1 (ATG6), ATG5, ATG7 and LC3-II (ATG8). The biomarkers were found to be at higher than basal levels, suggesting a higher rate of autophagic activity and thus, a link between autophagy and MSCs senescence [31]. Also, studies of the tumor suppressor p53 known to be involved in replicative senescence in mesenchymal stromal cells, show that p53 also upregulates autophagic activity [55], providing a molecular link between autophagy and replicative senescence [56]. Another study focused on a type of cellular senescence called Oncogene-Induced Senescence (OIS). Senescent cells induced by oncogenic stress exhibit proliferation arrest with metabolic reprogramming as well as senescence-associated inflammation. This research suggested that in OIS fibroblast cells, autophagy was upregulated. Still moreover, autophagy was regulating the SASP by providing the biochemical building blocks needed to synthesize the inflammatory proteins and cytokines for secretion [57]. All this evidence suggests that autophagy, probably general autophagy versus selective autophagy, supports cellular senescence under certain circumstances. Thus, autophagy has a dual role in regulating senescence in MSCs and likely in bone and muscle homeostasis. Autophagy as an antisenescence process is predicted to help promote bone and muscle growth. Still, autophagy could also aid senescent-based bone and muscle loss as a prosenescence facilitator.

Reconciliation regarding autophagy and senescence

While there is evidence supporting a dual role of autophagy in cellular senescence, the molecular details of autophagy-mediated regulation of pro- versus antisenescence are limited. The current standing regarding the intricate relationship between autophagy and senescence is that it depends on whether a cell undergoes general or selective autophagy and on the triggering stimulus. Evidence suggests that under certain stimuli, i.e., D-galactose and oxidative stress, or mitophagy, selective autophagy has antisenescence capabilities [43,49,51–56,58,59]. Whereas under stimuli-like glucose and hypoxia, general autophagy showed prosenescence capabilities [43,49,51–56,58,59]. However, autophagy induced by replicative exhaustion has been linked to both anti- and prosenescence. The fact that replicative exhaustion as an autophagy stimulus has been found to drive senescence and reduce senescence underscores the need for continued research to molecularly define the effects of replicative exhaustion on autophagy and senescence. Currently, we believe that the timing of induction of general autophagy also plays an important role in determining if replicative exhaustion promotes or reduces senescence. When general autophagy acts early to maintain homeostasis, it exhibits antisenescence properties. In contrast, when general autophagy acts late to maintain homeostasis, it shows prosenescence properties [43,49,51–56,58,59].

Depending on the cell type, selective autophagy can have antisenescence or prosenescence capabilities. In fibroblasts, selective autophagy tends to exhibit antisenescence capabilities, whereas, in primary lung cells, selective autophagy exerts prosenescence capabilities. However, in MSCs, selective autophagy presents antisenescence as well as prosenescence properties [43,60–64]. For example, there is evidence suggesting that under normal conditions, p62 (autophagy receptor, sequestosome 1 [SQSTM 1]), binds strongly to GATA4, a central regulator of the SASP, which triggers GATA4 catabolism (selective autophagy) and prevents senescence in MSCs [43,60–64]. In contrast, under senescence stimuli, p62 cannot bind to GATA4, and its selective degradation does not occur, resulting in the expression of cellular senescence (Fig. 3). Ultimately, it seems that whether autophagy acts to induce or prevent cellular senescence depends on the type of autophagy, the timing, the stimuli triggering it and the cell type. Based on these complexities, additional research is needed to establish the role(s) of general and selective autophagy in MSCs and bone homeostasis and to potentially identify specific molecular targets for increasing health-span.

One caveat to many of the published studies addressing the role of autophagy in senescence is that the approach has been to typically target components of the autophagic core machinery such as Beclin (ATG6), LC3 (ATG8), or mTOR activity. As such, effects on general autophagy cannot be easily discerned from effects on selective autophagy pathways such as mitophagy. In order to fully elucidate whether autophagy is a prosenescence or antisenescence

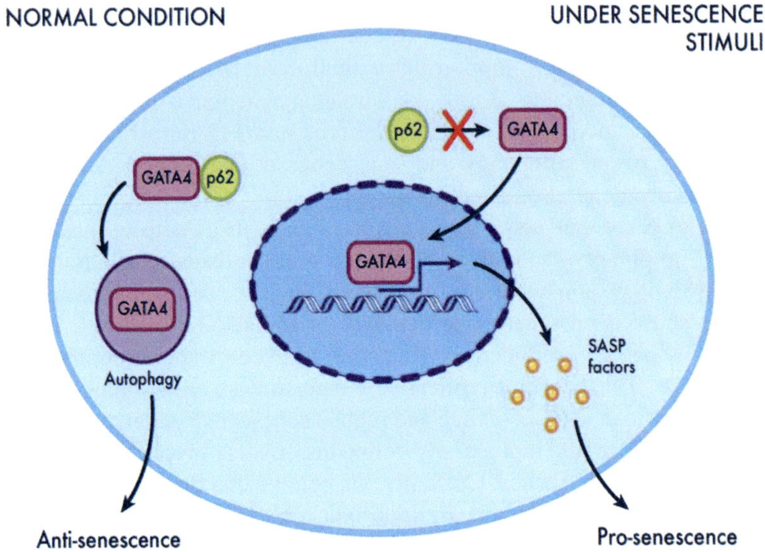

FIG. 3 Effect of senescent stimuli on the autophagic receptor p62 and selective autophagy. The autophagic receptor p62 binds strongly to GATA4 (a main transcription factor complex element regulator of the SASP molecule expression), shunting it into the autophagosome for degradation triggering selective autophagy and preventing senescence under normal conditions. When exposed to senescent stimuli, the autophagic receptor p62 cannot bind to GATA4 drives SASP factor expression promoting senescence.

process will require a determination of the specific autophagy pathway and its functional role in the cells being studied. For example, during mitophagy, the core autophagic machinery is needed to catabolize damaged mitochondria and reduce ROS generation. Therefore, targeting any of the genes required for the core machinery would affect both general and selective autophagy. Thus, it would be necessary to target proteins that are dedicated to mitophagy, such as PTEN-induced putative kinase PINK1 and Parkin, an E3 ligase. The PINK1/Parkin axis is involved in targeting mitochondria with reduced membrane potential with polyubiquitin chains required for mitochondria targeting to autophagic vesicles [40] (Fig. 3). Once ubiquitinated, specific receptor proteins, including optineurin, NDP52, and TaxBP1, will recruit autophagic membranes to engulf these tagged mitochondria. The importance of PINK1 and Parkin in regulating mitochondrial function via mitophagy to prevent senescence also has been demonstrated in familial-age related diseases like Parkinson's [65]. However, not all mitophagy is dependent on PINK1/Parkin function. A recent study conducted in skeletal muscle cells identified AMPK as the key regulator of mitophagy by enhancing mitochondrial fission (via MFF phosphorylation) and mitochondrial autophagosome engulfment (via TBK1 phosphorylation) in a PINK1/Parkin independent manner [66]. A role for AMPK in the regulation of mitophagy was previously indicated [67], and involves its role in inducing mitochondrial fission, a required event that precedes mitophagy, and in activating ULK1 which recruits damaged mitochondria to the lysosome [68,69]. In addition to regulation of mitophagy, AMPK has many cellular functions, including regulation of metabolism and cellular homeostasis, cell survival and death, and general autophagy. All of these AMPK functions have the potential to impact aging. Therefore, it is not surprising that AMPK activation has been shown to delay aging and increase life span in *Drosophila melanogaster* and protect against senescence in aged rats by induction of autophagy that ultimately reduced oxidative damage [70].

AMPK and cellular senescence of MSCs

Multiple studies have indicated that AMPK activation prevents senescence in various cell types and that the mechanism involves AMPK-mediated activation of autophagy. In fibroblasts, AMPK activators like metformin prevented the development of oxidative stress-induced senescence. The prevention of senescence in the fibroblasts was due in part to increased autophagic flux NAD+ homeostasis [71]. Mechanistically, the results of the study by Han et al. are entirely consistent with the roles of AMPK in the regulation of cellular metabolism, general autophagy and mitochondrial homeostasis by mitophagy [72]. AMPK is essentially a cellular energy sensor. It is a heterotrimeric complex composed of a catalytic α subunit and regulatory β and γ (gamma) subunits with multiple isoforms of each subunit encoded by different genes. The gamma subunit is responsible for the ability of AMPK to respond to changes in the ATP-to-AMP ratio via its ability to bind adenine nucleotides. The binding of AMP or ADP stimulates AMPK, to the gamma subunit via multiple mechanisms that have been recently reviewed [72]. Once bound by AMP, activated AMPK will typically stimulate catabolic pathways such as glycolysis and fatty acid oxidation and autophagy, and block anabolic pathways such that ATP production is stimulated [72]. Concerning general autophagy there may be multiple mechanisms whereby active AMPK can initiate autophagy or regulate autophagic flux. One of these mechanisms involves AMPK-mediated phosphorylation and activation of ULK1, a major effector of autophagy initiation. Of interest, the PGC-1α/AMPK pathway appears to play a critical role in preventing cellular senescence in MSCs.

PGC-1α is a master regulator of mitochondrial biogenesis that can be finely tuned in response to cellular metabolic fluctuations. AMPK α is one of the metabolic sensors that affect PGC1α activity and ultimately mitochondrial activity, defining a critical regulatory network for metabolic homeostasis [73,74]. Further studies have identified C1q and tumor necrosis factor-related protein 9 (CTRP9) as a novel cytoprotective cytokine with antioxidant effects that may play a critical role in preventing cellular senescence and facilitating stem cell rejuvenation. Specifically, CTRP9 ameliorates cellular senescence via PGC-1α/AMPK signaling in the MSCs [73].

Overall it is clear that AMPK can play a central role in retarding senescence, most likely via its participation in cellular autophagy, and mitophagy pathways. Although activating AMPK with drugs such as metformin may be an attractive approach toward postponing senescence in cells of tissues, some caution is advised. For example, AMPK activation has been shown to support the viability of dormant breast cancer cells [75].

Antiaging effects of senostatics (senomorphics) in the musculoskeletal system

Not long ago, senescent cells were viewed as merely dormant cells which posed no noxious effects to human health. However, recent studies have demonstrated that senescent cells cause detrimental effects like systemic inflammation due to their SASP proinflammatory and prosenescent products. These have been shown to induce aging-related changes and are associated with many chronic diseases that come with age itself, such as osteoporosis and sarcopenia. Nonetheless, senescent cells also provide beneficial actions like protecting against cancer and assisting in wound healing [76–78]. Indeed, it would not be wise to eliminate every senescent cell because they do serve a beneficial role in maintaining homeostasis. Rather a less drastic approach might be preferable and more helpful to increase the human health-span [77]. Recently, agents have been identified with the capacity to inhibit proinflammatory products produced by the SASP. These include senostatics or senomorphics, which target processes in senescent cells which help drive the SASP or target subsets of SASP molecules directly. Among these targets are the rapamycin receptor (mTORC1) and the JAK1/JAK2-STAT3 pathway.

A few senostatics are already being studied with mouse models, including rapamycin inhibitors, Ruxolitinib (JAK1/JAK2-STAT3 inhibitor), glucocorticoids and metformin (commonly used to treat type 2 diabetes) [25,79–83]. These agents have been shown to reduce frailty, heart failure and cognitive impairment in mouse models, suggesting the possibility of being able to increase health-span [45,84–88]. Ruxolitinib, for example, is a JAK1/JAK2-STAT3 inhibitor. It is used clinically to treat polycythemia vera, myelofibrosis and graft versus host disease [81]. In recent studies done with 22 and 24 months old C57BL/6 mice, it was found that Ruxolitinib has senostatic properties capable of attenuating insulin resistance, reduce osteoporosis, and decreased stem cell dysfunction [81,89], all effects with major significance in osteosarcopenia. Another study confirmed these results when mice treated with Ruxolitinib presented higher bone mass, better bone microstructure and improved cardiovascular function, suggesting the senotherapeutic agent may even be beneficial in multiple age-related comorbidities [89]. Notably, the drug has proven to reduce frailty in human patients, confirming that the senomorphic properties of the drug are not only seen in mouse models [90].

The effectiveness of Ruxolitinib as a senostatic agent lies in its ability to inhibit the JAK/STAT pathway. This pathway can be overexpressed in senescent cells, and its inhibition leads to the suppression of the SASP proinflammatory products, ultimately reducing chronic systemic inflammation [91]. It appears that the SASP between different cell types tends to be relatively similar [11,92]. This is advantageous because it facilitates the development of new senotherapeutic agents that can simultaneously target SASP in multiple cell types. More importantly, it is possible that future senostatics can effectively reduce polypharmacy, one of modern medicine's most significant drawbacks, by targeting and treating multiple chronic diseases concurrently.

Senolytics antiaging effects in bone

In 2015, additional senotherapeutic agents were discovered that killed senescent cells instead of inhibiting the SASP proinflammatory products [93]. These agents were termed senolytics and included small molecules, peptides, and antibodies that target the senescence-associated antiapoptotic pathways (SCAPs) [18,26,94]. Several SCAPs include the dependence receptors/tyrosine kinases, the BCL-2 family, the PI3K/AKT metabolic network, p53/p21/serpins, and HIF1 α [18]. Interestingly, HIF1α competes against the aryl hydrocarbon receptor that is activated by kynurenine in MSCs, inducing senescence [50]. These SCAPs inhibit the proapoptotic pathways of senescent cells, hence, blocking apoptotic cell death [93,95]. Apoptosis, defined as programmed cell death, is a homeostatic mechanism that cells employ to regulate cell populations in tissues [96]. Interestingly, researchers found that SCAPs can involve protein families, which are essential for maintaining the antiapoptotic pathways like tyrosine kinases (or dependence receptors) and the BCL-2 protein family [18]. Thus, SCAPs reflect the diversity of composition of SASP that can depend on the senescent cell type, the stimulus triggering senescence, and the hormonal and growth factor milieu. Although SCAPs are cell and context dependent, the targeting (blocking) of the functioning SCAPs permit the proapoptotic pathways to be expressed and ultimately induce apoptosis of the senescent cells [5,93].

The first effective senolytic drug recipe (D+Q) combines Dasatinib, an FDA approved antibody-based tyrosine kinase inhibitor, and Quercetin, a flavanol present in many fruits and vegetables [93,97,98]. Independently, Dasatinib works by inhibiting the dependence receptors/tyrosine kinase SCAP and Quercetin by targeting the BCL-2/BCL-XL, PI3K/AKT, and p53/p21/serpine SCAPs. Initial studies showed that Dasatinib was able to block the SCAP of primary human senescent preadipocytes but not the SCAP of primary human embryonic venous endothelial cells HUVECs. In contrast, Quercetin effectively blocked the SCAP in the senescent HUVECs, but not the SCAP of the senescent preadipocytes. Importantly, D+Q used in combination eliminated both the senescent preadipocytes and HUVECs. A similar synergistic senolytic outcome was noted when D+Q was used to treat cultured senescent mouse embryonic fibroblasts, compared to the complete lack of senolytic activity when D+Q were used separately [93].

Research on human adipose tissue explants found that the senescent cells could be eliminated after 18h of continuous exposure to D+Q treatment [28]. Even more astonishing is the fact that albeit D+Q has a half-life of only a few hours, it was able to diminish the detrimental effects of exposing a mouse leg to a 10-Gy dose of radiation, even 7 months after injury [93]. In more recent studies, D+Q treatment has been shown to alleviate osteoporosis in mice; however, this outcome required intermittent dosing of the D+Q combination [89]. This may occur because intermittent senolytic treatment effectively allowed osteoprogenitors cells like osteoblasts to maintain function. It is known that SASP produced by senescent cells disrupts the balance between bone deposition and resorption, with more bone degradation and, ultimately, calcium in the bloodstream. Over time, this disruption in bone homeostasis can lead to degenerative bone diseases like osteoporosis. Thus, by eliminating the senescent osteocytes with senolytic drugs, the SASP molecules are also eradicated. Consequently, the quantity of osteoblasts increases and bone formation follows shortly after [13]. The fact that intermittent dosing was required to effectively treat osteoporosis in this murine model underscores the fact that the exact dosing of a senolytic drug will depend at least in part on the rate of senescent cell accumulation [99].

Recently, two additional senolytic agents were discovered. One is a powerful flavonoid called Fisetin, while the other is an antitumor agent named navitoclax, which is a BCL-2 family inhibitor. Bcl2 family molecules are part of the larger binding homology domain (BH3) family because each member of this family contains a BH3 domain critical for regulating apoptosis. Navitoclax is a BH3 mimetic that potently binds to the BH3 domain of Bcl2 and BCLXL [100], and effectively inhibits the BCL-2/BCLXL SCAP allowing the proapoptotic pathways to kill the senescent cells expressing these BH3 family members [93,101–104].

A major setback in the development of new senolytic drugs is the fact that SCAPs tend to differ between cell types [93]. This makes individual senolytic drugs somewhat specific and only effective toward subsets of senescent cells. An example of this is navitoclax, which is effective against senescent HUVECs, but ineffective against primary human adipocyte progenitors [93,101,105]. However, in advanced states of tissue senescence, the effectiveness of senolytics may be an issue. For example, we have recently shown that with advanced age in mice, the degree of senescence in bone may be so high that treatment with a senolytic like navitoclax may actually increase bone loss due to killing too many osteogenic cells leading to further inhibition of bone formation/repair [106]. Therefore, in clinical practice, it may be problematic to use senolytics or careful dose titration and targeting earlier phases of the disease process with a lower degree of overall senescence may be needed. In addition, whether these therapies also work in sarcopenia remains unknown.

The field of senolytics has drawn much attention from the scientific community, given the potential antiaging properties of these senotherapeutic drugs. This interest only grew more intense following research with the INK-ATTAC mouse model. These mice allow systemic knockout of the $p16^{Ink4a}$ tumor suppressor gene after treatment with AP20187, a drug with senolytic properties [107]. This pharmacological approach produced the elimination of both senescent and nonsenescent cells. In comparison, the other two experimental groups were treated with the senolytic D + Q and the senostatic Ruxolitinib [89]. These latter two approaches also improved bone microarchitecture and strength, suppressed bone resorption, and promoted bone formation [89]. Furthermore, the data collected from the study demonstrated an increase in osteoblast numbers and a decrease in bone marrow adipose tissue in old INK-ATTAC mice after treatment with AP20187 compared with vehicle-treated mice. These results are consistent with stem cells in bone tissue committing to the osteoblastic lineage instead of the adipocyte lineage, a phenomenon which tends to happen with aging and is thought to decrease the size of the osteogenic cell pool, consequently reducing the rate of bone formation leading to homeostatic imbalance and bone loss [89].

Senolytic drugs continue to be identified, and their use supports the concept that the elimination of senescent cells is a viable approach to treating chronic diseases of aging. An example is UBX0101, a senolytic agent that targets the BCL-2 family and can eliminate senescent cells in articular cartilage and synovium following anterior cruciate ligament transection (ACLT). This senolytic agent proved to alleviate osteoarthritis in mice [108]. Another example is the combination of curcumin and 0-vanillin, which proved to reduce senescent intervertebral disk cells, reduce back pain and increase matrix synthesis [109]. While there is ample evidence supporting the beneficial effects of senolytics, there is also evidence suggesting that many also pose cytotoxic effects, as is the case of the BCL-2 inhibitors [11]. Moreover, many senolytic drugs lack specificity toward senescent cells and kill nonsenescent cells as well. Recently, however, a group of researchers identified a promising senolytic drug capable of selectively killing senescent cells. The drug, 17-DMAG, inhibits the heat shock protein (HSP90) [5]. This chaperone protein is ubiquitously expressed in mammalian cells and assists in maintaining cellular senescence. It is critical for protein stabilization, including that of antiapoptotic proteins. For example, 17-DMAG disrupts the interaction of HSP90-AKT, hindering the antiapoptotic pathway PI3K/AKT [110]. Without this essential survival pathway, many senescent cells are no longer viable and enter apoptosis. Importantly, 17-DMAG was found to have senolytic activity in-vivo as well as in-vitro. Furthermore, the compound has the capacity to selectively kill senescent cells induced to undergo senescence by different types of stimuli like DNA damage, genotoxic stress, oxidative stress, and inflammatory stress. Even more, the compound can broadly kill senescent cells from different sources, such as mouse fibroblasts, mesenchymal stem cells, and human lung fibroblasts. Of particular advantage, intermittent dosing was enough to reduce the symptoms of various age-related chronic diseases like neurodegeneration, frailty, ataxia, gait disorder, kyphosis, and osteoporosis. While there is still much to learn regarding senotherapeutics, senolytic drugs are potential candidates for treating bone degenerative diseases like osteoporosis, increasing health-span, and reducing polypharmacy.

Senostatics or senolytics

Senotherapeutic agents have drawn interest among the scientific community given their antiaging effects. Nonetheless, questions of whether senostatics (AKA senomorphics) should be used over senolytics, or in combination and the timing remain. In order to better understand if one has an advantage over the other, it is essential to understand the mechanisms of action for each and how they interact with senescent cells (Fig. 4A and B). Evidence suggests that utilizing SASP inhibitors can alleviate many chronic diseases such as osteoporosis

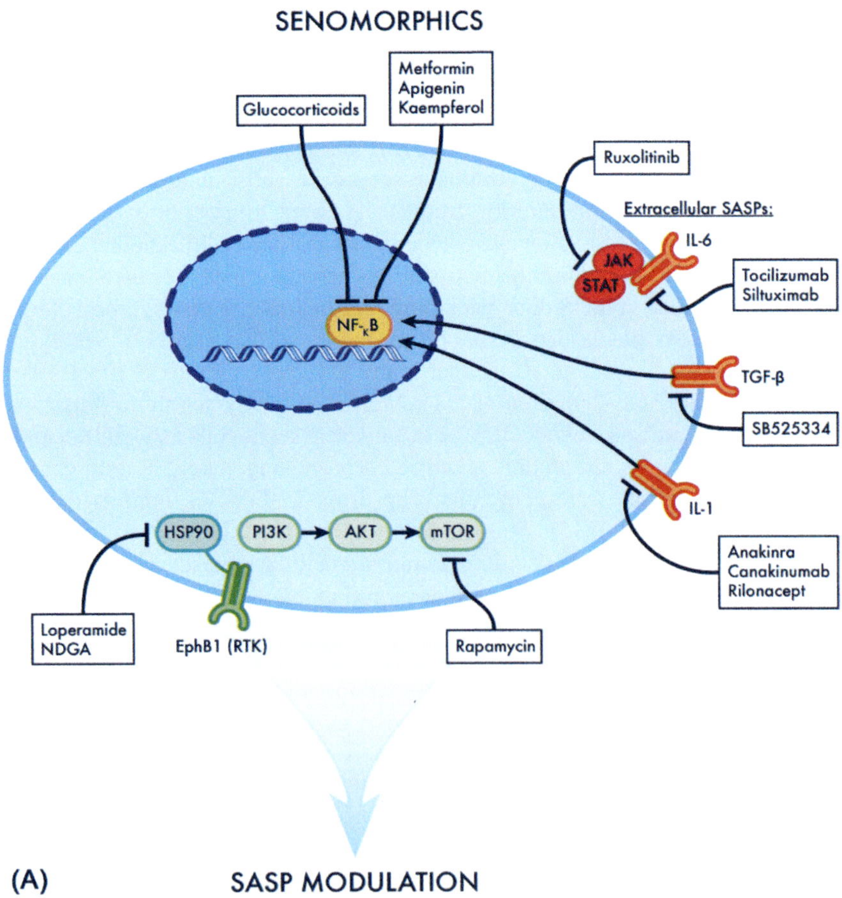

FIG. 4 Senostatics versus senolytics (A) senostatics drugs interfering with SASP proinflammatory products like cytokines.

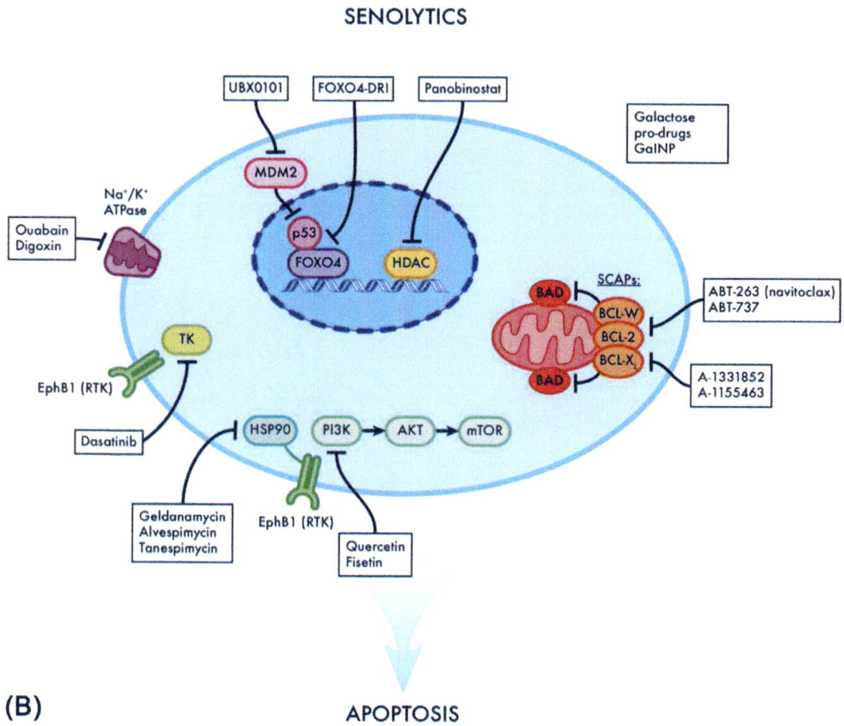

FIG. 4, Cont'd (B) Senolytic drugs interfere with pathways essential for the survival of the senescent cells like the PI3K/Akt and Bcl2 family pathways. The different agents in current use as senostatics and senolytics and the pathways they target are shown.

and sarcopenia, where age is a primary underlying risk, by inhibiting their proinflammatory products and reducing stem cell dysfunction (Fig. 5). A few like Ruxolitinib (JAK/STAT pathway inhibitor) and metformin, most commonly used to treat Type II Diabetes have already shown favorable results in preclinical trials [11,99]. Additional evidence suggests that utilizing senostatics over senolytics has the advantage of leaving the previously senescent cells intact, which sustain tissue structure and physiological integrity when a very high percentage of the tissue's cells undergo senescence [8,80].

Another advantage of senostatics is that they can target multiple types of senescent cells because the type of SASP tends to be similar across a broad range of cell types [11,92]. They might also reduce polypharmacy by allowing fewer drugs to be used when treating comorbidities. In terms of the disadvantages of senostatics, evidence suggests that their use as a therapeutic drug to treat a degenerative bone disease such as osteoporosis, may require regular doses of the therapeutic agent [99], a disadvantage compared to current treatments. If the senescent cell is not being killed, but rather its proinflammatory products are being inhibited, then the mechanisms driving the induction of senescence

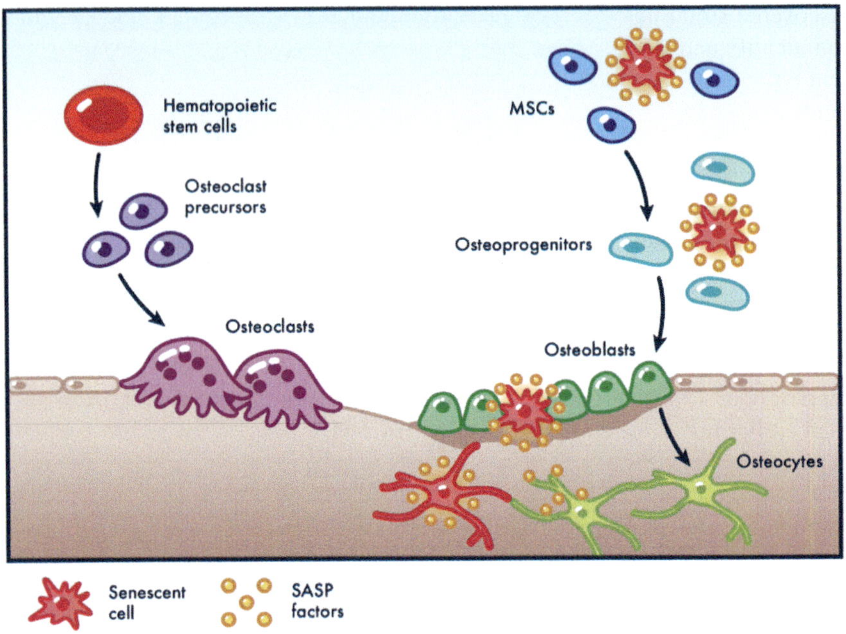

FIG. 5 Senescent cells and their SASP proinflammatory products that target MSCs, osteoblasts, and osteocytes. The SASP produced by senescent cells prefers targeting osteoprogenitor cells like MSCs and osteoblasts over osteoclasts (unpublished data from the Hill laboratory). The age-associated induction of senescence in osteogenic cells disrupts the balance between bone formation and resorption, by driving osteogenic cell dysfunction, secretion of SASP factors and blocking osteogenic cell proliferation. Over time, this can lead to osteoporosis.

may not be constitutively targeted by the senostatic. Therefore, senostatic therapy may require long-term management of the senescent population by regular administration of these agents rather than one time or intermittent treatment as with senolytics. This potentially increases the risk of harmful off-target effects, which is an area currently under study [11,99]. In contrast, the benefits of utilizing senolytics potentially include the capacity to reduce excessive bone resorption and increase bone formation with only intermittent dosing. This is a favorable treatment approach because it reduces the probability of developing off-target effects, which is also the problem with many of the drugs currently used to treat osteoporosis [13,99]. Further, evidence suggests that senolytic therapy is immune to proliferation dependent drug resistance since senescent cells do not divide and proliferate, and hence, cannot acquire potentially problematic mutations.

There is great clinical translational interest in senolytic agents with a number currently in preclinical and clinical trials including Dasatinib , Quercetin , navitoclax, and Fisetin [13,99]. Nonetheless, senolytics have their downside. Reports suggest that besides the HSP90 inhibitor 17-DMAG, the senolytics discovered so far act in a highly specific manner in terms of the cell type they can identify and kill [5]. Thus, further research is needed to find more universal senolytic agents. Another disadvantage of senolytic drugs, specifically BCL-2 inhibitors like Navitoclax, is that they exhibit cytotoxic effects, which can be detrimental to the host, such as a dose-dependent, but reversible thrombocytopenia in healthy subjects. [11,13,99]. In addition, Navitoclax's in vivo effects are still not completely understood. In a study done on 6-week-old INK-ATTAC mice, a mouse model which expresses accelerated aging, the senolytic agent showed increased bone density and formation. In contrast, in a study from our group using older mice (24-month-old), navitoclax induced bone loss most likely due to the advanced already significant loss of bone and the high percentage of the total osteocyte population undergoing senescence, leaving few surviving cells to support bone formation [5,106]. These data suggest that senolytics may be best used earlier in disease processes before significant tissue loss or high numbers of senescent cells. So in degenerative diseases like osteoporosis, senolytics may prove optimally beneficial when administered at earlier stages of the disease or in combination with senostatics in a phase-specific manner [5,106].

In addition, the timing of therapy and whether senolytics are delivered alone or in combination with other drugs is an area of intense interest. It may be possible that the preferable treatments will be case dependent, ultimately reliant on the type of chronic disease and stage of the disease. Whichever the case, it is critical to continue research to discover better senescent biomarkers, given those currently available lack specificity and accuracy when used individually. If methods for detecting senescent cells improve, studying the beneficial effects of senotherapeutic agents as well as their off-target effects would also become more feasible. Without a doubt, senostatics and senolytics have the potential of alleviating or postponing many chronic diseases which tend to appear with age and are associated with alterations in cell differentiation, including osteoporosis and sarcopenia, but further research is still needed before establishing therapies.

Conclusion

The geroscience hypothesis is gaining strength and credibility among the scientific community. The hypothesis poses that age seems to be the primary underlying cause of most chronic diseases. Hence, by addressing aging physiology, the prevention or mitigation of chronic diseases may be approached [111]. There has been an alarming increase in patients with chronic diseases over the years, which is expected to keep growing. Importantly, the chronic state of most conditions, in part, is correlated to an increase in the number of senescent (nondividing and permanently growth-arrested) cells in the tissue of interest. Thus, targeting this nonfunctional cell population is a novel approach to the treatment of chronic disease.

This chapter discussed the role(s) of autophagy, senescence, AMPK linkages, and the potential of senostatics and senolytics as treatment approaches.

Studies suggest that these treatment options have great promise in treating or at least partially alleviating elements of degenerative diseases like osteoporosis and sarcopenia [11,13,43,49,51–56,58,59,99]. Indeed, evidence supports targeting autophagy to decrease the senescent cell burden on bone tissue and increase bone formation. Moreover, the use of senostatics has proven to inhibit the SASP proinflammatory products, while maintaining intact the senescent cells for tissue structure and physiological integrity [11,13,99]. At the same time, the use of senolytics proved able to reverse one of the hallmarks of aging, stem cell disfunction. Stem cell aging with induction of stem cell senescence hinders bone and muscle formation by altering the lineage commitment of stem cells toward the adipocyte lineage, instead of the osteoblastic or myoblastic lineages, as well as inhibiting osteoprogenitor differentiation and osteogenic function [11,13,99]. Although autophagy regulation, senostatics and senolytics have the potential to treat various chronic diseases, many vital questions remain unanswered. Information is lacking regarding which stimuli lead autophagy into being antisenescence or prosenescence. Furthermore, the type of cell also seems to play a major role in determining the anti- or prosenescence properties of autophagy [43,49,51–56,58,59]. This context- and cell-type-dependent role of autophagy function is complex, but needs to be delineated mechanistically to successfully target specific chronic musculoskeletal diseases. In addition, the off-target effects of using senostatics and senolytics have been poorly studied. Hence, more research is needed to prevent or mitigate potential harmful side effects. Moreover, current biomarkers for detecting senescent cells are not individually specific or selective, requiring multiple approaches to identify senescent cells. Thus, there is a great need for novel biomarkers with the ability to detect senescent cells with greater accuracy and precision [11,13,99]. Nonetheless, appropriate autophagy regulation, senostatics, and senolytics have the potential of increasing health-span while reducing polypharmacy by targeting the aging physiology, ultimately reducing senescent cell burden, and postponing or alleviating chronic diseases like osteoporosis.

References

[1] Riedel S. Edward Jenner and the history of smallpox and vaccination. Proc (Baylor Univ Med Cent) 2005;18(1):21–5.

[2] Barberis I, et al. History and evolution of influenza control through vaccination: from the first monovalent vaccine to universal vaccines. J Prev Med Hyg 2016;57(3):E115–e120.

[3] Ribeiro da Cunha B, Fonseca LP, Calado CRC. Antibiotic discovery: where have we come from, where do we go? Antibiotics (Basel) 2019;8(2):45.

[4] Prevention, CfDCA. Health and economic costs of chronic diseases; 2019.

[5] Fuhrmann-Stroissnigg H, et al. Identification of HSP90 inhibitors as a novel class of senolytics. Nat Commun 2017;8(1):422.

[6] Organization WH. Global Health Observatory (GHO) data: life expectancy. WHO; 2020.

[7] Herranz N, Gil J. Mechanisms and functions of cellular senescence. J Clin Invest 2018;128(4):1238–46.

[8] Lopes-Paciencia S, et al. The senescence-associated secretory phenotype and its regulation. Cytokine 2019;117:15–22.
[9] van Deursen JM. The role of senescent cells in ageing. Nature 2014;509(7501):439–46.
[10] Toussaint O, Medrano EE, von Zglinicki T. Cellular and molecular mechanisms of stress-induced premature senescence (SIPS) of human diploid fibroblasts and melanocytes. Exp Gerontol 2000;35(8):927–45.
[11] Song S, et al. Senescent cells: emerging targets for human aging and age-related diseases. Trends Biochem Sci 2020;45(7):578–92.
[12] Jun JI, Lau LF. The matricellular protein CCN1 induces fibroblast senescence and restricts fibrosis in cutaneous wound healing. Nat Cell Biol 2010;12(7):676–85.
[13] Farr JN, Khosla S. Cellular senescence in bone. Bone 2019;121:121–33.
[14] Wang J, Geiger H, Rudolph KL. Immunoaging induced by hematopoietic stem cell aging. Curr Opin Immunol 2011;23(4):532–6.
[15] Tchkonia T, et al. Cellular senescence and the senescent secretory phenotype: therapeutic opportunities. J Clin Invest 2013;123(3):966–72.
[16] Campisi J, d'Adda di Fagagna F. Cellular senescence: when bad things happen to good cells. Nat Rev Mol Cell Biol 2007;8(9):729–40.
[17] Muñoz-Espín D, Serrano M. Cellular senescence: from physiology to pathology. Nat Rev Mol Cell Biol 2014;15(7):482–96.
[18] Kirkland JL, Tchkonia T. Cellular senescence: a translational perspective. EBioMedicine 2017;21:21–8.
[19] Ren J-L, et al. Inflammatory signaling and cellular senescence. Cell Signal 2009;21(3):378–83.
[20] Kim KS, et al. Induction of cellular senescence by insulin-like growth factor binding protein-5 through a p53-dependent mechanism. Mol Biol Cell 2007;18(11):4543–52.
[21] Ghosh K, Capell BC. The senescence-associated secretory phenotype: critical effector in skin cancer and aging. J Investig Dermatol 2016;136(11):2133–9.
[22] Catherine Hagan DVM. When are mice considered old?; 2017.
[23] Sieber CC. The elderly patient—who is that? Internist (Berl) 2007;48(11):1190. 1192–4.
[24] LeBrasseur NK, Tchkonia T, Kirkland JL. Cellular senescence and the biology of aging, disease, and frailty. Nestle Nutr Inst Workshop Ser 2015;83:11–8.
[25] Xu M, et al. Targeting senescent cells enhances adipogenesis and metabolic function in old age. elife 2015;4, e12997.
[26] Tchkonia T, Kirkland JL. Aging, cell senescence, and chronic disease: emerging therapeutic strategies. JAMA 2018;320(13):1319–20.
[27] Coppé JP, et al. Secretion of vascular endothelial growth factor by primary human fibroblasts at senescence. J Biol Chem 2006;281(40):29568–74.
[28] Xu M, et al. Senolytics improve physical function and increase lifespan in old age. Nat Med 2018;24(8):1246–56.
[29] Sözen T, Özışık L, Başaran NÇ. An overview and management of osteoporosis. Eur J Rheumatol 2017;4(1):46–56.
[30] Burge R, et al. Incidence and economic burden of osteoporosis-related fractures in the United States, 2005-2025. J Bone Miner Res 2007;22(3):465–75.
[31] Debacq-Chainiaux F, et al. Protocols to detect senescence-associated beta-galactosidase (SA-betagal) activity, a biomarker of senescent cells in culture and in vivo. Nat Protoc 2009;4(12):1798–806.
[32] Itahana K, Campisi J, Dimri GP. Methods to detect biomarkers of cellular senescence: the senescence-associated beta-galactosidase assay. Methods Mol Biol 2007;371:21–31.

[33] Hewitt G, et al. Telomeres are favoured targets of a persistent DNA damage response in ageing and stress-induced senescence. Nat Commun 2012;3:708.
[34] Swanson EC, et al. Higher-order unfolding of satellite heterochromatin is a consistent and early event in cell senescence. J Cell Biol 2013;203(6):929–42.
[35] Davalos AR, et al. p53-dependent release of Alarmin HMGB1 is a central mediator of senescent phenotypes. J Cell Biol 2013;201(4):613–29.
[36] Lee BY, et al. Senescence-associated beta-galactosidase is lysosomal beta-galactosidase. Aging Cell 2006;5(2):187–95.
[37] Kirkin V. History of the selective autophagy research: how did it begin and where does it stand today? J Mol Biol 2020;432(1):3–27.
[38] Klionsky DJ, et al. Guidelines for the use and interpretation of assays for monitoring autophagy (3rd edition). Autophagy 2016;12(1):1–222.
[39] Glick D, Barth S, Macleod KF. Autophagy: cellular and molecular mechanisms. J Pathol 2010;221(1):3–12.
[40] Korolchuk VI, et al. Mitochondria in cell senescence: is mitophagy the weakest link? EBioMedicine 2017;21:7–13.
[41] López-Otín C, et al. The hallmarks of aging. Cell 2013;153(6):1194–217.
[42] Dikic I, Elazar Z. Mechanism and medical implications of mammalian autophagy. Nat Rev Mol Cell Biol 2018;19(6):349–64.
[43] Rastaldo R, Vitale E, Giachino C. Dual role of autophagy in regulation of mesenchymal stem cell senescence. Front Cell Dev Biol 2020;8:276.
[44] Simonsen A, et al. Promoting basal levels of autophagy in the nervous system enhances longevity and oxidant resistance in adult Drosophila. Autophagy 2008;4(2):176–84.
[45] Harrison DE, et al. Rapamycin fed late in life extends lifespan in genetically heterogeneous mice. Nature 2009;460(7253):392–5.
[46] García-Prat L, et al. Autophagy maintains stemness by preventing senescence. Nature 2016;529(7584):37–42.
[47] Kang HT, et al. Autophagy impairment induces premature senescence in primary human fibroblasts. PLoS One 2011;6(8), e23367.
[48] Kang C, Elledge SJ. How autophagy both activates and inhibits cellular senescence. Autophagy 2016;12(5):898–9.
[49] Zhang D, et al. Autophagy inhibits the mesenchymal stem cell aging induced by D-galactose through ROS/JNK/p38 signalling. Clin Exp Pharmacol Physiol 2020;47(3):466–77.
[50] Kondrikov D, et al. Kynurenine inhibits autophagy and promotes senescence in aged bone marrow mesenchymal stem cells through the aryl hydrocarbon receptor pathway. Exp Gerontol 2020;130, 110805.
[51] Ma Y, et al. Autophagy controls mesenchymal stem cell properties and senescence during bone aging. Aging Cell 2018;17(1), e12709.
[52] Zheng Y, et al. Inhibition of autophagy alleviates the senescent state of rat mesenchymal stem cells during long-term culture. Mol Med Rep 2014;10(6):3003–8.
[53] Yang M, et al. Knockdown of insulin-like growth factor 1 exerts a protective effect on hypoxic injury of aged BM-MSCs: role of autophagy. Stem Cell Res Ther 2018;9(1):284.
[54] Chang T-C, Hsu M-F, Wu KK. High glucose induces bone marrow-derived mesenchymal stem cell senescence by upregulating autophagy. PLoS One 2015;10(5), e0126537.
[55] Zheng Y, et al. p53 regulates autophagic activity in senescent rat mesenchymal stromal cells. Exp Gerontol 2016;75:64–71.
[56] Fafián-Labora JA, Morente-López M, Arufe MC. Effect of aging on behaviour of mesenchymal stem cells. World J Stem Cells 2019;11(6):337–46.

[57] Young AR, et al. Autophagy mediates the mitotic senescence transition. Genes Dev 2009;23(7):798–803.

[58] Song C, Song C, Tong F. Autophagy induction is a survival response against oxidative stress in bone marrow-derived mesenchymal stromal cells. Cytotherapy 2014;16(10):1361–70.

[59] Capasso S, et al. Changes in autophagy, proteasome activity and metabolism to determine a specific signature for acute and chronic senescent mesenchymal stromal cells. Oncotarget 2015;6(37):39457–68.

[60] Lee JY, et al. GATA4-dependent regulation of the secretory phenotype via MCP-1underlies Lamin A-mediated human mesenchymal stem cell aging. Exp Mol Med 2018;50(5):1–12.

[61] Infante A, et al. Prelamin a accumulation and stress conditions induce impaired Oct-1 activity and autophagy in prematurely aged human mesenchymal stem cell. Aging (Albany NY) 2014;6(4):264–80.

[62] Kang C, et al. The DNA damage response induces inflammation and senescence by inhibiting autophagy of GATA4. Science 2015;349(6255), aaa5612.

[63] Narita M, et al. Spatial coupling of mTOR and autophagy augments secretory phenotypes. Science 2011;332(6032):966.

[64] Dou Z, et al. Autophagy mediates degradation of nuclear lamina. Nature 2015;527(7576): 105–9.

[65] Deas E, Wood NW, Plun-Favreau H. Mitophagy and Parkinson's disease: the PINK1-parkin link. Biochim Biophys Acta 2011;1813(4):623–33.

[66] Seabright AP, et al. AMPK activation induces mitophagy and promotes mitochondrial fission while activating TBK1 in a PINK1-Parkin independent manner. FASEB J 2020;34(5): 6284–301.

[67] Laker RC, et al. Ampk phosphorylation of Ulk1 is required for targeting of mitochondria to lysosomes in exercise-induced mitophagy. Nat Commun 2017;8(1):548.

[68] Ducommun S, et al. Motif affinity and mass spectrometry proteomic approach for the discovery of cellular AMPK targets: identification of mitochondrial fission factor as a new AMPK substrate. Cell Signal 2015;27(5):978–88.

[69] Toyama EQ, et al, Metabolism. AMP-activated protein kinase mediates mitochondrial fission in response to energy stress. Science 2016;351(6270):275–81.

[70] Ulgherait M, et al. AMPK modulates tissue and organismal aging in a non-cell-autonomous manner. Cell Rep 2014;8(6):1767–80.

[71] Han X, et al. AMPK activation protects cells from oxidative stress-induced senescence via autophagic flux restoration and intracellular NAD(+) elevation. Aging Cell 2016;15(3):416–27.

[72] Herzig S, Shaw RJ. AMPK: guardian of metabolism and mitochondrial homeostasis. Nat Rev Mol Cell Biol 2018;19(2):121–35.

[73] Li Q, et al. CTRP9 ameliorates cellular senescence via PGC-1α/AMPK signaling in mesenchymal stem cells. Int J Mol Med 2018;42(2):1054–63.

[74] Cantó C, Auwerx J. PGC-1alpha, SIRT1 and AMPK, an energy sensing network that controls energy expenditure. Curr Opin Lipidol 2009;20(2):98–105.

[75] Hampsch RA, et al. AMPK activation by metformin promotes survival of dormant ER(+) breast cancer cells. Clin Cancer Res 2020;26(14):3707–19.

[76] Menon R. Initiation of human parturition: signaling from senescent fetal tissues via extracellular vesicle mediated paracrine mechanism. Obstet Gynecol Sci 2019;62(4):199–211.

[77] Faget DV, Ren Q, Stewart SA. Unmasking senescence: context-dependent effects of SASP in cancer. Nat Rev Cancer 2019;19(8):439–53.

[78] Demaria M, et al. An essential role for senescent cells in optimal wound healing through secretion of PDGF-AA. Dev Cell 2014;31(6):722–33.

[79] Laberge RM, et al. Glucocorticoids suppress selected components of the senescence-associated secretory phenotype. Aging Cell 2012;11(4):569–78.
[80] Moiseeva O, et al. Metformin inhibits the senescence-associated secretory phenotype by interfering with IKK/NF-κB activation. Aging Cell 2013;12(3):489–98.
[81] Xu M, et al. JAK inhibition alleviates the cellular senescence-associated secretory phenotype and frailty in old age. Proc Natl Acad Sci U S A 2015;112(46):E6301–10.
[82] Singh M, et al. Effect of low-dose rapamycin on senescence markers and physical functioning in older adults with coronary artery disease: results of a pilot study. J Frailty Aging 2016;5(4):204–7.
[83] Herranz N, et al. mTOR regulates MAPKAPK2 translation to control the senescence-associated secretory phenotype. Nat Cell Biol 2015;17(9):1205–17.
[84] Li J, Kim SG, Blenis J. Rapamycin: one drug, many effects. Cell Metab 2014;19(3):373–9.
[85] Majumder S, et al. Lifelong rapamycin administration ameliorates age-dependent cognitive deficits by reducing IL-1β and enhancing NMDA signaling. Aging Cell 2012;11(2):326–35.
[86] Wilkinson JE, et al. Rapamycin slows aging in mice. Aging Cell 2012;11(4):675–82.
[87] Zhang Y, et al. Rapamycin extends life and health in C57BL/6 mice. J Gerontol A Biol Sci Med Sci 2014;69(2):119–30.
[88] Mannick JB, et al. mTOR inhibition improves immune function in the elderly. Sci Transl Med 2014;6(268). 268ra179.
[89] Farr JN, et al. Targeting cellular senescence prevents age-related bone loss in mice. Nat Med 2017;23(9):1072–9.
[90] Verstovsek S, et al. Safety and efficacy of INCB018424, a JAK1 and JAK2 inhibitor, in myelofibrosis. N Engl J Med 2010;363(12):1117–27.
[91] Xu M, Tchkonia T, Kirkland JL. Perspective: targeting the JAK/STAT pathway to fight age-related dysfunction. Pharmacol Res 2016;111:152–4.
[92] Hernandez-Segura A, et al. Unmasking transcriptional heterogeneity in senescent cells. Curr Biol 2017;27(17):2652–2660.e4.
[93] Zhu Y, et al. The Achilles' heel of senescent cells: from transcriptome to senolytic drugs. Aging Cell 2015;14(4):644–58.
[94] Kirkland JL, et al. The clinical potential of senolytic drugs. J Am Geriatr Soc 2017;65(10):2297–301.
[95] Wang E. Senescent human fibroblasts resist programmed cell death, and failure to suppress bcl2 is involved. Cancer Res 1995;55(11):2284–92.
[96] Elmore S. Apoptosis: a review of programmed cell death. Toxicol Pathol 2007;35(4): 495–516.
[97] Yi JS, et al. Low-dose dasatinib rescues cardiac function in Noonan syndrome. JCI Insight 2016;1(20), e90220.
[98] D'Andrea G. Quercetin: a flavonol with multifaceted therapeutic applications? Fitoterapia 2015;106:256–71.
[99] Khosla S, et al. The role of cellular senescence in ageing and endocrine disease. Nat Rev Endocrinol 2020;16(5):263–75.
[100] Mohamad Anuar NN, et al. Clinical review: navitoclax as a pro-apoptotic and anti-fibrotic agent. Front Pharmacol 2020;11, 564108.
[101] Zhu Y, et al. Identification of a novel senolytic agent, navitoclax, targeting the Bcl-2 family of antiapoptotic factors. Aging Cell 2016;15(3):428–35.
[102] Chang J, et al. Clearance of senescent cells by ABT263 rejuvenates aged hematopoietic stem cells in mice. Nat Med 2016;22(1):78–83.

[103] Zhu Y, et al. New agents that target senescent cells: the flavone, Fisetin, and the BCL-X(L) inhibitors, A1331852 and A1155463. Aging (Albany NY) 2017;9(3):955–63.
[104] Yousefzadeh MJ, et al. Fisetin is a senotherapeutic that extends health and lifespan. EBioMedicine 2018;36:18–28.
[105] Schafer MJ, et al. Cellular senescence mediates fibrotic pulmonary disease. Nat Commun 2017;8:14532.
[106] Sharma AK, et al. The senolytic drug navitoclax (ABT-263) causes trabecular bone loss and impaired osteoprogenitor function in aged mice. Front Cell Dev Biol 2020;8:354.
[107] Baker DJ, et al. Clearance of p16Ink4a-positive senescent cells delays ageing-associated disorders. Nature 2011;479(7372):232–6.
[108] Jeon OH, et al. Local clearance of senescent cells attenuates the development of post-traumatic osteoarthritis and creates a pro-regenerative environment. Nat Med 2017;23(6):775–81.
[109] Cherif H, et al. Curcumin and o-vanillin exhibit evidence of senolytic activity in human IVD cells in vitro. J Clin Med 2019;8(4):433.
[110] Karkoulis PK, et al. Targeted inhibition of heat shock protein 90 disrupts multiple oncogenic signaling pathways, thus inducing cell cycle arrest and programmed cell death in human urinary bladder cancer cell lines. Cancer Cell Int 2013;13(1):11.
[111] Felipe Sierra P. What is geroscience? American Federation for Aging Research (AFAR); 2020.

Chapter 5

Osteosarcopenia as a lifetime syndrome: Could it be prevented?

Charikleia Stefanaki[a,b,c]

[a]*University Research Institute of Maternal and Child Health & Precision Medicine, National and Kapodistrian University of Athens, "Aghia Sophia" Children's Hospital, Athens, Greece,* [b]*UNESCO Chair on Adolescent Health Care, National and Kapodistrian University of Athens, "Aghia Sophia" Children's Hospital, Athens, Greece,* [c]*Unit of Endocrinology, Diabetes mellitus, and Metabolism, School of Medicine, National and Kapodistrian University of Athens, Aretaieion Hospital, Athens, Greece*

Introduction

Osteosarcopenia is an entity relatively unknown to the medical sciences, but an old notion to the body composition analysis studies. In 1989, Zheng and Rosenberg first introduced the term "sarcopenia" in older persons, referring to the loss of skeletal muscle mass with aging based on a set of assessments [1]. In 1996, Heber et al. recognized an entity called "sarcopenic obesity" by employing bio-impedance body composition analysis (BIA), and then concluded that "additional studies are needed to determine the metabolic and clinical significance of sarcopenic obesity." [2].

It was not until 2014 that Professor J. Ilich introduced the term "osteosarcopenic obesity," referring to the loss of bone mass along with the muscular muscle mass in the presence of obesity in older populations [3]. And finally, Professor G. Duque, in 2015, coined the term "osteosarcopenia" in an older population with history of falling where loss of skeletal muscle and bone mass were present, along with frailty [4]. Others have also shown that postmenopausal women with osteopenia and/or osteoporosis evaluated by DEXA had decreased fat, skeletal, and bone mass compared with normal bone density women, suggesting concordance in the change of these three organ masses in postmenopausal women [5], and in lean polycystic ovary syndrome patients of reproductive age [6].

From then, till now, many studies have been published about osteosarcopenia, whether accompanied by obesity or not. They all have concluded that osteosarcopenia is an independent risk factor of the human health status [7],

Osteosarcopenia. https://doi.org/10.1016/B978-0-12-820088-9.00012-3

while also demonstrating that osteosarcopenic phenotypes were part of the clinical presentation of many metabolic disorders such as metabolic syndrome (MetS) [8], polycystic ovary syndrome (PCOS) [6], osteoporosis [9], in the form of cachexia in the presence of neoplasias [10], and as a result of stress system imbalance, and thus, as a result of low-grade, subclinical inflammation [11,12].

To date, very few studies have addressed the conundrum on the onset of this new condition. This chapter will focus on the osteosarcopenia as an entity during the human lifespan.

Definitions

There is no commonly used definition of the term "osteosarcopenia" just yet. Osteosarcopenia is regarded as a syndrome, characterized by progressive and generalized loss of bone and skeletal muscle mass and strength with a higher risk of adverse outcomes, such as physical disability, poor quality of life and death [13,14].

Regarding the definition of sarcopenia, several consensus papers have been published recommending different diagnostic approaches. The most commonly cited are those written under the auspices of the Second European Working Group on Sarcopenia in Older People (EWGSOP2) [15–17], the European Society for Clinical Nutrition and Metabolism Special Interest Groups (ESPEN-SIG) [18], and the International Working Group on Sarcopenia (IWGS) [19], respectively.

The aforementioned definitions proposed different diagnostic approaches. The presence of low skeletal muscle mass, and either low muscle strength or low muscle performance is diagnostic of sarcopenia, and when all three conditions are present, severe sarcopenia may be diagnosed (EWGSOP) [16]. In contrast, a second definition (ESPEN-SIG) proposed diagnosing sarcopenia only with the presence of low skeletal muscle mass and low muscle strength (which they advised could be assessed by walking speed) [18]. A third definition (IWGS) proposed the presence of low skeletal muscle mass and low muscle function, which they advised could be assessed by walking speed, and "that sarcopenia is associated with muscle mass loss alone, or in conjunction with increased fat mass" [19]. Except for the latter, the first consensus, developed by the EWGSOP separated muscle strength, and muscle performance, and allowed for a slightly broader definition, providing a classification of a severe condition [17,20].

Moreover, the diagnosis of sarcopenia can then be carried out by assessing the following parameters:

1. Measure walking speed in older persons (>65 years): If walking speed is below 0.8 m/s at the 4-m walking test, measure the muscle mass.
2. A low muscle mass, i.e., a percentage of muscle mass divided by height squared is below two standard deviations of the normal young mean (<7.23 kg/m^2 and in women at <5.67 kg/m^2) as defined using dual energy X-ray absorptiometry. If the walking speed at the 4-m walking test is higher than 0.8 m/s the handgrip strength should be tested; if this value is lower than 20 kg in women and 30 kg in man the muscle mass must be analyzed

as described previously. In any of the aforementioned definitions, and when combined with a T-score in the BMD below − 1 SD in the femoral neck, osteosarcopenia could be identified in older persons as a newly described geriatric syndrome that takes its great toll in the health status of these populations [16,21,22]. However, the variety of definitions for sarcopenia has limited consensus on how to define osteosarcopenia, a situation that also occurs in osteosarcopenic obesity. Nevertheless, the several features of these syndromes seem to be present in the youth also [23]. Therefore, the burning questions are: Does osteopenia and/or sarcopenia exist in the young populations? Can we define osteosarcopenia in the young populations? and when, or how? Or, is it a strictly geriatric syndrome? [10,24].

Pathophysiology

Muscle, fat, and bone cell masses derive from mesenchymal stem cells (MSCs). The differentiation between muscle, fat and bone is influenced by numerous environmental cues, such as hormones [25]. Sarcopenia implicates both loss of muscle mass and subsequent dysfunction, such as impairment of contraction, metabolic, and endocrine abnormalities. It affects metabolism, immune, and inflammatory responses, and includes parameters related to force, functional capacity, and the amount of body fat [26,27].

In subjects in development, such as children or adolescents, and in adult humans, appetite regulation and physical activity affect energy balance. More specifically, in children and adolescents, appetite regulation seems to be dysregulated in excess body fat mass, and certain types of exercise favor muscle health, depending on the age. In some individuals, inflammation induces anorexia and fat loss in combination with sarcopenia. However, in others, appetite is maintained, despite activation of systemic, subclinical low-grade inflammation, leading to sarcopenia with seemingly normal or increased fat content [26].

Sarcopenia is accompanied by infiltration of muscle tissue by lipids, leading to increased adipocyte number and lipid deposition within muscle fibers. Lipid deposition in muscle is called myosteatosis and seems to be the result of the reduced oxidative capacity of muscle fibers with aging. Elevated fat mass in combination with low muscle mass, or increased fat mass together with decreased muscle strength are termed as sarcopenic obesity [28]. Sarcopenia is a diagnosis made by means of dual X-ray absorptiometry (DXA), bioelectric impedance (BIA), or cross-sectional imaging with CT or MRI. However, normative data for skeletal muscle mass are absent, especially in pediatrics. Last, but not least, studies of evaluation of skeletal muscle mass by cross-sectional imaging in children are limited [29,30].

Although mechanical forces clearly have a significant role in the pathogenesis of osteosarcopenia, more recent research suggests paracrine, or endocrine crosstalk is implicated. Important hormones mediating this crosstalk include growth hormone/insulin-like growth factor-1 (GH/IGF-1), gonadal sex hormones, and vitamin D, with age-related decreases contributing to the development of osteosarcopenia. Muscle and bone, also, secrete certain factors, known as myokines, and osteokines respectively, which aid the communication between muscle, and bone [31]. An extensively researched myokine is myostatin, a member of the transforming growth factor beta (TGF-β) superfamily, which inhibits skeletal muscle growth, but also has effects on bone and tendon [32].

Bone-muscle crosstalk is mediated by several important signaling pathways. For example, the canonical Wnt-β-catenin signaling pathway controls osteoblastic activity and is, also, involved in muscle regeneration, the GH/IGF-1 axis is a key regulator of bone and muscle growth, mediating its effects via several signaling pathways. There is hope that exploiting these pathways will facilitate the development of new therapeutic agents in the future [31,33].

Genetic polymorphisms of various genes also contribute to the pathogenesis of osteosarcopenia. As reviewed by Kaji et al., these include androgen receptor, estrogen receptor, catechol-*O*-methyltransferase, IGF-I, vitamin D receptor and low-density-lipoprotein receptor-related protein [32].

Conclusively, the pathogenesis of osteosarcopenia is multifactorial, with an array of mechanical, biochemical, genetic and lifestyle factors all contributing to involution of the "bone-muscle unit" [24,31].

Osteopenia, osteoporosis, and sarcopenia in the young populations

Body composition analysis in the young populations drew interest of many researchers, during the last 10 years. Osteoporosis is defined as a skeletal disorder characterized by compromised bone density and strength, predisposing a person to an increased risk of fracture. Traditionally, osteoporosis is considered as a disease of aged populations. Nevertheless, it occurs in patients of all ages, and is seems to be increasingly identified in the pediatric populations. Patients, of both sexes, including children with chronic diseases, are at risk for bone fragility.

There are several forms of osteoporosis that implicate genetic factors and that should be identified at early stages to ensure adequate treatment. The diagnosis of osteoporosis in the young aged populations is tricky since their bone mineral density (BMD) is affected by growth and pubertal development. In addition to low BMD, an individual in development should present with a significant tendency to fractures before the osteoporosis diagnosis can be made.

Typically, primary osteoporosis is defined as a condition, characterized by global skeletal fragility that develops in association with menopause and advancing age. Secondary osteoporosis may be caused by specific disorders, including endocrinopathies, drugs and genetic diseases that cause low BMD, either by interfering with attainment of peak bone mass or by increasing rates of involutional bone loss [34]. Osteoporosis in children and adolescents may be primary, or secondary (Table 1) [35].

TABLE 1 Causes of osteoporosis in children and adolescents.

Primary osteoporosis
Ehlers-Danlos
Homocystinuria
Marfan's
Osteogenesis imperfecta
Idiopathic osteoporosis
Genetic osteoporosis
Secondary osteoporosis
JIA[a]
SLE[b]
IBD[c]
Cerebral palsy
Meningomyelocele
Myopathies
Malabsorption syndromes
Shwachman-Diamond
Cystic fibrosis
Gaucher disease type 1 or 3
Niemann Pick A/B
Inborn errors of calcium and phosphorus homeostasis
Malnutrition
Leukemias
Thalassemia
Growth hormone deficiency
Hypogonadism
Turner's
Hyperthyroidism
Hyperparathyroidism
Cushing's
Vitamin D deficiency

TABLE 1 Causes of osteoporosis in children and adolescents.—cont'd

Anorexia nervosa
Chemotherapy for malignancy
Chemotherapy following solid organ transplant
Glucocorticoids
Anticonvulsants
Heparin
Calcineurin inhibitors
Chronic kidney disease
Liver disease

[a] *Juvenile idiopathic arthritis.*
[b] *Systemic lupus erythematosus.*
[c] *Inflammatory bowel disease.*

The definition for osteoporosis in children and adolescents includes: (1) A clinically significant fracture history (one or more of the following) (a) Long bone fracture of the lower extremities; (b) Vertebral compression fracture; (c) Two or more long-bone fractures of the upper extremities; (2) Low spinal or total body less head areal bone mineral density or bone mineral content, defined as a *Z*-score less than or equal to −2.0 adjusted for age, gender and body size, as appropriate [36,37].

Skeletal muscle is a modifiable tissue that presents with plasticity and is capable of altering its structure and its metabolism. Though, the total number of muscle fibers seem to be set during fetal life, between the 6–8th and 8–18th week of pregnancy, as studies have shown [38]. Postpartum, the mass of muscle fibers exhibit more hypertrophy than hyperplasia, meaning that they grow mainly in size and to a lesser degree in number [39]. Thus, defects in muscle development, occurring during fetal development may be maintained postpartum throughout adult life [40]. There are several factors affecting skeletal muscle mass development, such as intrauterine and genetic influences [40], dietary protein [41], physical activity [42], chronic diseases [43], and obesity [44], leading to sarcopenia in children and adolescents.

There are many studies that have demonstrated the susceptibility of IUGR, SGA children to reduced myoblast replication and thus, to the development of sarcopenia, later in life [45,46]. Also, many patients with myopathies, or other neurologic diseases [47], apart from developing osteopenia and osteoporosis, are prone to sarcopenia, due to the defects in the function of the muscle mass innervation [48,49]. Growing evidence suggests that osteosarcopenia and osteosarcopenic obesity is on the rise in the pediatric and adolescent populations in the developed countries, probably due to diminished intake of protein, which was below the highest acceptable macronutrient distribution range of 35% for an age/sex group [50].

Sedentary lifestyle, increased screen time and lack of physical activity and exercise lead to prompt underdevelopment of skeletal muscle mass in children and adolescents [51]. Chronic diseases, such as liver, kidney and intestinal failure cause sarcopenia, due to disruption of ammonia metabolism, subsequent increased muscle mass inflammation, and impaired muscle growth, with grave implications in the prognosis [52,53]. Obesity in children and adolescents complicate the clinical presentation of sarcopenia. Especially in the case of MetS and prediabetic patients [54], it seems that they seem to combine early elements of osteopenia/osteoporosis and sarcopenia, exhibiting a mixed phenotype of adult type osteosarcopenic obesity [23,55] (Fig. 1), as described in the next paragraph.

Sarcopenia is an underestimated entity by the clinicians, a fact partially explained by the lack of consensus and the lack of means of evaluation. Additionally, larger scale studies and available reference ranges for other specific populations, including children, are lacking [29]. Reference ranges exist for DXA- and BIA-derived muscle mass parameters in children. Still, the aforementioned studies were not able to provide normative reference ranges per age year since they were not powered [56].

Outcome studies in pediatric populations have demonstrated that, similar to adults, sarcopenia in children is associated with increased morbidity and mortality. Studies employing computed-tomography (CT) or magnetic resonance imaging (MRI) quantification of skeletal muscle mass have been performed in subjects with pediatric malignancies, such as neuroblastomas, acute

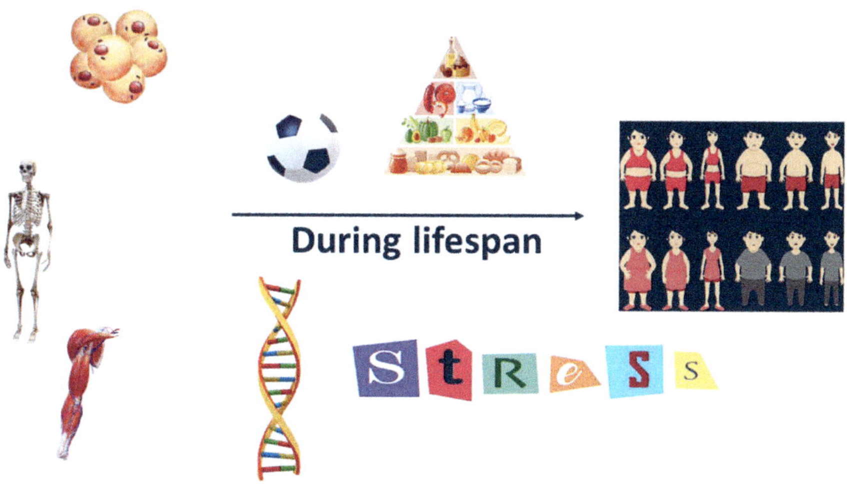

FIG. 1 Osteosarcopenia during lifespan.

lymphocytic leukemia, appendicitis, IBD [57], and end-stage liver, kidney, intestine failure and have shown lower skeletal muscle areas and worse outcomes compared to controls. These findings suggested that sarcopenia is not exclusive to older adults but rather is present in children with a variety of pathologies, including pediatric-specific pathologies, such as neurologic and neoplastic disorders [58–60].

Osteosarcopenic obesity

Osteosarcopenic obesity has been identified for many years [61]. It is another aspect of the osteosarcopenia (reviewed in Chapter 10 of this book), and it is roughly divided in osteosarcopenic visceral obesity, and osteosarcopenic subcutaneous obesity. Individuals presenting with the osteosarcopenic visceral obesity phenotype seem to demonstrate a higher risk of fractures, inflammation, and a worse metabolic profile. These conditions in individuals with the osteosarcopenic subcutaneous obesity exhibit an increase of visceral adipose tissue, while those with osteosarcopenic subcutaneous obesity seem to benefit related to the "obesity paradox" [62].

Early osteosarcopenic features have been also observed in young populations in the past. Most of the studies evaluated healthy children and adolescents, but there are also studies about young adult patients with various disorders that demonstrate early osteosarcopenic phenotypes [6,23]. As the trend of pediatric and adolescent obesity is constantly increasing, the prevalence of metabolic syndrome in this specific population is on the rise and is greatly influenced by the degree of adiposity measured as BMI, or waist circumference. Studies of representative adolescent samples in Greece have reported abdominal obesity prevalence of 9.1%–9.5% [63–66]; and in obese adolescents metabolic syndrome prevalence of 31.6% [64].

Data from a recent study revealed that osteosarcopenia along with obesity and metabolic syndrome (MetS) was found in populations of male and female adolescents, aged 12–17 years of life [67,68]. The study of Ayvaz et al. in 2011 had similar results, since they had found higher basal metabolic rate and fat mass percentage, but lower fat-free mass and total body water percentages in obese Turkish adolescents with MetS compared with those without MetS [69]. In 2016, Stefanaki et al. revealed features of osteosarcopenia in obese youngsters, aged 18–21 years. The sample in this study included clinically healthy overweight/obese participants, either males or females that demonstrated decreased muscle and bone masses [23].

Prevention

Osteosarcopenic features in childhood and adolescence seem to follow the individual throughout the adult lifespan. Prevention measures should start as early as in pregnancy, or a year before conception, to ensure optimal maternal health, in order to diminish any risk of complications in pregnancy outcomes, such as premature birth, IUGR, or SGA neonates. These prevention measures include a healthy lifestyle, avoidance of unhealthy habits, and frequent, regular health check-ups, before, and after birth. Any maternal health issue should be addressed according to the current guidelines and should be improved and managed accordingly. Any genetic disease of the mother should be accompanied by proper genetic counseling.

Every medical condition, predisposing to osteosarcopenia should be also addressed and managed, so that the developing individual should enter into adulthood in optimal health conditions. One crucial factor of prevention is a balanced nutrient intake through proper and healthy food choices, according to the age of the individual and the guidelines given by the scientific societies. The bioavailability of calcium in maternal milk is far superior to commercial formulas, making it the leading source for calcium during breastfeeding. Only in the case of infants should calcium intake be increased to the recommended supplementary levels using commercial formulas with higher calcium contents [70]. Proper quantities of protein, calcium, and vitamin D_3 intake seem to be extremely important in periods of development [71]. Early introduction of the individual to exercise practice, along with a healthy diet in the family is guaranteed to form solid, healthy daily routine and to provide the right start in life [72,73].

Also, imaging for osteosarcopenia prevention should be administered at an early age, especially in young populations at risk. Imaging may be performed by employing ultrasound (U/S), computed tomography (CT), magnetic resonance imaging (MRI), or bio-impedance (BIA). Pediatric studies of muscle mass quantification by CT or MRI have most commonly used the measures of psoas area, or psoas muscle index measured at L3 on CT, although some studies used L2, L4, or L5, MRI, paraspinous muscle area, or intramuscular adipose tissue area.

Future research should be directed at evaluating the correlation of estimates of skeletal muscle mass (by imaging, per spinal level) to total body skeletal muscle mass as well as nomograms for estimates of skeletal muscle mass in pediatric and adolescent populations across age groups and developmental stages. This would greatly facilitate additional sarcopenia-related imaging research in the area of pediatrics [74]. Last, but not least, new biomarkers, such as circulating osteoprogenitor (COP) cells have been identified in humans as osteosarcopenia biomarkers [75], or gut microbiome metabolites that may be employed in the prevention strategies against osteosarcopenia [76,77].

References

[1] Zheng JJ, Rosenberg IH. What is the nutritional status of the elderly? Geriatrics 1989;44(6):57–8. 60, 63-4.

[2] Heber D, Ingles S, Ashley JM, Maxwell MH, Lyons RF, Elashoff RM. Clinical detection of sarcopenic obesity by bioelectrical impedance analysis. Am J Clin Nutr 1996;64(3 Suppl):472S–7S. https://doi.org/10.1093/ajcn/64.3.472S.

[3] Ormsbee MJ, Prado CM, Ilich JZ, et al. Osteosarcopenic obesity: the role of bone, muscle, and fat on health. J Cachexia Sarcopenia Muscle 2014;5(3):183–92. https://doi.org/10.1007/s13539-014-0146-x.
[4] Huo YR, Suriyaarachchi P, Gomez F, et al. Phenotype of osteosarcopenia in older individuals with a history of falling. J Am Med Dir Assoc 2015;16(4):290–5. https://doi.org/10.1016/j.jamda.2014.10.018.
[5] Peppa M, Stefanaki C, Papaefstathiou A, Boschiero D, Dimitriadis G, Chrousos GP. Bioimpedance analysis vs. DEXA as a screening tool for osteosarcopenia in lean, overweight and obese Caucasian postmenopausal females. Hormones 2017;16(2):181–93. https://doi.org/10.14310/horm.2002.1732.
[6] Stefanaki C, Bacopoulou F, Kandaraki E, Boschiero D, Diamandi-Kandarakis E. Lean women on metformin and oral contraceptives for polycystic ovary syndrome demonstrate a dehydrated osteosarcopenic phenotype: A pilot study. Nutrients 2019;11(9). https://doi.org/10.3390/nu11092055.
[7] Drey M, Sieber CC, Bertsch T, Bauer JM, Schmidmaier R, Fi ATig. Osteosarcopenia is more than sarcopenia and osteopenia alone. Aging Clin Exp Res 2016;28(5):895–9. https://doi.org/10.1007/s40520-015-0494-1.
[8] Rubio-Ruiz ME, Guarner-Lans V, Perez-Torres I, Soto ME. Mechanisms underlying metabolic syndrome-related sarcopenia and possible therapeutic measures. Int J Mol Sci 2019;20(3). https://doi.org/10.3390/ijms20030647.
[9] Reiss J, Iglseder B, Alzner R, et al. Sarcopenia and osteoporosis are interrelated in geriatric inpatients. Z Gerontol Geriatr 2019;52(7):688–93. Sarkopenie und Osteoporose sind bei geriatrischen Krankenhauspatienten miteinander assoziiert https://doi.org/10.1007/s00391-019-01553-z.
[10] Hassan EB, Duque G. Osteosarcopenia: a new geriatric syndrome. Aust Fam Physician 2017;46(11):849–53.
[11] Ilich JZ, Gilman JC, Cvijetic S, Boschiero D. Chronic stress contributes to osteosarcopenic adiposity via inflammation and immune modulation: the case for more precise nutritional investigation. Nutrients 2020;12(4). https://doi.org/10.3390/nu12040989.
[12] Stefanaki C, Pervanidou P, Boschiero D, Chrousos GP. Chronic stress and body composition disorders: implications for health and disease. Hormones 2018;17(1):33–43. https://doi.org/10.1007/s42000-018-0023-7.
[13] Santilli V, Bernetti A, Mangone M, Paoloni M. Clinical definition of sarcopenia. Clin Cases Miner Bone Metab 2014;11(3):177–80.
[14] Goodpaster BH, Park SW, Harris TB, et al. The loss of skeletal muscle strength, mass, and quality in older adults: the health, aging and body composition study. J Gerontol A Biol Sci Med Sci 2006;61(10):1059–64. https://doi.org/10.1093/gerona/61.10.1059.
[15] Cruz-Jentoft AJ, Bahat G, Bauer J, et al. Sarcopenia: revised European consensus on definition and diagnosis. Age Ageing 2019;48(1):16–31. https://doi.org/10.1093/ageing/afy169.
[16] Cruz-Jentoft AJ, Baeyens JP, Bauer JM, et al. Sarcopenia: European consensus on definition and diagnosis: report of the European working group on sarcopenia in older people. Age Ageing 2010;39(4):412–23. https://doi.org/10.1093/ageing/afq034.
[17] Davalos-Yerovi V, Marco E, Sanchez-Rodriguez D, et al. Sarcopenia according to the revised European consensus on definition and diagnosis (EWGSOP2) criteria predicts hospitalizations and long-term mortality in rehabilitation patients with stable chronic obstructive pulmonary disease. J Am Med Dir Assoc 2019;20(8):1047–9. https://doi.org/10.1016/j.jamda.2019.03.019.

[18] Muscaritoli M, Anker SD, Argiles J, et al. Consensus definition of sarcopenia, cachexia and pre-cachexia: joint document elaborated by special interest groups (SIG) "cachexia-anorexia in chronic wasting diseases" and "nutrition in geriatrics". Clin Nutr 2010;29(2):154–9. https://doi.org/10.1016/j.clnu.2009.12.004.

[19] Fielding RA, Vellas B, Evans WJ, et al. Sarcopenia: an undiagnosed condition in older adults. Current consensus definition: prevalence, etiology, and consequences. International working group on sarcopenia. J Am Med Dir Assoc 2011;12(4):249–56. https://doi.org/10.1016/j.jamda.2011.01.003.

[20] Rizzoli R, Reginster JY, Arnal JF, et al. Quality of life in sarcopenia and frailty. Calcif Tissue Int 2013;93(2):101–20. https://doi.org/10.1007/s00223-013-9758-y.

[21] Olde Rikkert MG, Rigaud AS, van Hoeyweghen RJ, de Graaf J. Geriatric syndromes: medical misnomer or progress in geriatrics? Neth J Med 2003;61(3):83–7.

[22] Cruz-Jentoft AJ, Landi F, Topinkova E, Michel JP. Understanding sarcopenia as a geriatric syndrome. Curr Opin Clin Nutr Metab Care 2010;13(1):1–7. https://doi.org/10.1097/MCO.0b013e328333c1c1.

[23] Stefanaki C, Peppa M, Boschiero D, Chrousos GP. Healthy overweight/obese youth: early osteosarcopenic obesity features. Eur J Clin Invest 2016;46(9):767–78. https://doi.org/10.1111/eci.12659.

[24] Paintin J, Cooper C, Dennison E. Osteosarcopenia. Br J Hosp Med 2018;79(5):253–8. https://doi.org/10.12968/hmed.2018.79.5.253.

[25] Ilich JZ, Kelly OJ, Inglis JE, Panton LB, Duque G, Ormsbee MJ. Interrelationship among muscle, fat, and bone: connecting the dots on cellular, hormonal, and whole body levels. Ageing Res Rev 2014;15:51–60. https://doi.org/10.1016/j.arr.2014.02.007.

[26] Biolo G, Cederholm T, Muscaritoli M. Muscle contractile and metabolic dysfunction is a common feature of sarcopenia of aging and chronic diseases: from sarcopenic obesity to cachexia. Clin Nutr 2014;33(5):737–48. https://doi.org/10.1016/j.clnu.2014.03.007.

[27] Jensen GL, Hsiao PY. Obesity in older adults: relationship to functional limitation. Curr Opin Clin Nutr Metab Care 2010;13(1):46–51. https://doi.org/10.1097/MCO.0b013e32833309cf.

[28] Scott D, Sanders KM, Aitken D, Hayes A, Ebeling PR, Jones G. Sarcopenic obesity and dynapenic obesity: 5-year associations with falls risk in middle-aged and older adults. Obesity (Silver Spring) 2014;22(6):1568–74. https://doi.org/10.1002/oby.20734.

[29] Gilligan LA, Towbin AJ, Dillman JR, Somasundaram E, Trout AT. Quantification of skeletal muscle mass: sarcopenia as a marker of overall health in children and adults. Pediatr Radiol 2020;50(4):455–64. https://doi.org/10.1007/s00247-019-04562-7.

[30] Weber DR, Boyce A, Gordon C, et al. The utility of DXA assessment at the forearm, proximal femur, and lateral distal femur, and vertebral fracture assessment in the pediatric population: 2019 ISCD official position. J Clin Densitom 2019;22(4):567–89. https://doi.org/10.1016/j.jocd.2019.07.002.

[31] Girgis CM, Mokbel N, Digirolamo DJ. Therapies for musculoskeletal disease: can we treat two birds with one stone? Curr Osteoporos Rep 2014;12(2):142–53. https://doi.org/10.1007/s11914-014-0204-5.

[32] Kaji H. Interaction between muscle and bone. J Bone Metab 2014;21(1):29–40. https://doi.org/10.11005/jbm.2014.21.1.29.

[33] Oliveira A, Vaz C. The role of sarcopenia in the risk of osteoporotic hip fracture. Clin Rheumatol 2015;34(10):1673–80. https://doi.org/10.1007/s10067-015-2943-9.

[34] Lorentzon M, Cummings SR. Osteoporosis: the evolution of a diagnosis. J Intern Med 2015;277(6):650–61. https://doi.org/10.1111/joim.12369.

[35] Langeveld M, Hollak CEM. Bone health in patients with inborn errors of metabolism. Rev Endocr Metab Disord 2018;19(1):81–92. https://doi.org/10.1007/s11154-018-9460-5.

[36] Rauch F, Plotkin H, DiMeglio L, et al. Fracture prediction and the definition of osteoporosis in children and adolescents: the ISCD 2007 pediatric official positions. J Clin Densitom 2008;11(1):22–8. https://doi.org/10.1016/j.jocd.2007.12.003.

[37] Saraff V, Hogler W. Endocrinology and adolescence: osteoporosis in children: diagnosis and management. Eur J Endocrinol 2015;173(6):R185–97. https://doi.org/10.1530/EJE-14-0865.

[38] Fukada SI. The roles of muscle stem cells in muscle injury, atrophy and hypertrophy. J Biochem 2018;163(5):353–8. https://doi.org/10.1093/jb/mvy019.

[39] Verdijk LB, Snijders T, Drost M, Delhaas T, Kadi F, van Loon LJ. Satellite cells in human skeletal muscle; from birth to old age. Age 2014;36(2):545–7. https://doi.org/10.1007/s11357-013-9583-2.

[40] Sayer AA, Cooper C. Fetal programming of body composition and musculoskeletal development. Early Hum Dev 2005;81(9):735–44. https://doi.org/10.1016/j.earlhumdev.2005.07.003.

[41] Costa-Orvay JA, Figueras-Aloy J, Romera G, Closa-Monasterolo R, Carbonell-Estrany X. The effects of varying protein and energy intakes on the growth and body composition of very low birth weight infants. Nutr J 2011;10:140. https://doi.org/10.1186/1475-2891-10-140.

[42] Wackerhage H, Rennie MJ. How nutrition and exercise maintain the human musculoskeletal mass. J Anat 2006;208(4):451–8. https://doi.org/10.1111/j.1469-7580.2006.00544.x.

[43] Martinez EE, Smallwood CD, Quinn NL, et al. Body composition in children with chronic illness: accuracy of bedside assessment techniques. J Pediatr 2017;190:56–62. https://doi.org/10.1016/j.jpeds.2017.07.045.

[44] Wu H, Ballantyne CM. Skeletal muscle inflammation and insulin resistance in obesity. J Clin Invest 2017;127(1):43–54. https://doi.org/10.1172/JCI88880.

[45] Soto SM, Blake AC, Wesolowski SR, et al. Myoblast replication is reduced in the IUGR fetus despite maintained proliferative capacity in vitro. J Endocrinol 2017;232(3):475–91. https://doi.org/10.1530/JOE-16-0123.

[46] Sayer AA, Syddall H, Martin H, Patel H, Baylis D, Cooper C. The developmental origins of sarcopenia. J Nutr Health Aging 2008;12(7):427–32. https://doi.org/10.1007/BF02982703.

[47] Shortland A. Muscle deficits in cerebral palsy and early loss of mobility: can we learn something from our elders? Dev Med Child Neurol 2009;51(Suppl. 4):59–63. https://doi.org/10.1111/j.1469-8749.2009.03434.x.

[48] Palmio J, Udd B. Borderlines between sarcopenia and mild late-onset muscle disease. Front Aging Neurosci 2014;6:267. https://doi.org/10.3389/fnagi.2014.00267.

[49] Pestronk A, Keeling R, Choksi R. Sarcopenia, age, atrophy, and myopathy: mitochondrial oxidative enzyme activities. Muscle Nerve 2017;56(1):122–8. https://doi.org/10.1002/mus.25442.

[50] Fulgoni 3rd VL. Current protein intake in America: analysis of the National Health and Nutrition Examination Survey, 2003–2004. Am J Clin Nutr 2008;87(5):1554S–7S. https://doi.org/10.1093/ajcn/87.5.1554S.

[51] Nguyen VH. School-based exercise interventions effectively increase bone mineralization in children and adolescents. Osteoporos Sarcopenia 2018;4(2):39–46. https://doi.org/10.1016/j.afos.2018.05.002.

[52] Rezende IFB, Conceicao-Machado MEP, Souza VS, Santos EMD, Silva LR. Sarcopenia in children and adolescents with chronic liver disease. J Pediatr (Rio J) 2019. https://doi.org/10.1016/j.jped.2019.02.005.

[53] Mangus RS, Bush WJ, Miller C, Kubal CA. Severe sarcopenia and increased fat stores in pediatric patients with liver, kidney, or intestine failure. J Pediatr Gastroenterol Nutr 2017;65(5):579–83. https://doi.org/10.1097/MPG.0000000000001651.

[54] Kawada T. Insulin resistance and sarcopenia are closely related to metabolic syndrome in male and female adolescents. Public Health Nutr 2016;19(8):1528. https://doi.org/10.1017/S1368980015002475.

[55] Bauer JM, Cruz-Jentoft AJ, Fielding RA, et al. Is there enough evidence for osteosarcopenic obesity as a distinct entity? A critical literature review. Calcif Tissue Int 2019;105(2):109–24. https://doi.org/10.1007/s00223-019-00561-w.

[56] Shuhart CR, Yeap SS, Anderson PA, et al. Executive summary of the 2019 ISCD position development conference on monitoring treatment, DXA cross-calibration and least significant change, spinal cord injury, peri-prosthetic and orthopedic bone health, transgender medicine, and pediatrics. J Clin Densitom 2019;22(4):453–71. https://doi.org/10.1016/j.jocd.2019.07.001.

[57] Scaldaferri F, Pizzoferrato M, Lopetuso LR, et al. Nutrition and IBD: malnutrition and/or sarcopenia? A practical guide. Gastroenterol Res Pract 2017;2017:8646495. https://doi.org/10.1155/2017/8646495.

[58] Wren TA, Ponrartana S, Van Speybroeck A, Ryan DD, Chia JM, Hu HH. Heterogeneity of muscle fat infiltration in children with spina bifida. Res Dev Disabil 2014;35(1):215–22. https://doi.org/10.1016/j.ridd.2013.10.002.

[59] Mueske NM, Mittelman SD, Wren TAL, Gilsanz V, Orgel E. Myosteatosis in adolescents and young adults treated for acute lymphoblastic leukemia. Leuk Lymphoma 2019;60(13):-3146–53. https://doi.org/10.1080/10428194.2019.1623889.

[60] Lorenzana DJ, Mueske NM, Ryan DD, Van Speybroeck AL, Wren TA. Quantitative analysis of lower leg adipose tissue distribution in youth with myelomeningocele. J Child Neurol 2016;31(8):979–84. https://doi.org/10.1177/0883073816634858.

[61] Roubenoff R. Sarcopenic obesity: does muscle loss cause fat gain? Lessons from rheumatoid arthritis and osteoarthritis. Ann N Y Acad Sci 2000;904:553–7. https://doi.org/10.1111/j.1749-6632.2000.tb06515.x.

[62] Perna S, Spadaccini D, Nichetti M, Avanzato I, Faliva MA, Rondanelli M. Osteosarcopenic visceral obesity and osteosarcopenic subcutaneous obesity, two new phenotypes of sarcopenia: prevalence, metabolic profile, and risk factors. J Aging Res 2018;2018:6147426. https://doi.org/10.1155/2018/6147426.

[63] Bacopoulou F, Efthymiou V, Landis G, Rentoumis A, Chrousos GP. Waist circumference, waist-to-hip ratio and waist-to-height ratio reference percentiles for abdominal obesity among Greek adolescents. BMC Pediatr 2015;15:50. https://doi.org/10.1186/s12887-015-0366-z.

[64] Bacopoulou F, Efthymiou V, Palaiologos G, et al. Telemedicine screening adolescent metabolic syndrome in Greek schools. Eur J Clin Invest 2019;49(4). https://doi.org/10.1111/eci.13075, e13075.

[65] Grammatikopoulou MG, Maraki MI, Giannopoulou D, Poulimeneas D, Sidossis LS, Tsigga M. Similar Mediterranean diet adherence but greater central adiposity is observed among Greek diaspora adolescents living in Istanbul, compared to Athens. Ethn Health 2018;23(2):221–32. https://doi.org/10.1080/13557858.2016.1258043.

[66] Grammatikopoulou MG, Poulimeneas D, Gounitsioti IS, et al. Prevalence of simple and abdominal obesity in Greek adolescents: the ADONUT study. Clin Obes 2014;4(6):303–8. https://doi.org/10.1111/cob.12070.

[67] Bacopoulou F, Landis GN, Palasz A, et al. Identifying early abdominal obesity risk in adolescents by telemedicine: a cross-sectional study in Greece. Food Chem Toxicol 2020;144. https://doi.org/10.1016/j.fct.2020.111532, 111532.

[68] Bacopoulou F, Landis G, Pałasz A, et al. Body composition in abdominal obesity and/or metabolic syndrome: A cross-sectional telemedicine study of 1,578 adolescent students. Athens 11527, Attica, Greece: First Department of Pediatrics, School of Medicine, National and Kapodistrian University of Athens, Aghia Sophia Children's Hospital; 2020.

[69] Ayvaz D, Kilinç F, Pac F, Çakal E. Anthropometric measurements and body composition analysis of obese adolescents with and without metabolic syndrome. Turk J Med Sci 2011;41:267–74.

[70] Vierucci F, Saggese G, Cimaz R. Osteoporosis in childhood. Curr Opin Rheumatol 2017;29(5):535–46. https://doi.org/10.1097/BOR.0000000000000423.

[71] Earl S, Cole ZA, Holroyd C, Cooper C, Harvey NC. Session 2: other diseases: dietary management of osteoporosis throughout the life course. Proc Nutr Soc 2010;69(1):25–33. https://doi.org/10.1017/S0029665109991765.

[72] Saggese G, Baroncelli GI, Bertelloni S. Osteoporosis in children and adolescents: diagnosis, risk factors, and prevention. J Pediatr Endocrinol Metab 2001;14(7):833–59. https://doi.org/10.1515/jpem.2001.14.7.833.

[73] Weaver CM, Gordon CM, Janz KF, et al. The National Osteoporosis Foundation's position statement on peak bone mass development and lifestyle factors: a systematic review and implementation recommendations. Osteoporos Int 2016;27(4):1281–386. https://doi.org/10.1007/s00198-015-3440-3.

[74] Orsso CE, Tibaes JRB, Oliveira CLP, et al. Low muscle mass and strength in pediatrics patients: why should we care? Clin Nutr 2019;38(5):2002–15. https://doi.org/10.1016/j.clnu.2019.04.012.

[75] Gunawardene P, Al Saedi A, Singh L, et al. Age, gender, and percentage of circulating osteoprogenitor (COP) cells: the COP study. Exp Gerontol 2017;96:68–72. https://doi.org/10.1016/j.exger.2017.06.004.

[76] You L, Zhu L, Li PZ, et al. Dysbacteriosis-derived lipopolysaccharide causes embryonic osteopenia through retinoic-acid-regulated DLX5 expression. Int J Mol Sci 2020;21(7). https://doi.org/10.3390/ijms21072518.

[77] Stefanaki C, Bacopoulou F, Michos A. The impact of probiotics' administration on glycemic control, body composition, gut microbiome, mitochondria, and other hormonal signals in adolescents with prediabetes - a randomized, controlled trial study protocol. Contem Clin Trials Commun 2018;11:55–62. https://doi.org/10.1016/j.conctc.2018.06.002.

Chapter 6

Inflammation and osteosarcopenia

Yushu Huang[a], Yukang Li[b], and Sean X. Leng[b]
[a]*Brandeis University, Waltham, MA, United States,* [b]*Division of Geriatric Medicine & Gerontology, Department of Medicine, Johns Hopkins University School of Medicine, Baltimore, MD, United States*

Introduction

Osteoporosis and sarcopenia are two common age-related conditions well known to clinicians and researchers in geriatrics and gerontology. These two conditions often co-exist in an older and frail subset of the elderly population, giving rise to a new geriatric syndrome termed osteosarcopenia [1–5]. While osteoporosis and sarcopenia are common and important clinical syndromes individually, osteosarcopenia has been increasingly recognized for its prevalence and significance as frail individuals are the fastest-growing subset of the older adult population. Osteosarcopenia entails significantly higher risks of physical functional impairment as measured by reduced grip strength and sit-to-stand power as well as chair rising time [6], falls, fractures, institutionalization [7], and mortality [8] than osteoporosis or sarcopenia alone. These observations highlight the importance of advancing our understanding of the pathogenesis of this new geriatric syndrome and developing effective preventative and therapeutic interventions for it.

Muscle and bone are neighbors with close ties and crosstalk. They interact not only mechanically, but also through biological mediators and processes [9,10]. Muscle and bone as an integrated unit represent a large portion of body mass and play a critical role in mobility and metabolic health in humans. At the same time, systemic biological processes, including metabolic disturbances, hormonal dysregulations, chronic inflammation, and aging, have a major impact on muscle and bone homeostasis. When such homeostasis is perturbed over time, it leads to the development of osteopenia/osteoporosis, sarcopenia, or both, i.e., osteosarcopenia. The shared or overlapping pathophysiology between osteoporosis and sarcopenia may serve as the pathophysiological basis for osteosarcopenia and point to exciting possibilities for potential interventions. As mechanobiology and a number of systemic biological processes are discussed

Osteosarcopenia. https://doi.org/10.1016/B978-0-12-820088-9.00013-5

elsewhere in the book, this chapter focuses on chronic inflammation. It will first provide an overview of age-related chronic low-grade inflammatory phenotype (CLIP) or inflammaging, termed CLIP-inflammaging. It will then present current evidence supporting the role of CLIP-inflammaging in contributing to osteoporosis, sarcopenia, and osteosarcopenia in older adults and discuss potential interventional strategies.

Age-related CLIP-inflammaging: Conceptual evolution and etiologic factors

Traditionally, inflammation, either acute or chronic, is regarded as a protective response that kills, inactivates, or walls off the insulting agent, such as an infectious agent or traumatic injury. Like many other immune reactions, this physiological response is highly regulated with prompt initiation and timely resolution [11,12]. While too little or too late of this response would not provide effective protection, an uncontrolled or unresolved one would potentially lead to harm and pathologies.

CLIP, initially coined by Krabbe and colleagues [13], defines a low-grade, systemic, unresolved, and smoldering chronic inflammation clearly demonstrated by a two- to four-fold increase in circulating levels of inflammatory mediators such as interleukin-6 (IL-6) and C-reactive protein (CRP) in the absence of evident immediate triggers [14]. "Inflammaging," a term originally proposed by Claudio Franceschi [15], describes a chronic, systemic, low-grade inflammatory status that occurs during aging. Therefore, CLIP and inflammaging can be used interchangeably in the context of aging. As such, the two are combined that gives rise to the term CLIP-inflammaging. In addition to IL-6 and CRP, a large number of cellular (i.e., leukocytes and subpopulations, e.g., granulocytes and monocytes) and molecular inflammatory components are involved in CLIP-inflammaging or are produced as a result of inflammatory processes that lead to CLIP-inflammaging [14–16]. For example, a plethora of pro- and antiinflammatory mediators have been described in the literature, including: (1) cytokines and their soluble receptors or associated molecules, such as IL-1, IL-1 receptor antagonist (IL-1ra), IL-6, IL-13, IL-18, interferon (IFN)-α and IFN-γ, tumor necrosis factor (TNF)-α and its soluble receptors 1 (sTNFR-1) and 2 (sTNFR-2); (2) chemokines including CCL2, CCL3, CCL5, IL-8, and CXCL10; (3) adhesion molecules, such as vascular cell adhesion molecule (VCAM)-1, intercellular adhesion molecule (ICAM)-1, and E-selectin; and (4) acute-phase reactants, such as CRP, serum amyloid A, and fibrinogen. This is not an exhaustive list and it continues to grow rapidly.

Etiologic factors and mechanisms of CLIP-inflammaging are likely multifaceted and remain to be fully elucidated. As a result, the concept itself continues to evolve. For example, "garb-aging" is a term in which endogenous, inappropriately exposed and misplaced, or misfolded or otherwise altered molecules or substances (collectively labeled as waste materials or "garbage") were considered to be main sources or triggers of CLIP-inflammaging [17]. These materials originate from damaged and/or dead cells accumulated during aging and are recognized by receptors of the innate immune system, suggesting an auto-inflammatory process [17]. A related concept is "senescence-associated secretary phenotype" (SASP), suggesting that senescent cells can survive and accumulate in the circulation and tissues throughout the body during aging. While they no longer proliferate or perform much of their designated physiologic functions, they secret a wide range of pro-inflammatory mediators, thus contributing to CLIP-inflammaging [18,19]. Another concept is "metainflammation," which is literally translated as inflammation accompanying metabolic dysregulation, such as one associated with obesity, and suggests fat tissue as a major source of CLIP-inflammaging [20]. Despite differences in terminology, these concepts emphasize multiple sources known to contribute to elevated levels of inflammatory biomediators in CLIP-inflammaging. Other potentially important etiologic factors that have been proposed include persistent viral infections, such as chronic cytomegalovirus (CMV) and human immune deficiency virus (HIV) infections, and dysregulated microbiota and gut permeability or gut dysbiosis [14,21–25]. Finally, emerging evidence suggests defects in inflammation resolution, the final phase of any acute inflammatory response, as a potentially important mechanism for unresolved, persistent inflammation, leading to age-related development of CLIP-inflammaging [12,26]. Understanding the key players in this active and dynamically regulated process will provide a basis for the potential development of effective interventional strategies for the prevention and treatment of CLIP-inflammaging, which will be further discussed later in this chapter.

CLIP-inflammaging: Clinical significance and potential underlying mechanisms

A large body of literature supports the notion that CLIP-inflammaging is a major risk factor for almost all age-related pathophysiological processes and chronic diseases, such as atherosclerosis and cardiovascular diseases, neurodegeneration and Alzheimer's disease, insulin resistance and type 2 diabetes mellitus, tumorigenesis and cancer, as well as osteoporosis, sarcopenia, and frailty [15,16,27]. The unique features of the clinical implication include (1) these chronic conditions are almost all age-related; and (2) they are otherwise seemingly unrelated pathophysiological processes and chronic conditions. The clinical significance is immediately evident because these chronic diseases are highly prevalent, often coexisting, and frequently lead to disability and early mortality in older adults.

Despite CLIP-inflammaging being recognized for the contribution to the aforementioned age-related pathophysiological processes and chronic diseases, the underlying mechanisms are far from being elucidated and likely context-dependent. One example is frailty, a common and important geriatric syndrome characterized by depletion of physiologic reserve and multiorgan system dysregulation. Substantial evidence suggests that CLIP-inflammaging contributes to the development of frailty in older adults directly and/or indirectly through other intermediate pathophysiologic processes [28]. This is supported by a large number of studies documenting direct associations between frailty and CLIP-inflammaging as marked by increased counts of circulating white blood cells (WBC) and specific subpopulations (neutrophils, monocytes, $CD8^{+}CD28^{-}$ and $CCR5^{+}$ T lymphocytes) and elevated levels of molecular mediators of inflammation and immune activation (CRP, IL-6, TNF-α, neopterin, chemokine CXCL-10, etc.) [29–41]. Moreover, studies have shown that circulating IL-6 levels have inverse associations with hemoglobin concentration and serum insulin-like growth factor-1 (IGF-1) levels only in frail older adults rather than in nonfrail controls, and WBC counts were inversely associated with IGF-1 levels; low hemoglobin and IGF-1 levels were each independently associated with frailty, as well. These and other studies suggest that CLIP-inflammaging may impact frailty through other intermediate pathophysiologic processes [33,42–44]. In the context of cardiovascular diseases, atherosclerosis is regarded as a condition or pathophysiological process primarily caused by the accumulation of cholesterol-containing, oxidized LDL particles, seemingly unrelated to CLIP-inflammaging. However, oxidized LDL particles trigger an inflammatory response that can persist without timely resolution [45]. Immune activation and subsequent CLIP-inflammaging can actively contribute to the initiation and progression of atherosclerosis, from early or further endothelial damage and dysfunction, acute thrombotic complications triggered by plaque rupture, to arterial wall fibrosis, calcification, stiffness, and stenosis, leading to the development of acute and chronic cardiovascular diseases. Therefore, CLIP-inflammaging contributes to the initiation and/or acceleration of this vicious cascade of events in the pathogenesis of atherosclerosis and cardiovascular diseases [46].

The following sections provide a brief summary of current evidence supportive of the role of CLIP-inflammaging in contributing to osteoporosis, sarcopenia, and osteosarcopenia.

Osteoimmunology and role of CLIP-inflammaging in contributing to osteoporosis

Osteoimmunology, initially coined by Aaron and Choi in the year 2000 [47], is an emerging interdisciplinary research field on the interactions between the bone and immune systems. These two seemingly unrelated systems not only have extensive reciprocal interactions, but also appear to be integrated with shared signaling pathways and regulatory mechanisms [48]. A major focus of osteoimmunology is to investigate how the immune system impacts bone turnover in physiological and pathological conditions through the immunoskeletal interface [48]. Understanding this interface will provide novel insights and help establish a framework for developing innovative preventative and therapeutic strategies for diseases related to both bone and immune systems.

Osteoporosis is a common geriatric syndrome characterized by loss of bone mass and bone mineral density (BMD) and disruption of bone microarchitecture to the extent that the skeleton becomes fragile, exposing the individual to increased risk of fractures [49]. Osteoporosis is highly prevalent in postmenopausal women. As such, it was long considered simply as a result of postmenopausal estrogen decline. However, studies have shown that estrogen also has its receptor on immune cells, bone and bone marrow precursors, and that estrogen deficiency in postmenopausal women increases class II major histocompatibility complex human (MHCH) antigen expression on antigen-presenting cells (APCs) and inhibits T cell apoptosis, leading to T cell proliferation and activation. These effects result in the expansion of activated T cells, hyperproduction of pro-inflammatory cytokines, and chronic osteoclast stimulation, leading to bone loss and osteoporosis [50–52]. Therefore, while postmenopausal estrogen decline is an important etiologic factor for osteoporosis, this estrogen deficiency may trigger or accelerate age-related CLIP-inflammaging, which, in turn, likely serves as the main underlying mechanism for bone tissue alteration and loss of BMD in postmenopausal women [53,54].

Substantial and growing evidence in the field of osteoimmunology indicates extensive sharing of signal transduction pathways and regulatory mechanisms between the bone and immune systems, which not only demonstrates resounding crosstalk and tight regulation between the two systems, but also firmly establishes the role of CLIP-inflammaging in the pathogenesis of osteoporosis with therapeutic implications [55–58]. One key example is the receptor activator of nuclear factor-kB (RANK) and its ligand (RANKL). In the immune system, RANK/RANKL binding, through the adapter protein TNF-receptor-associated factor 6 (TRAF6), activates a number of key transcriptional factors, including nuclear factor 1 of activated T cells (NFATc1), activator proteins 1 (AP1), c-fos, and MAP kinases (MAPKs), the major hub of signaling pathways that govern immune activation and regulation [59,60]. Importantly, RANK/RANKL also activates nuclear factor-κB (NF-κB) signaling, the canonical pathway for activation of the inflammatory cascade, leading to the production of a large number of pro- and antiinflammatory cytokines [61], many of which are main cytokine mediators involved in bone remodeling (Table 1) [57,62,63]. In the bone tissue, osteoblasts, osteocytes, and osteoclasts of the basic multicellular unit continuously communicate with each other through RANK/RANKL. For example, osteoblasts produce RANKL and macrophage colony-stimulating factor (M-CSF). The binding of RANKL to its receptor RANK on osteoclasts and their precursors is the main activation signal for bone resorption. This RANK/RANKL activation signal is further enabled by the binding of M-CSF and its receptor c-fms on these cells. Osteoprotegerin (OPG) inhibits osteoclastogenesis by acting as a decoy receptor of RANKL, thus preventing bone resorption [56,57]. Therefore, RANK/RANKL is not only a crucial factor in immune

TABLE 1 Main cytokine mediators involved in bone remodeling.

Cytokine	Proresorptive effects	Antiresorptive effects
IL-1	• TRAF6 expression stimulation, NF-κB induction and MAPK activation • OC maturation induction • PGE2 and RANKL expression induction on OB • Enhancement of RANKL induced osteoclastogenesis • Amplification of RANKL secretion by stromal cells induced by TNF-α	
IL-4	• Induction of TNF-α expression on macrophages through IL-6 action • IL-1 increase	• Inhibition of RANKL and TNF-α induced osteoclastogenesis • Decrease of COX-2 activity and PG production • IL-1 signaling inhibition • c-Fos and NFATc1 expression inhibition via STAT6 • RANKL expression inhibition and OPG expression stimulation
IL-6	• Inhibition of SHP2/MEK2/ERK and SHP2/PI3K/Akt2 mediated OB differentiation • RANKL production by synovial and bone marrow stromal cells • Synergy with IL-1, TNF-α and PGE • Generalized inflammatory effects	• OPG increase
IL-7	• T and B cell activation • Promotion of RANKL and osteoclastogenic cytokine production by T cells • Synergy with IL-1, TNF-α and IFN-γ	• Osteoclastogenesis decrease directly acting on OC
IL-8	• RANKL increase	• NO increase
IL-10	• Induction of TNF-α expression (in synergy with IL-4)	• NO increase • Increase of OPG and decrease of RANKL expression • Inhibition of NFATC1, cFos and cJun downstream RANK signaling • Antiinflammatory Th1 cell differentiation • Inflammatory and osteoclastogenic cytokine inhibition

TABLE 1 Main cytokine mediators involved in bone remodeling—cont'd

Cytokine	Proresorptive effects	Antiresorptive effects
IL-11	• Increase of RANKL/OPG ratio	• Antagonism with IL-6
IL-12	• IL-1 and Th1 derived cytokine induction	• Decrease of T cell induced osteoclastogenesis • Direct inhibitory effect on osteoclasts • Synergy with IFN-γ and IL-18
IL-13	• OB inhibition • Mineralization blocking	• OC inhibition
IL-15	• OC differentiation • Synergy with TNF-α	
IL-17	• Induction of RANKL expression on OB, synovial cells and fibroblasts • Synthesis induction of bone matrix degrading enzymes (MMP) • Induction of TNF-α and IL6 production by inflammatory cells • Synergy with TNF-α, IL-1 and PGE	
IL-18		• Induction of OPG production from stromal cells • Induction of GM-CSF and IFN-γ production from T cells • RANKL signaling inhibition
IL-23	• OC activation in inflammatory pathologies • Th17 increase • IL-17 and RANKL induction	• OC inhibition in physiological condition • Fusion inhibition of OCP • Inhibition of OC survival • Decrease OC maturation via T cells • Synergy with IL-18 in inhibiting osteoclastogenesis
IL-31	• Stimulation of proinflammatory cytokine, chemokine and matrix metalloproteinase secretion (TNF-α, IL-1β, IL-8, MMP)	
IL-32	• Proinflammatory cytokine production stimulation • OCP differentiation induction	• OC maturation blocking

(Continued)

TABLE 1 Main cytokine mediators involved in bone remodeling—cont'd

Cytokine	Proresorptive effects	Antiresorptive effects
IL-33	• TNF-α expression induction • Bone resorption induction (in synergy with IL-6)	• Synergy with IL-4 • OCP and OC inhibition
TNF-α	• M-CSF and RANKL expression induction and inflammation • OC transcription factor (TRAF2, NF-κB) activation through TNF-R1 • OBP maturation inhibition, OB activity inhibition and OB apoptosis induction • Induction of negative regulators of the Wnt pathway expression • Inhibition of genes involved in bone formation (APH, 1,25-(OH)2 D3 receptor, PTH receptor)	
TGF-β	• Promotion of RANKL induced osteoclastogenesis	• Inhibition of T cell activation and bone resorption • Proinflammatory cytokine production down-modulation • Induction of OC apoptosis and OPG production by OB • OBP migration to sites of bone resorption and OBP differentiation
INF-γ	• MHCII antigen expression induction on APC • Antigen presentation enhancement and T cell activation • Osteoclastogenic cytokine production enhancement • Synergy with IL-12	• TRAF6 proteasomal degradation through specific OC receptors • Cathepsin K decrease • Decrease of 1,25-(OH)2 D3, PTH and IL-1 mediated osteoclastogenesis • Antagonism with TNF-α
SOFAT	• Direct promotion of osteoclastogenesis in a RANKL-independent manner • Induction of IL-6 production by OB	
M-CSF	• RANK expression upregulation on OCP • OCP pool expansion • OC formation (in synergy with RANKL) • Monocyte/macrophage lineage differentiation	

TABLE 1 Main cytokine mediators involved in bone remodeling—cont'd

Cytokine	Proresorptive effects	Antiresorptive effects
G-CSF	• OB apoptosis • MSC apoptosis	• RANKL signaling inhibition • Granulocyte differentiation
HMGB1	• RAGE-dependent RANKL-induced OC differentiation	

Abbreviations: *GM-CSF*, granulocyte-macrophage colony-stimulating factor; *M-CSF*, monocyte/macrophage colony-stimulating factor; *IFN*, interferon; *IL*, interleukin; *RANK*, receptor activator of nuclear factor-κB; *RANKL*, receptor activator of nuclear factor-κB ligand; *Th*, T-helper; *TNF*, tumor necrosis factor; *TGF*, transforming growth factor; *OC*, osteoclast; *OCP*, osteoclast precursor; *OB*, osteoblast; *OBP*, osteoblast precursor; *SOFAT*, secreted osteoclastogenic factor of activated T cells; *NFATc*, nuclear factor of activated T cells; *OPG*, osteoprotegerin; *NO*, nitric oxide; *TRAF*, TNF receptor associated factor; *STAT*, signal transducer and activator of transcription; *PTH*, parathyroid hormone; *PG*, prostaglandin; *MHCII*, major histocompatibility complex-class II; *APC*, antigen presenting cells; *1,25-(OH)2 D3*, dihydroxyvitamin D3; *APH*, alkaline phosphatase; *MMP*, matrix metalloproteinase; *NF-κB*, nuclear factor kappa-light-chain-enhancer of activated B cells; *TNF-R*, TNF-receptor; *MAPK*, mitogen-activated protein kinase; *ERK*, extracellular signal-regulated kinases; *PI3K*, phosphatidylinositol-3-kinase; *Wnt*, wingless pathway; *HMGB1*, high mobility group box 1.
Reproduced from Ginaldi L, De MM. Osteoimmunology and beyond. Curr Med Chem 2016;23(33):3754–3774 with permission.

regulation, but also the principle osteoclastogenic mediator [64,65]. The clinical and translational implication of this mechanistic understanding is the development of an anti-RANKL monoclonal antibody, denosumab, as an effective therapy for osteoporosis with confirmed antiresorption activity of the bone [66–68].

The so-called secondary osteoporosis observed in patients with rheumatoid arthritis (RA) provides additional evidence supporting the role of inflammation in the pathogenesis of osteoporosis outside of the context of aging. In this autoimmune and inflammatory disease, increased bone resorption is a major pathophysiologic process leading to juxta-articular bone erosions, irreversible joint damage, and systemic osteoporosis, including decreased BMD in the spine and hip as well as a higher prevalence of fractures [69]. Bisphosphonates, a class of potent inhibitors of osteoclast activity that are standard therapy for primary osteoporosis, are also effective for treating secondary osteoporosis in RA patients. Furthermore, monoclonal antibodies against various pro-inflammatory cytokines and their receptors, including those against TNF-α, are beneficial in preventing and reversing bone erosions and systemic osteoporosis in RA [70].

Of note, while most pro-inflammatory cytokines are osteoclastogenic mediators, there are cytokines that counteract bone resorption and exert osteoblastogenic properties, forming a complex bone remodeling cytokine network [56,57,63]. Moreover, many cytokine mediators are pleiotropic and can exert different and, at times, contrasting effects, both pro-resorptive and antiresorptive effects, as listed in Table 1. These pleiotropic effects largely depend on the specific context in which the cytokine mediators operate, the maturation stage of target cells, and the influence of other factors in the microenvironment, including cytokines. For example, in physiological bone remodeling, IFN-γ, a well-known pleiotropic cytokine, exerts antiosteoclastogenic effects by inducing TRAF6 proteasomal degradation with consequent inhibition of RANK/RNAKL signaling. However, in age-related, particularly postmenopausal osteoporosis, the overall effect of IFN-γ is skewed toward pro-osteoclastogenic/bone resorption through T-cell activation and RANKL expression. Studies have shown that IFN-γ is a powerful inducer of MHCH antigen expression on APCs, which, in turn, activates T cells along with specific antigen stimulation via T-cell receptors, inducing further immune activation and production of osteoclastogenic pro-inflammatory cytokines [57,71,72]. These findings further suggest the level of complexity of this cytokine network as well as a heightened level of caution necessary in searching for therapeutic targets and designing interventional studies.

Role of CLIP-inflammaging in contributing to sarcopenia

Sarcopenia, defined by the loss of muscle mass and strength [73,74], is the key component or contributing factor of the syndrome of frailty [28,75], functional disability, and early mortality in older adults [76–78]. An individual's baseline muscle mass and function and their age-related rate of decline are influenced by one's genetic background, i.e., the complex interplay of genetic and epigenetic factors [79,80]. Major detrimental factors also include lack of exercise and physical inactivity, malnutrition, age-associated decline in systemic hormones (e.g., IGF-1, testosterone, and estrogen), alteration in muscle growth regulators (e.g., myostatin, etc.), and neuromuscular junction dysfunction [81–83].

Epidemiological studies have shown strong associations between CLIP-inflammaging and sarcopenia. For example, circulating levels of IL-6 and TNF-α are significantly elevated in older adults with sarcopenia [84]. A large number of studies, including a meta-analysis, demonstrate a strong association of sarcopenia with increased circulating levels of various pro-inflammatory mediators, particularly CRP, IL-6, and soluble TNF-α receptors, compared to those in nonsarcopenic older individuals [85–88]. In addition, systemic inflammation is considered as one of the primary mediators of skeletal muscle wasting in many chronic inflammatory conditions, such as RA, acquired immune deficiency syndrome (AIDS), chronic obstructive pulmonary disease (COPD), Crohn's disease, and congestive heart failure [89–91]. Moreover, data from longitudinal studies suggest that these associations may be causal. For instance, elevated serum IL-6 levels predict the development of sarcopenia, and high levels of IL6 and CRP at baseline are associated with a two- to -threefold greater risk of losing more than 40% of grip strength over 3 years [92,93]. Furthermore, in a study that followed community-dwelling older women for 3.5 years, increased IL-6 levels were shown to predict a significant reduction of muscle strength and motor performance [76]. Taken together, these and other longitudinal studies suggest that CLIP-inflammaging contributes, at least in part, to the onset and/or progression of age-related sarcopenia [94,95].

At the physiological level, CLIP-inflammaging impacts systemic hormones, such as IGF-1 and testosterone, major influencing factors of sarcopenia, similar to the associations between inflammatory mediators and IGF-1 levels in the syndrome of frailty cited above [33,40]. At the molecular level, studies suggest that sarcopenia is associated with activation of catabolic pathways in the skeletal muscle governed mainly by three protein degradation systems, namely, the ubiquitin-proteasome system (UPS), the autophagy-lysosome system, and apoptosis. Activation of these protein degradation pathways leads to proteolysis, mitochondrial dysfunction, muscle fiber reorganization and denervation, and myofibril degeneration and myocyte death [96–98]. On the anabolic side, mechanistic targeting of the rapamycin (mTOR) pathway is the key regulator of protein synthesis in skeletal muscle. Its activation increases protein translation, primarily myofibrillar proteins, and promotes transport of branched-chain amino acids (BCAAs) into the muscle cells whose adequate intracellular level is critical for continuous protein synthesis/recycling and expression of sirtuin 1 (SIRT1) and genes that are important for energy production. Taken together, activation of the mTOR pathway and its downstream molecules is important for stimulating cell growth and mitochondrial biogenesis as well as preventing "wear and tear" protein damage from accumulating, all of which facilitate muscle injury repair, prevent muscle atrophy, and maintain muscle quality and function [97–100]. However, activation of the NOD-like receptor family pyrin domain containing 3 (NLRP3) inflammasome, typically triggered by cell debris and misfolded or damaged proteins, causes increased production of reactive oxygen species (ROS) and secretion of pro-inflammatory cytokines IL-1, IL18, and IL-33 [101,102], which in turn, can lead to not only activation of catabolic pathways, but also disturbed BCAA transport across cell membranes and impaired protein synthesis and mitochondrial biogenesis, resulting in muscle atrophy and dysfunction.

Perhaps the most direct evidence is from studies of animal models of acute inflammation. In rodents, inject of lipopolysaccharide (LPS), an endotoxin from Gram (−) bacteria, was shown to induce a systemic inflammatory response, increased expression of IL-6 and TNF-α mRNA in skeletal muscle, and activation of muscle catabolism through inflammatory signaling, resulting in loss of muscle mass and strength [103,104]. Exogenous administration of TNF-α was shown to cause myofiber atrophy and muscle loss via several aforementioned mechanisms, such as activation of the canonical master regulator of inflammation pathway NF-κB, activation of UPS catabolic pathway, as well as a reduction in intracellular concentration of BCAAs and suppression of mTOR pathway of protein synthesis in the muscle [105–110]. One interventional study in humans has demonstrated that blunting an acute infection-induced inflammation improved muscle performance in older adults [111]. While limited translation potential of these findings from acute inflammation models to the setting of CLIP-inflammaging is recognized, it is conceivable that chronic elevation of these inflammatory mediators will likely adversely impact muscle mass and quality, leading to the development and/or progression of sarcopenia.

Role of CLIP-inflammaging in contributing to osteosarcopenia

As osteosarcopenia is a syndrome that encompasses both osteoporosis and sarcopenia, it is likely that CLIP-inflammaging contributes similarly to the underlying mechanisms, at least partially. Since osteosarcopenia is a recently defined syndrome, data from studies of osteosarcopenia as an integrated entity rather than its components are still scarce but rapidly growing. For example, the very first study of osteosarcopenia identified significantly higher circulating levels of uric acid, a well-established mediator of inflammation and endothelial dysfunction [112], in participants with osteosarcopenia compared to those with either of the two components or none [7].

Investigation into muscle, bone, and adipose tissue crosstalk, a recent line of research, may also provide novel insights into the role of CLIP-inflammaging in contributing to osteosarcopenia [113]. Skeletal muscle, bone, and adipose tissue all produce cytokine mediators, namely, myokines, osteokines, and adipokines, respectively. These cytokine mediators exert autocrine/paracrine effects and establish a complex network that facilitates close interactions among the three seemingly unrelated organ/tissues. At the same time, many of these cytokine mediators have potent pro-inflammatory properties, exerting systemic effects as part of the CLIP-inflammaging. For instance, aging is associated with changes in body composition and increased adiposity. Adipocyte hypertrophy augments insulin resistance, perpetuating metabolic dysregulation. It recruits infiltrating immune cells, including macrophages that produce pro-inflammatory cytokines, further promoting CLIP-inflammaging [114,115]. In addition, adipokines such as leptin upregulate IL-6 and TNF-α, and together downregulate adiponectin, the adipokine with antiinflammatory property. This metabolic and inflammatory vicious cycle of obesity not only promotes fatty infiltrates in the muscle tissue and bone marrow, but also feeds the catabolism and results in aberrant crosstalk of the bone, muscle, and fat tissue, initiating or exacerbating osteosarcopenia in older adults [116,117].

Tumor necrosis factor (TNF)-related weak inducer of apoptosis (TWEAK) is a pro-inflammatory and immune regulatory mediator that is increasingly recognized for its role in contributing to osteosarcopenia. TWEAK is a TNF superfamily member that is primarily produced by circulating immune cells, including resting and activated monocytes, dendritic cells (DCs), NK cells, as well as T and B lymphocytes [118]. Its only known signaling receptor, fibroblast growth factor-inducible 14 (Fn14), is not expressed by these circulating immune cells, but mainly by epithelial cells, endothelial cells, and other cells in the periphery, including the skeletal muscle and bone. Fn14 is normally expressed at relatively low levels in healthy tissues, and TWEAK triggers its inducible expression. Therefore, the TWEAK/Fn14 pathway has been recognized as a critical "immune switch" that plays an important role in mediating the impact of inflammation and immune activation on the function and regulation of peripheral organ systems [119–121]. For example, the TWEAK/Fn14 pathway may serve as an important underlying mechanism mediating the contributing role of CLIP-inflammaging to cardiovascular diseases and their severity. This is supported by the data from a clinical study of patients who were hospitalized for cardiovascular diseases in which TWEAK levels that were measured within 24 h after hospital admission were significantly higher in those with ST-elevation myocardial infarction (STEMI) than in healthy controls or patients with stable cardiovascular diseases [122]. High TWEAK levels were also a predictor of adverse short-term outcome after STEMI [122]. Several groups have also shown that TWEAK/Fn-14 pathway activation stimulates the production of pro-inflammatory cytokines and chemokines, such as IL-6, IL-17, matrix metalloproteinase (MMP)-3 and MMP-9, and Regulated upon Activation, Normal T Cell Expressed and presumably Secreted (RANTES or CCL-5), triggering or perpetuating CLIP-inflammaging [121,123–125]. In animal studies, genetic deletion of the gene encoding Fn14 was shown to be protective against myocardial hypertrophy, fibrosis, and heart failure; deletion of the gene encoding TWEAK or treatment with a TWEAK blocking antibody in atherosclerosis-prone mice resulted in the reduction of atherosclerosis burden and lesion size in the aorta with enhanced plaque stability [126,127], providing direct evidence supportive of the mediating role of the TWEAK/Fn14 pathway in contributing to cardiovascular diseases. Interestingly, recent data demonstrate that influenza immunization significantly reduced circulating TWEAK levels in older adults, particularly those who are frail, suggesting a potential underlying molecular mechanism for the observed cardiovascular protective effect of influenza immunization [128,129]. While the TWEAK/Fn14 pathway may indirectly contribute to osteosarcopenia through the aforementioned cardiovascular pathologies with impaired blood supply, TWEAK has been shown to exert a direct detrimental impact on the skeletal muscle and bone. High TWEAK levels suppressed the self-renewal of progenitor cells and inhibited the differentiation of myoblasts. Upon injury and in disease conditions, TWEAK was observed to attenuate regeneration of damaged myofibers and promote fibrosis, leading to the impairment of skeletal muscle regeneration, differentiation, and repair, as well as its adequate structural and functional maintenance [130,131]. The TWEAK/Fn14 pathway has also been recognized for its role in contributing to dysregulated bone remodeling. TWEAK/Fn14 activation was shown to inhibit osteoblast differentiation and promote its apoptosis [132,133]. On the other hand, TWEAK/Fn14 was observed to induce RANKL expression, osteoclastogenesis, and poor bone mineralization, all of which lead to accelerated bone loss and destruction [134,135]. Blocking TWEAK/Fn14 signaling either by monoclonal antibody against TWEAK or Fn14 or by Fn14-Fc suppressed expression of RANKL and IL-17 as well as osteoclast differentiation, providing further supportive evidence [136,137]. Together, these studies suggest the important role of the TWEAK/Fn14 pathway in contributing to osteosarcopenia, both directly through its adverse impact on the skeletal muscle and bone and indirectly through its cardiovascular pathologies. The therapeutic implications are significant because not only biologicals specific to TWEAK and Fn14 for careful manipulation of the TWEAK/Fn14 signaling are available and appear to be safe in humans [138,139], but also TWEAK/Fn14 activities appear to be regulated by other immune interventions such as routine influenza vaccination [128]. Vaccines are known to have nonspecific immunomodulatory effects [140].

CLIP-inflammaging in osteosarcopenia: Consideration of preventative and therapeutic interventions

Exercise and high levels of physical activities are believed to be the best nonpharmacological intervention with a wide range of health benefits for cardiovascular function and endurance, cognitive function, as well as metabolism and musculoskeletal system, and thus exercise is recommended for the prevention and treatment of almost all chronic conditions in older adults including osteosarcopenia [81,141–143]. The importance of exercise and physical activity in maintaining musculoskeletal health and preventing osteosarcopenia in older adults is further emphasized by a 5-day bed rest study among well-characterized healthy young and old individuals, which demonstrates reduction of leg lean mass and strength along with increased markers of muscle proteolysis and osteoclastogenesis only in old participants [144].

Exercise is also known to exert major positive impacts on the immune system [145–147]. Substantial and growing evidence indicates that exercise imparts a potent antiinflammatory effect, which serves as an important mechanism underlying its preventative and therapeutic benefits for bone loss, sarcopenia, and osteosarcopenia [147–149]. However, it is worth mentioning that an acute bout of exercise is known to induce a substantial increase in the production and circulating levels of IL-6, a seemingly paradoxical pro-inflammatory response [147,148]. In this setting, IL-6, a pleiotropic cytokine mediator, is believed to reduce TNF-α production whose levels only increase locally within the skeletal muscle and remain undetectable or unchanged in the circulation [148]. IL-6 also stimulates M2-type macrophages, the type of resident macrophages that are antiinflammatory in nature and involved in muscle regeneration, to produce antiinflammatory mediators, such as IL-10 and IL-1ra (Fig. 1) [143,145,149]. Regular (chronic) exercises, both endurance (aerobic) and resistance training, are known to suppress CLIP-inflammaging. While exercise reduces fat mass and pro-inflammatory adipokines, there is a significant phenotypic shift of resident macrophages in this setting, from the pro-inflammatory M1 type to the antiinflammatory M2 type, creating an antiinflammatory microenvironment within the skeletal muscle (Fig. 1) [143,149,150]. Consequently, exercise appears to exert its preventative and therapeutic effects on osteosarcopenia and other chronic geriatric conditions, at least in part, through its induced suppression of CLIP-inflammaging.

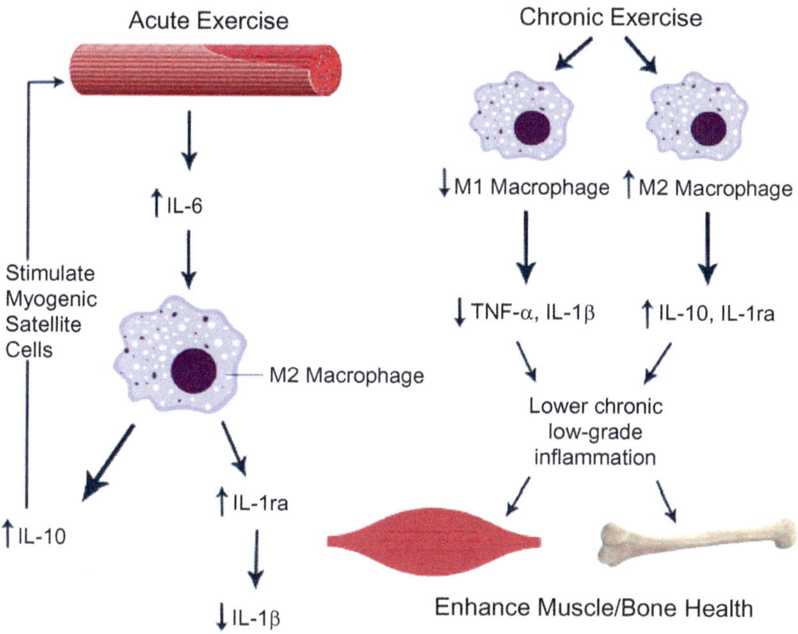

FIG. 1 Acute and chronic effects of exercise on mediators of CLIP or inflammating as underlying mechanisms for the prevention and treatment of osteosarcopenia. *(Reproduced from Cornish SM, Chilibeck PD, Candow DG. Potential importance of immune system response to exercise on aging muscle and bone. Curr Osteoporos Rep 2020;18(4):350–356 with permission.)*

Vitamin D supplementation has been widely recommended for the prevention and treatment of osteoporosis in older adults based on its established beneficial effects on calcium metabolism and bone homeostasis, and that vitamin D deficiency is highly prevalent in older adults [151]. Studies have also demonstrated that vitamin D is an immune modulator that can downregulate TNF-α production and inflammation through the NF-κB pathway [152,153]. These and other studies suggest vitamin D as a promising therapeutic modality for osteosarcopenia via its antiinflammatory effects. However, studies thus far have shown beneficial effects only on muscle strength, not muscle mass, and only in older adults with vitamin D deficiency [154–157]. Further research is needed.

Whether antiinflammatory agents have the potential as a treatment modality for osteosarcopenia is far less clear and is dependent on the specific individual agents. As discussed earlier, monoclonal antibodies against TNF-α and RANKL have a great potential to be applied for such purpose if further testing proves their clinical efficacy [66–68,70]. One of the biologics targeted to the TWEAK/Fn14 pathway appears to be safe in a human study, but its clinical efficacy has yet to be reported [139]. Glucocorticoids are some of the most potent antiinflammatory agents that have been recommended to treat severe acute inflammatory responses such as the 2019 coronavirus infectious disease (COVID-19)-associated acute respiratory distress syndrome (ARDS) and cytokine storm [157]. They also serve as the standard therapy for a number of chronic inflammatory and autoimmune diseases, such as RA, systemic lupus erythematosus, and inflammatory bowel disease in their severe form. However, glucocorticoids should not be used to treat osteosarcopenia as they cause systemic osteoporosis and muscle wasting through their potent catabolic and antianabolic effects [158]. In addition, TNF-α and other pro-inflammatory cytokine mediators can activate an enzyme 11βHSD1 to convert inactive cortisone to cortisol in the local tissue of the skeletal muscle and bone; cortisol as a local glucocorticoid further promotes detrimental effects of CLIP-inflammaging on the skeletal muscle and bone [159,160]. The utility of nonsteroidal antiinflammatory drugs (NSAIDs) as a therapeutic agent for osteosarcopenia is unclear at the present time. For example, a cross-sectional study in community-dwelling older adults over 80 years of age showed that the group with chronic use of NSAIDs had a significantly lower prevalence of sarcopenia than the nonuser group (9% vs 32%) [161]. In addition, recent data from the Physicians' Health Study showed a protective effect of long-term aspirin use against the geriatric syndrome of frailty, a distal surrogate of osteosarcopenia [162]. However, animal studies have shown that inhibition of cyclooxygenase (COX)-1 and -2 as well as the concomitant prostaglandin synthesis, which are the major mechanism for the antiinflammatory effects, resulted in decreased muscle fiber regeneration following injury and poor ex vivo muscle satellite cell proliferation, differentiation and fusion [163,164]. Such inhibition also led to decreased intramuscular macrophage accumulation, cell proliferation and subsequent compensatory hypertrophic response in a synergist muscle ablation model [165]. In addition, NSAIDs are known for their gastric, cardiovascular and hepato-renal adverse side effects [166], which are particularly a high risk for older adults. Therefore, considering long-term use of NSAIDs as a potential treatment modality for osteosarcopenia requires a heightened level of caution and further research.

Two emerging yet exciting lines of research deserve mentioning. The first one is the potential to target inflammation resolution. As discussed earlier in this chapter, resolution of any inflammatory response, either acute or chronic, is an active and highly regulated dynamic process [26]. It involves small lipid molecules that physiologically derived from the metabolism of dietary polyunsaturated fatty acids, giving rise to four families of specialized, pro-resolving mediators (SPMs), including lipoxins, resolvins, protectins, and maresins [167]. SPMs suppress neutrophil infiltration, promote neutrophil apoptosis by macrophages termed efferocytosis, and reduce excessive oxidative stress [167–169]. Giannakis and colleagues have recently shown that SPMs enhanced the functional activity of muscle infiltrating macrophages that could mediate postdamage skeletal muscle regeneration [170]. Interestingly, acute resistance exercise transiently stimulates skeletal muscle production of metabolites involved in the biosynthesis of SPMs [171], further suggesting the potential of SPMs as a novel group of therapeutic agents for sarcopenia. Whether SPMs are involved in bone health requires further investigation. The second one is the geroscience approach. Geroscience is a new area of translational research that targets aging itself and its underlying mechanisms [172,173]. Osteosarcopenia has been proposed as a case for potential geroscience intervention [4]. While this research is still in its infancy, N-3 polyunsaturated fatty acids (PUFAs) and metformin are among potential therapeutic agents that typically have antiinflammatory properties, target the mTOR pathway with significant regulation over metabolism, and exert beneficial effects on skeletal muscle and bone [174–179]. Stem cell senescence and exhaustion, as well as SASP-associated CLIP-inflammaging, are all overlapping features of both sarcopenia, osteoporosis, and thus of osteosarcopenia. As such, stem cell therapy and senolytic drugs can also be promising candidate therapeutic interventions for osteosarcopenia [180–182]. Further development in this nascent yet exciting field will require international collaborations among government entities, academic biomedical research centers and nonprofit organizations, as well as partnerships between public and private sectors [183].

Acknowledgment

This work was supported, in part, by grants from National Institutes of Health (NIH), United States (R01 AI108907, R42AG054322, U54 AG062333, and R21 AG059742), and funding from Irma and Paul Milstein Program for Senior Health, Milstein Medical Asian American Partnership (MMAAP) Foundation, United States (www.mmaapf.org) to SXL.

References

[1] Binkley N, Buehring B. Beyond FRAX: it's time to consider "sarco-osteopenia". J Clin Densitom 2009;12(4):413–6.

[2] Hassan EB, Duque G. Osteosarcopenia: a new geriatric syndrome. Aust Fam Physician 2017;46(11):849–53.

[3] Paintin J, Cooper C, Dennison E. Osteosarcopenia. Br J Hosp Med (Lond) 2018;79(5):253–8.

[4] Kirk B, Al SA, Duque G. Osteosarcopenia: a case of geroscience. Aging Med (Milton) 2019;2(3):147–56.

[5] Zanker J, Duque G. Osteosarcopenia: the path beyond controversy. Curr Osteoporos Rep 2020;18(2):81–4.

[6] Drey M, Sieber CC, Bertsch T, Bauer JM, Schmidmaier R. Osteosarcopenia is more than sarcopenia and osteopenia alone. Aging Clin Exp Res 2016;28(5):895–9.

[7] Huo YR, Suriyaarachchi P, Gomez F, Curcio CL, Boersma D, Muir SW, et al. Phenotype of osteosarcopenia in older individuals with a history of falling. J Am Med Dir Assoc 2015;16(4):290–5.

[8] Yoo JI, Kim H, Ha YC, Kwon HB, Koo KH. Osteosarcopenia in patients with hip fracture is related with high mortality. J Korean Med Sci 2018;33(4), e27.

[9] Girgis CM, Mokbel N, Digirolamo DJ. Therapies for musculoskeletal disease: can we treat two birds with one stone? Curr Osteoporos Rep 2014;12(2):142–53.

[10] Karsenty G, Mera P. Molecular bases of the crosstalk between bone and muscle. Bone 2018;115:43–9.

[11] Chovatiya R, Medzhitov R. Stress, inflammation, and defense of homeostasis. Mol Cell 2014;54(2):281–8.
[12] Lawrence T, Willoughby DA, Gilroy DW. Anti-inflammatory lipid mediators and insights into the resolution of inflammation. Nat Rev Immunol 2002;2(10):787–95.
[13] Krabbe KS, Pedersen M, Bruunsgaard H. Inflammatory mediators in the elderly. Exp Gerontol 2004;39(5):687–99.
[14] Chen Y, Liu S, Leng SX. Chronic low-grade inflammatory phenotype (CLIP) and senescent immune dysregulation. Clin Ther 2019;41(3):400–9.
[15] Franceschi C, Bonafe M, Valensin S, Olivieri F, De LM, Ottaviani E, et al. Inflamm-aging. An evolutionary perspective on immunosenescence. Ann N Y Acad Sci 2000;908:244–54.
[16] Ferrucci L, Fabbri E. Inflammageing: chronic inflammation in ageing, cardiovascular disease, and frailty. Nat Rev Cardiol 2018;15(9):505–22.
[17] Franceschi C, Garagnani P, Vitale G, Capri M, Salvioli S. Inflammaging and 'Garb-aging'. Trends Endocrinol Metab 2017;28(3):199–212.
[18] Borodkina AV, Deryabin PI, Giukova AA, Nikolsky NN. "Social life" of senescent cells: what is SASP and why study it? Acta Nat 2018;10(1):4–14.
[19] Campisi J, Kapahi P, Lithgow GJ, Melov S, Newman JC, Verdin E. From discoveries in ageing research to therapeutics for healthy ageing. Nature 2019;571(7764):183–92.
[20] Chen G, Yung R. Meta-inflammaging at the crossroad of geroscience. Aging Med (Milton) 2019;2(3):157–61.
[21] Leng SX, Margolick JB. Understanding frailty, aging, and inflammation in HIV infection. Curr HIV/AIDS Rep 2015;12(1):25–32.
[22] Li H, Weng P, Najarro K, Xue QL, Semba RD, Margolick JB, et al. Chronic CMV infection in older women: longitudinal comparisons of CMV DNA in peripheral monocytes, anti-CMV IgG titers, serum IL-6 levels, and CMV pp65 (NLV)-specific CD8(+) T-cell frequencies with twelve year follow-up. Exp Gerontol 2014;54:84–9.
[23] Margolick JB, Bream JH, Nilles TL, Li H, Langan SJ, Deng S, et al. Relationship between T-cell responses to CMV, markers of inflammation, and frailty in HIV-uninfected and HIV-infected men in the multicenter AIDS cohort study. J Infect Dis 2018;218(2):249–58.
[24] Rampelli S, Candela M, Turroni S, Biagi E, Collino S, Franceschi C, et al. Functional metagenomic profiling of intestinal microbiome in extreme ageing. Aging (Albany NY) 2013;5(12):902–12.
[25] Thevaranjan N, Puchta A, Schulz C, Naidoo A, Szamosi JC, Verschoor CP, et al. Age-associated microbial dysbiosis promotes intestinal permeability, systemic inflammation, and macrophage dysfunction. Cell Host Microbe 2017;21(4):455–66.
[26] Serhan CN, Chiang N, Dalli J. The resolution code of acute inflammation: novel pro-resolving lipid mediators in resolution. Semin Immunol 2015;27(3):200–15.
[27] Wang J, Leng SX. Inflammation and its role in ageing and disease. In: Michel JP, Beattie BL, Martin GE, Walston JD, editors. Oxford textbook of geriatric medicine. 3rd ed. Atlanta: Oxford University Press; 2018. p. 323–9.
[28] Chen X, Mao G, Leng SX. Frailty syndrome: an overview. Clin Interv Aging 2014;9:433–41.
[29] Qu T, Walston JD, Yang H, Fedarko NS, Xue QL, Beamer BA, et al. Upregulated ex vivo expression of stress-responsive inflammatory pathway genes by LPS-challenged CD14(+) monocytes in frail older adults. Mech Ageing Dev 2009;130(3):161–6.
[30] Semba RD, Margolick JB, Leng S, Walston J, Ricks MO, Fried LP. T cell subsets and mortality in older community-dwelling women. Exp Gerontol 2005;40(1–2):81–7.

[31] Collerton J, Martin-Ruiz C, Davies K, Hilkens CM, Isaacs J, Kolenda C, et al. Frailty and the role of inflammation, immunosenescence and cellular ageing in the very old: cross-sectional findings from the Newcastle 85+ study. Mech Ageing Dev 2012;133(6):456–66.
[32] Schmaltz HN, Fried LP, Xue QL, Walston J, Leng SX, Semba RD. Chronic cytomegalovirus infection and inflammation are associated with prevalent frailty in community-dwelling older women. J Am Geriatr Soc 2005;53(5):747–54.
[33] Leng S, Chaves P, Koenig K, Walston J. Serum interleukin-6 and hemoglobin as physiological correlates in the geriatric syndrome of frailty: a pilot study. J Am Geriatr Soc 2002;50(7):1268–71.
[34] Walston J, McBurnie MA, Newman A, Tracy R, Kop WJ, Hirsch CH, et al. Frailty and activation of the inflammation and coagulation systems with and without clinical morbidities: results from the cardiovascular health study. Arch Intern Med 2002;162:2333–41.
[35] Leng S, Yang H, Walston J. Decreased cell proliferation and altered cytokine production in frail older adults. Aging Clin Exp Res 2004;16:249–52.
[36] Hubbard RE, O'Mahony MS, Savva GM, Calver BL, Woodhouse KW. Inflammation and frailty measures in older people. J Cell Mol Med 2009;13(9B):3103–9.
[37] Leng SX, Tian X, Matteini A, Li H, Hughes J, Jain A, et al. IL-6-independent association of elevated serum neopterin levels with prevalent frailty in community-dwelling older adults. Age Ageing 2011;40(4):475–81.
[38] Leng SX, Xue QL, Tian J, Walston JD, Fried LP. Inflammation and frailty in older women. J Am Geriatr Soc 2007;55(6):864–71.
[39] De FU, Wang GC, Fedarko NS, Walston JD, Casolaro V, Leng SX. T-lymphocytes expressing CC chemokine receptor-5 are increased in frail older adults. J Am Geriatr Soc 2008;56(5):904–8.
[40] Leng S, Xue Q, Tian J. Association of neutrophil and monocyte counts with fraily in community-dwelling older women. Exp Gerontol 2009;44:511–6.
[41] Qu T, Yang H, Walston JD, Fedarko NS, Leng SX. Upregulated monocytic expression of CXC chemokine ligand 10 (CXCL-10) and its relationship with serum interleukin-6 levels in the syndrome of frailty. Cytokine 2009;46(3):319–24.
[42] Leng SX, Hung W, Cappola AR, Yu Q, Xue QL, Fried LP. White blood cell counts, insulin-like growth factor-1 levels, and frailty in community-dwelling older women. J Gerontol A Biol Sci Med Sci 2009;64(4):499–502.
[43] Leng SX, Cappola AR, Andersen RE, Blackman MR, Koenig K, Blair M, et al. Serum levels of insulin-like growth factor-I (IGF-I) and dehydroepiandrosterone sulfate (DHEA-S), and their relationships with serum interleukin-6, in the geriatric syndrome of frailty. Aging Clin Exp Res 2004;16(2):153–7.
[44] Chaves PH, Semba RD, Leng SX, Woodman RC, Ferrucci L, Guralnik JM, et al. Impact of anemia and cardiovascular disease on frailty status of community-dwelling older women: the Women's health and aging studies I and II. J Gerontol A Biol Sci Med Sci 2005;60(6):729–35.
[45] Libby P, Ridker PM, Hansson GK. Progress and challenges in translating the biology of atherosclerosis. Nature 2011;473(7347):317–25.
[46] Guarner V, Rubio-Ruiz ME. Low-grade systemic inflammation connects aging, metabolic syndrome and cardiovascular disease. Interdiscip Top Gerontol 2015;40:99–106.
[47] Arron JR, Choi Y. Bone versus immune system. Nature 2000;408(6812):535–6.
[48] Okamoto K, Takayanagi H. Osteoimmunology. Cold Spring Harb Perspect Med 2019;9:1.
[49] Geusens P, Lems WF. Osteoimmunology and osteoporosis. Arthritis Res Ther 2011;13(5):242.

[50] Mansoori MN, Tyagi AM, Shukla P, Srivastava K, Dev K, Chillara R, et al. Methoxyisoflavones formononetin and isoformononetin inhibit the differentiation of Th17 cells and B-cell lymphopoesis to promote osteogenesis in estrogen-deficient bone loss conditions. Menopause 2016;23(5):565–76.
[51] Li H, Lu Y, Qian J, Zheng Y, Zhang M, Bi E, et al. Human osteoclasts are inducible immunosuppressive cells in response to T cell-derived IFN-γ and CD40 ligand in vitro. J Bone Miner Res 2014;29(12):2666–75.
[52] Weitzmann MN. T-cells and B-cells in osteoporosis. Curr Opin Endocrinol Diabetes Obes 2014;21(6):461–7.
[53] Weitzmann MN, Pacifici R. T cells: unexpected players in the bone loss induced by estrogen deficiency and in basal bone homeostasis. Ann N Y Acad Sci 2007;1116:360–75.
[54] D'Amelio P. The immune system and postmenopausal osteoporosis. Immunol Investig 2013;42(7):544–54.
[55] Takayanagi H. Osteoimmunology: shared mechanisms and crosstalk between the immune and bone systems. Nat Rev Immunol 2007;7(4):292–304.
[56] De MM, Di Benedetto MC, Mengoli LP, Ginaldi L. Senile osteoporosis: is it an immune-mediated disease? Inflamm Res 2006;55(10):399–404.
[57] Khosla S. Pathogenesis of age-related bone loss in humans. J Gerontol A Biol Sci Med Sci 2013;68(10):1226–35.
[58] Zupan J, Jeras M, Marc J. Osteoimmunology and the influence of pro-inflammatory cytokines on osteoclasts. Biochem Med (Zagreb) 2013;23(1):43–63.
[59] Takayanagi H. Osteoimmunology in 2014: two-faced immunology-from osteogenesis to bone resorption. Nat Rev Rheumatol 2015;11(2):74–6.
[60] Sobacchi C, Menale C, Villa A. The RANKL-RANK axis: a bone to thymus round trip. Front Immunol 2019;10:629.
[61] Lawrence T. The nuclear factor NF-kappaB pathway in inflammation. Cold Spring Harb Perspect Biol 2009;1(6), a001651.
[62] Ginaldi L, De MM. Osteoimmunology and beyond. Curr Med Chem 2016;23(33):3754–74.
[63] Weitzmann MN. The role of inflammatory cytokines, the RANKL/OPG axis, and the immunoskeletal interface in physiological bone turnover and osteoporosis. Scientifica (Cairo) 2013;2013, 125705.
[64] Walsh MC, Choi Y. Biology of the RANKL-RANK-OPG system in immunity, bone, and beyond. Front Immunol 2014;5:511.
[65] Teitelbaum SL. Bone resorption by osteoclasts. Science 2000;289(5484):1504–8.
[66] Klontzas ME, Kenanidis EI, MacFarlane RJ, Michail T, Potoupnis ME, Heliotis M, et al. Investigational drugs for fracture healing: preclinical & clinical data. Expert Opin Investig Drugs 2016;25(5):585–96.
[67] Schwarz P, Jorgensen NR, Abrahamsen B. Status of drug development for the prevention and treatment of osteoporosis. Expert Opin Drug Discovery 2014;9(3):245–53.
[68] Chang B, Quan Q, Li Y, Qiu H, Peng J, Gu Y. Treatment of osteoporosis, with a focus on 2 monoclonal antibodies. Med Sci Monit 2018;24:8758–66.
[69] Jones D, Glimcher LH, Aliprantis AO. Osteoimmunology at the nexus of arthritis, osteoporosis, cancer, and infection. J Clin Invest 2011;121(7):2534–42.
[70] Brown JP, Roux C, Ho PR, Bolognese MA, Hall J, Bone HG, et al. Denosumab significantly increases bone mineral density and reduces bone turnover compared with monthly oral ibandronate and risedronate in postmenopausal women who remained at higher risk for fracture despite previous suboptimal treatment with an oral bisphosphonate. Osteoporos Int 2014;25(7):1953–61.

[71] Ginaldi L, De MM, Ciccarelli F, Saitta S, Imbesi S, Mannucci C, et al. Increased levels of interleukin 31 (IL-31) in osteoporosis. BMC Immunol 2015;16:60.
[72] Salem S, Gao C, Li A, Wang H, Nguyen-Yamamoto L, Goltzman D, et al. A novel role for interferon regulatory factor 1 (IRF1) in regulation of bone metabolism. J Cell Mol Med 2014;18(8):1588–98.
[73] Fuggle N, Shaw S, Dennison E, Cooper C. Sarcopenia. Best Pract Res Clin Rheumatol 2017;31(2):218–42.
[74] von Haehling S, Morley JE, Anker SD. An overview of sarcopenia: facts and numbers on prevalence and clinical impact. J Cachexia Sarcopenia Muscle 2010;1(2):129–33.
[75] Walston J, Buta B, Xue QL. Frailty screening and interventions: considerations for clinical practice. Clin Geriatr Med 2018;34(1):25–38.
[76] Ferrucci L, Penninx BW, Volpato S, Harris TB, Bandeen-Roche K, Balfour J, et al. Change in muscle strength explains accelerated decline of physical function in older women with high interleukin-6 serum levels. J Am Geriatr Soc 2002;50(12):1947–54.
[77] Murphy RA, Ip EH, Zhang Q, Boudreau RM, Cawthon PM, Newman AB, et al. Transition to sarcopenia and determinants of transitions in older adults: a population-based study. J Gerontol A Biol Sci Med Sci 2014;69(6):751–8.
[78] Filippin LI, Teixeira VN, da Silva MP, Miraglia F, da Silva FS. Sarcopenia: a predictor of mortality and the need for early diagnosis and intervention. Aging Clin Exp Res 2015;27(3):249–54.
[79] Livshits G, Gao F, Malkin I, Needhamsen M, Xia Y, Yuan W, et al. Contribution of heritability and epigenetic factors to skeletal muscle mass variation in United Kingdom twins. J Clin Endocrinol Metab 2016;101(6):2450–9.
[80] Shafiee G, Asgari Y, Soltani A, Larijani B, Heshmat R. Identification of candidate genes and proteins in aging skeletal muscle (sarcopenia) using gene expression and structural analysis. PeerJ 2018;6, e5239.
[81] Kaeberlein M, Rabinovitch PS, Martin GM. Healthy aging: the ultimate preventative medicine. Science 2015;350(6265):1191–3.
[82] Kalinkovich A, Livshits G. Sarcopenia—the search for emerging biomarkers. Ageing Res Rev 2015;22:58–71.
[83] Gonzalez-Freire M, de Cabo R, Studenski SA, Ferrucci L. The neuromuscular junction: aging at the crossroad between nerves and muscle. Front Aging Neurosci 2014;6:208.
[84] Bian AL, Hu HY, Rong YD, Wang J, Wang JX, Zhou XZ. A study on relationship between elderly sarcopenia and inflammatory factors IL-6 and TNF-α. Eur J Med Res 2017;22(1):25.
[85] Felicio DC, Pereira DS, Assumpção AM, Jesus-Moraleida FR, Queiroz BZ, Silva JP, et al. Inflammatory mediators, muscle and functional performance of community-dwelling elderly women. Arch Gerontol Geriatr 2014;59(3):549–53.
[86] Soysal P, Stubbs B, Lucato P, Luchini C, Solmi M, Peluso R, et al. Inflammation and frailty in the elderly: a systematic review and meta-analysis. Ageing Res Rev 2016;31:1–8.
[87] Lustosa LP, Batista PP, Pereira DS, Pereira LSM, Scianni A, Ribeiro-Samora GA. Comparison between parameters of muscle performance and inflammatory biomarkers of non-sarcopenic and sarcopenic elderly women. Clin Interv Aging 2017;12:1183–91.
[88] Schaap LA, Pluijm SM, Deeg DJ, Harris TB, Kritchevsky SB, Newman AB, et al. Higher inflammatory marker levels in older persons: associations with 5-year change in muscle mass and muscle strength. J Gerontol A Biol Sci Med Sci 2009;64(11):1183–9.
[89] Sakuma K, Aoi W, Yamaguchi A. Current understanding of sarcopenia: possible candidates modulating muscle mass. Pflugers Arch 2015;467(2):213–29.

[90] Biolo G, Cederholm T, Muscaritoli M. Muscle contractile and metabolic dysfunction is a common feature of sarcopenia of aging and chronic diseases: from sarcopenic obesity to cachexia. Clin Nutr 2014;33(5):737–48.

[91] Evans WJ. Skeletal muscle loss: cachexia, sarcopenia, and inactivity. Am J Clin Nutr 2010;91(4):1123S–7S.

[92] Payette H, Roubenoff R, Jacques PF, Dinarello CA, Wilson PW, Abad LW, et al. Insulin-like growth factor-1 and interleukin 6 predict sarcopenia in very old community-living men and women: the Framingham heart study. J Am Geriatr Soc 2003;51(9):1237–43.

[93] Schaap LA, Pluijm SM, Deeg DJ, Visser M. Inflammatory markers and loss of muscle mass (sarcopenia) and strength. Am J Med 2006;119(6):526.e9–526.e17.

[94] Beyer I, Mets T, Bautmans I. Chronic low-grade inflammation and age-related sarcopenia. Curr Opin Clin Nutr Metab Care 2012;15(1):12–22.

[95] Argiles JM, Busquets S, Stemmler B, Lopez-Soriano FJ. Cachexia and sarcopenia: mechanisms and potential targets for intervention. Curr Opin Pharmacol 2015;22:100–6.

[96] von Haehling S, Ebner N, Dos Santos MR, Springer J, Anker SD. Muscle wasting and cachexia in heart failure: mechanisms and therapies. Nat Rev Cardiol 2017;14(6):323–41.

[97] Gonzalez-Freire M, Adelnia F, Moaddel R, Ferrucci L. Searching for a mitochondrial root to the decline in muscle function with ageing. J Cachexia Sarcopenia Muscle 2018;9(3):435–40.

[98] Hood DA, Memme JM, Oliveira AN, Triolo M. Maintenance of skeletal muscle mitochondria in health, exercise, and aging. Annu Rev Physiol 2019;81:19–41.

[99] Foure A, Bendahan D. Is branched-chain amino acids supplementation an efficient nutritional strategy to alleviate skeletal muscle damage? A systematic review. Nutrients 2017;9(10):1047.

[100] Coen PM, Musci RV, Hinkley JM, Miller BF. Mitochondria as a target for mitigating sarcopenia. Front Physiol 2018;9:1883.

[101] Yu JW, Lee MS. Mitochondria and the NLRP3 inflammasome: physiological and pathological relevance. Arch Pharm Res 2016;39(11):1503–18.

[102] Kufer TA, Nigro G, Sansonetti PJ. Multifaceted functions of NOD-like receptor proteins in myeloid cells at the intersection of innate and adaptive immunity. Microbiol Spectr 2016;4(4):1–9.

[103] Schakman O, Dehoux M, Bouchuari S, Delaere S, Lause P, Decroly N, et al. Role of IGF-I and the TNFa/NF-lB pathway in the induction of muscle atrogenes by acute inflammation. Am J Physiol Endocrinol Metab 2012;303(6):E729–39.

[104] Crossland H, Constantin-Teodosiu D, Gardiner SM, Constantin D, Greenhaff PL. A potential role for Akt/FOXO signalling in both protein loss and the impairment of muscle carbohydrate oxidation during sepsis in rodent skeletal muscle. J Physiol 2008;586(22):5589–600.

[105] Thoma A, Lightfoot AP. NF-kB and inflammatory cytokine signalling: role in skeletal muscle atrophy. Adv Exp Med Biol 2018;1088:267–79.

[106] Li YP, Reid MB. NF-kappaB mediates the protein loss induced by TNF-alpha in differentiated skeletal muscle myotubes. Am J Phys Regul Integr Comp Phys 2000;279(4):R1165–70.

[107] Ladner KJ, Caligiuri MA, Guttridge DC. Tumor necrosis factor-regulated biphasic activation of NF-kappa B is required for cytokine-induced loss of skeletal muscle gene products. J Biol Chem 2003;278(4):2294–303.

[108] Cai D, Frantz JD, Tawa Jr NE, Melendez PA, Oh BC, Lidov HG, et al. IKKbeta/NF-kappaB activation causes severe muscle wasting in mice. Cell 2004;119(2):285–98.

[109] Sarraf P, Frederich RC, Turner EM, Ma G, Jaskowiak NT, Rivet III DJ, et al. Multiple cytokines and acute inflammation raise mouse leptin levels: potential role in inflammatory anorexia. J Exp Med 1997;185(1):171–5.

[110] Pijet B, Pijet M, Litwiniuk A, Gajewska M, Pająk B, Orzechowski A. TNF-α and IFN-s-dependent muscle decay is linked to NF-κB- and STAT-1α-stimulated Atrogin1 and MuRF1 genes in C2C12 myotubes. Mediat Inflamm 2013;2013, 171437.
[111] Beyer I, Bautmans I, Njemini R, Demanet C, Bergmann P, Mets T. Effects on muscle performance of NSAID treatment with piroxicam versus placebo in geriatric patients with acute infection-induced inflammation. A double blind randomized controlled trial. BMC Musculoskelet Disord 2011;12:292.
[112] Kanellis J, Kang DH. Uric acid as a mediator of endothelial dysfunction, inflammation, and vascular disease. Semin Nephrol 2005;25(1):39–42.
[113] Kirk B, Feehan J, Lombardi G, Duque G. Muscle, bone, and fat crosstalk: the biological role of myokines, osteokines, and adipokines. Curr Osteoporos Rep 2020;18(4):388–400.
[114] Olefsky JM, Glass CK. Macrophages, inflammation, and insulin resistance. Annu Rev Physiol 2010;72:219–46.
[115] Mraz M, Haluzik M. The role of adipose tissue immune cells in obesity and low-grade inflammation. J Endocrinol 2014;222(3):R113–27.
[116] Hirschfeld HP, Kinsella R, Duque G. Osteosarcopenia: where bone, muscle, and fat collide. Osteoporos Int 2017;28(10):2781–90.
[117] Ormsbee MJ, Prado CM, Ilich JZ, Purcell S, Siervo M, Folsom A, et al. Osteosarcopenic obesity: the role of bone, muscle, and fat on health. J Cachexia Sarcopenia Muscle 2014;5(3):183–92.
[118] Chicheportiche Y, Bourdon PR, Xu H, Hsu YM, Scott H, Hession C, et al. TWEAK, a new secreted ligand in the tumor necrosis factor family that weakly induces apoptosis. J Biol Chem 1997;272(51):32401–10.
[119] Wiley SR, Cassiano L, Lofton T, Davis-Smith T, Winkles JA, Lindner V, et al. A novel TNF receptor family member binds TWEAK and is implicated in angiogenesis. Immunity 2001;15(5):837–46.
[120] Winkles JA. The TWEAK-Fn14 cytokine-receptor axis: discovery, biology and therapeutic targeting. Nat Rev Drug Discov 2008;7(5):411–25.
[121] Kim SH, Kang YJ, Kim WJ, Woo DK, Lee Y, Kim DI, et al. TWEAK can induce pro-inflammatory cytokines and matrix metalloproteinase-9 in macrophages. Circ J 2004;68(4):396–9.
[122] Chorianopoulos E, Jarr K, Steen H, Giannitsis E, Frey N, Katus HA. Soluble TWEAK is markedly upregulated in patients with ST-elevation myocardial infarction and related to an adverse short-term outcome. Atherosclerosis 2010;211(1):322–6.
[123] Ando T, Ichikawa J, Wako M, Hatsushika K, Watanabe Y, Sakuma M, et al. TWEAK/Fn14 interaction regulates RANTES production, BMP-2-induced differentiation, and RANKL expression in mouse osteoblastic MC3T3-E1 cells. Arthritis Res Ther 2006;8(5):R146.
[124] Park JS, Park MK, Lee SY, Oh HJ, Lim MA, Cho WT, et al. TWEAK promotes the production of Interleukin-17 in rheumatoid arthritis. Cytokine 2012;60(1):143–9.
[125] Dharmapatni AA, Smith MD, Crotti TN, Holding CA, Vincent C, Weedon HM, et al. TWEAK and Fn14 expression in the pathogenesis of joint inflammation and bone erosion in rheumatoid arthritis. Arthritis Res Ther 2011;13(2):R51.
[126] Novoyatleva T, Janssen W, Wietelmann A, Schermuly RT, Engel FB. TWEAK/Fn14 axis is a positive regulator of cardiac hypertrophy. Cytokine 2013;64(1):43–5.
[127] Sastre C, Fernandez-Laso V, Madrigal-Matute J, Munoz-Garcia B, Moreno JA, Pastor-Vargas C, et al. Genetic deletion or TWEAK blocking antibody administration reduce atherosclerosis and enhance plaque stability in mice. J Cell Mol Med 2014;18(4):721–34.
[128] Keshtkar-Jahromi M, Ouyang M, Keshtkarjahromi M, Almed S, Li H, Walston JD, et al. Effect of influenza vaccine on tumor necrosis factor-like weak inducer of apoptosis (TWEAK) in older adults. Vaccine 2018;36(16):2220–5.

[129] Cheng Y, Cao X, Cao Z, Xu C, Sun L, Gao Y, et al. Effects of influenza vaccination on the risk of cardiovascular and respiratory diseases and all-cause mortality. Ageing Res Rev 2020;62, 101124.

[130] Tajrishi MM, Zheng TS, Burkly LC, Kumar A. The TWEAK-Fn14 pathway: a potent regulator of skeletal muscle biology in health and disease. Cytokine Growth Factor Rev 2014;25(2):215–25.

[131] Sato S, Ogura Y, Kumar A. TWEAK/Fn14 signaling axis mediates skeletal muscle atrophy and metabolic dysfunction. Front Immunol 2014;5:18.

[132] Matsui H, Fukuno N, Kanda Y, Kantoh Y, Chida T, Nagaura Y, et al. The expression of Fn14 via mechanical stress-activated JNK contributes to apoptosis induction in osteoblasts. J Biol Chem 2014;289(10):6438–50.

[133] Vincent C, Findlay DM, Welldon KJ, Wijenayaka AR, Zheng TS, Haynes DR, et al. Pro-inflammatory cytokines TNF-related weak inducer of apoptosis (TWEAK) and TNFalpha induce the mitogen-activated protein kinase (MAPK)-dependent expression of sclerostin in human osteoblasts. J Bone Miner Res 2009;24(8):1434–49.

[134] Park JS, Kwok SK, Lim MA, Oh HJ, Kim EK, Jhun JY, et al. TWEAK promotes osteoclastogenesis in rheumatoid arthritis. Am J Pathol 2013;183(3):857–67.

[135] Findlay DM, Atkins GJ. TWEAK and TNF regulation of sclerostin: a novel pathway for the regulation of bone remodelling. Adv Exp Med Biol 2011;691:337–48.

[136] Salzmann S, Seher A, Trebing J, Weisenberger D, Rosenthal A, Siegmund D, et al. Fibroblast growth factor inducible (Fn14)-specific antibodies concomitantly display signaling pathway-specific agonistic and antagonistic activity. J Biol Chem 2013;288(19):13455–66.

[137] Yepes M, Winkles JA. Inhibition of TWEAK activity as a new treatment for inflammatory and degenerative diseases. Drug News Perspect 2006;19(10):589–95.

[138] Pascoe AL, Johnston AJ, Murphy RM. Controversies in TWEAK-Fn14 signaling in skeletal muscle atrophy and regeneration. Cell Mol Life Sci 2020;77(17):3369–81.

[139] Wisniacki N, Amaravadi L, Galluppi GR, Zheng TS, Zhang R, Kong J, et al. Safety, tolerability, pharmacokinetics, and pharmacodynamics of anti-TWEAK monoclonal antibody in patients with rheumatoid arthritis. Clin Ther 2013;35(8):1137–49.

[140] de Bree LCJ, Koeken VACM, Joosten LAB, Aaby P, Benn CS, van Crevel R, et al. Non-specific effects of vaccines: current evidence and potential implications. Semin Immunol 2018;39:35–43.

[141] Galloza J, Castillo B, Micheo W. Benefits of exercise in the older population. Phys Med Rehabil Clin N Am 2017;28(4):659–69.

[142] Konopka AR, Harber MP. Skeletal muscle hypertrophy after aerobic exercise training. Exerc Sport Sci Rev 2014;42(2):53–61.

[143] Cornish SM, Chilibeck PD, Candow DG. Potential importance of immune system response to exercise on aging muscle and bone. Curr Osteoporos Rep 2020;18(4):350–6.

[144] Tanner RE, Brunker LB, Agergaard J, Barrows KM, Briggs RA, Kwon OS, et al. Age-related differences in lean mass, protein synthesis and skeletal muscle markers of proteolysis after bed rest and exercise rehabilitation. J Physiol 2015;593(18):4259–73.

[145] Walsh NP, Gleeson M, Shephard RJ, Gleeson M, Woods JA, Bishop NC, et al. Position statement. Part one: immune function and exercise. Exerc Immunol Rev 2011;17:6–63.

[146] Walsh NP, Gleeson M, Pyne DB, Nieman DC, Dhabhar FS, Shephard RJ, et al. Position statement. Part two: maintaining immune health. Exerc Immunol Rev 2011;17:64–103.

[147] Sellami M, Gasmi M, Denham J, Hayes LD, Stratton D, Padulo J, et al. Effects of acute and chronic exercise on immunological parameters in the elderly aged: can physical activity counteract the effects of aging? Front Immunol 2018;9:2187.

[148] Peake JM, Della GP, Suzuki K, Nieman DC. Cytokine expression and secretion by skeletal muscle cells: regulatory mechanisms and exercise effects. Exerc Immunol Rev 2015;21:8–25.

[149] Gleeson M, Bishop NC, Stensel DJ, Lindley MR, Mastana SS, Nimmo MA. The anti-inflammatory effects of exercise: mechanisms and implications for the prevention and treatment of disease. Nat Rev Immunol 2011;11(9):607–15.

[150] Tidball JG. Regulation of muscle growth and regeneration by the immune system. Nat Rev Immunol 2017;17(3):165–78.

[151] Forrest KY, Stuhldreher WL. Prevalence and correlates of vitamin D deficiency in US adults. Nutr Res 2011;31(1):48–54.

[152] Cohen-Lahav M, Shany S, Tobvin D, Chaimovitz C, Douvdevani A. Vitamin D decreases NFkappaB activity by increasing IkappaBalpha levels. Nephrol Dial Transplant 2006;21(4):889–97.

[153] Calton EK, Keane KN, Newsholme P, Soares MJ. The impact of vitamin D levels on inflammatory status: a systematic review of immune cell studies. PLoS One 2015;10(11), e0141770.

[154] Stockton KA, Mengersen K, Paratz JD, Kandiah D, Bennell KL. Effect of vitamin D supplementation on muscle strength: a systematic review and meta-analysis. Osteoporos Int 2011;22(3):859–71.

[155] Muir SW, Montero-Odasso M. Effect of vitamin D supplementation on muscle strength, gait and balance in older adults: a systematic review and meta-analysis. J Am Geriatr Soc 2011;59(12):2291–300.

[156] Beaudart C, Buckinx F, Rabenda V, Gillain S, Cavalier E, Slomian J, et al. The effects of vitamin D on skeletal muscle strength, muscle mass, and muscle power: a systematic review and meta-analysis of randomized controlled trials. J Clin Endocrinol Metab 2014;99(11):4336–45.

[157] Gkekas NK, Anagnostis P, Paraschou V, Stamiris D, Dellis S, Kenanidis E, et al. The effect of vitamin D plus protein supplementation on sarcopenia: a systematic review and meta-analysis of randomized controlled trials. Maturitas 2021;145:56–63.

[158] Ye Z, Wang Y, Colunga-Lozano LE, Prasad M, Tangamornsuksan W, Rochwerg B, et al. Efficacy and safety of corticosteroids in COVID-19 based on evidence for COVID-19, other coronavirus infections, influenza, community-acquired pneumonia and acute respiratory distress syndrome: a systematic review and meta-analysis. CMAJ 2020;192(27):E756–67.

[159] Webster JM, Fenton CG, Langen R, Hardy RS. Exploring the interface between inflammatory and therapeutic glucocorticoid induced bone and muscle loss. Int J Mol Sci 2019;20(22):5768.

[160] Tomlinson JW, Walker EA, Bujalska IJ, Draper N, Lavery GG, Cooper MS, et al. 11beta-hydroxysteroid dehydrogenase type 1: a tissue-specific regulator of glucocorticoid response. Endocr Rev 2004;25(5):831–66.

[161] Morgan SA, Sherlock M, Gathercole LL, Lavery GG, Lenaghan C, Bujalska IJ, et al. 11beta-hydroxysteroid dehydrogenase type 1 regulates glucocorticoid-induced insulin resistance in skeletal muscle. Diabetes 2009;58(11):2506–15.

[162] Landi F, Marzetti E, Liperoti R, Pahor M, Russo A, Martone AM, et al. Nonsteroidal anti-inflammatory drug (NSAID) use and sarcopenia in older people: results from the ilSIRENTE study. J Am Med Dir Assoc 2013;14(8):626.e9.

[163] Orkaby AR, Yang L, Dufour AB, Travison TG, Sesso HD, Driver JA, et al. Association between long-term aspirin use and frailty in men: the physicians health study. J Gerontol A Biol Sci Med Sci 2021;76(6):1077–83.

[164] Bondesen BA, Mills ST, Kegley KM, Pavlath GK. The COX-2 pathway is essential during early stages of skeletal muscle regeneration. Am J Phys Cell Phys 2004;287(2):C475–83.

[165] Mendias CL, Tatsumi R, Allen RE. Role of cyclooxygenase-1 and -2 in satellite cell proliferation, differentiation, and fusion. Muscle Nerve 2004;30(4):497–500.

[166] Novak ML, Billich W, Smith SM, Sukhija KB, McLoughlin TJ, Hornberger TA, et al. COX-2 inhibitor reduces skeletal muscle hypertrophy in mice. Am J Phys Regul Integr Comp Phys 2009;296(4):R1132–9.

[167] Greig CA, Atherton PJ, Rennie MJ. Can an NSAID a day keep muscle wasting away? J Physiol 2009;587(Pt 24):5799–800.

[168] Serhan CN. Treating inflammation and infection in the 21st century: new hints from decoding resolution mediators and mechanisms. FASEB J 2017;31(4):1273–88.

[169] Bennett M, Gilroy DW. Lipid mediators in inflammation. In: Myeloid cells in health and disease: a synthesis. Wiley; 2017. p. 343–66.

[170] Chiang N, Serhan CN. Structural elucidation and physiologic functions of specialized pro-resolving mediators and their receptors. Mol Asp Med 2017;58:114–29.

[171] Giannakis N, Sansbury BE, Patsalos A, Hays TT, Riley CO, Han X, et al. Dynamic changes to lipid mediators support transitions among macrophage subtypes during muscle regeneration. Nat Immunol 2019;20(5):626–36.

[172] Vella L, Markworth JF, Farnfield MM, Maddipati KR, Russell AP, Cameron-Smith D. Intramuscular inflammatory and resolving lipid profile responses to an acute bout of resistance exercise in men. Physiol Rep 2019;7(13), e14108.

[173] Kennedy BK, Berger SL, Brunet A, Campisi J, Cuervo AM, Epel ES, et al. Geroscience: linking aging to chronic disease. Cell 2014;159(4):709–13.

[174] Sierra F, Kohanski R. Geroscience and the trans-NIH geroscience interest group. Geroscience 2017;39(1):1–5.

[175] Gingras AA, White PJ, Chouinard PY, Julien P, Davis TA, Dombrowski L, et al. Long-chain omega-3 fatty acids regulate bovine whole-body protein metabolism by promoting muscle insulin signalling to the Akt-mTOR-S6K1 pathway and insulin sensitivity. J Physiol 2007;579(Pt 1):269–84.

[176] Barzilai N, Crandall JP, Kritchevsky SB, Espeland MA. Metformin as a tool to target aging. Cell Metab 2016;23(6):1060–5.

[177] Williams JA, Pontzer CH, Shacter E. Regulation of macrophage interleukin-6 (IL-6) and IL-10 expression by prostaglandin E2: the role of p38 mitogen-activated protein kinase. J Interf Cytokine Res 2000;20(3):291–8.

[178] Smith GI, Julliand S, Reeds DN, Sinacore DR, Klein S, Mittendorfer B. Fish oil-derived n-3 PUFA therapy increases muscle mass and function in healthy older adults. Am J Clin Nutr 2015;102(1):115–22.

[179] Smith GI. The effects of dietary omega-3s on muscle composition and quality in older adults. Curr Nutr Rep 2016;5(2):99–105.

[180] Kulkarni AS, Gubbi S, Barzilai N. Benefits of metformin in attenuating the hallmarks of aging. Cell Metab 2020;32(1):15–30.

[181] Chhetri JK, de Souto BP, Fougere B, Rolland Y, Vellas B, Cesari M. Chronic inflammation and sarcopenia: a regenerative cell therapy perspective. Exp Gerontol 2018;103:115–23.

[182] Kirkland JL, Tchkonia T. Senolytic drugs: from discovery to translation. J Intern Med 2020;288:518–36.

[183] Leng SX, Kennedy BK. International investment in geroscience. Public Policy Aging Rep 2019;29(4):134–8.

Chapter 7

Sex steroids and gender differences in muscle, bone, and fat

Rahul D. Barmanray[a,b] and Christopher J. Yates[a,b]
[a]*Department of Medicine, The University of Melbourne, Parkville, VIC, Australia,* [b]*Department of Diabetes & Endocrinology, The Royal Melbourne Hospital, Parkville, VIC, Australia*

Introduction

Sex steroids are fundamentally important to human sexual differentiation and maturation. Given the anatomical differences evident between the human male and female phenotype, it is thus no surprise that sex steroids have wide-ranging effects upon the body's structural tissues, including bone, muscle, and fat.

This chapter will consider postpubertal sex steroid production, peripheral effects, and changes across the life course, with a focus on how these changes affect structural tissues. The role of sex steroids in sexual maturation and prepubertal growth is beyond the scope of this text.

Sex steroid biology

The vast majority of sex steroids are produced in two main locations: the zona reticularis of the adrenal glands and the gonads; the testes in the male and ovaries in the female. The contribution of each of these varies over the life course. Sex steroids can be broadly categorized into three groups. The androgens are typically considered "male sex steroids," while the estrogens and progestogens are considered "female sex steroids." While the adrenal gland produces primarily androgens and a small quantity of progestogens, the gonads produce hormones from all three categories.

Adrenal sex steroid production

In both males and females the adrenal glands predominantly produce the androgen dehydroepiandrosterone-sulfate (DHEAS). As with many endocrine hormones, its production is under negative feedback control by a tripartite loop

Osteosarcopenia. https://doi.org/10.1016/B978-0-12-820088-9.00006-8

known as the hypothalamic-pituitary-adrenal axis. The relevant hormones and tissues in this pathway are as follows:

- Hypothalamic paraventricular nucleus—Corticotropin-releasing hormone (CRH)
- Anterior pituitary corticotrope cells—Adrenocorticotropic hormone (ACTH)
- Adrenal cortex zona reticularis—Dehydroepiandrosterone-sulfate (DHEAS)

CRH stimulates ACTH, which, in turn, stimulates the adrenal cortex to produce both DHEAS and cortisol, a glucocorticoid. While DHEAS exerts no negative feedback on CRH or ACTH, this feedback is exerted by cortisol, thus completing a feedback loop that regulates DHEAS concentrations.

In addition to DHEAS, smaller concentrations of other weak androgens such as androstenedione and progestogens are also produced by the adrenal gland. Their production is similarly under the control of ACTH and ultimately CRH (Fig. 1).

Changes across the lifespan

Adrenal androgen production does not commence until the period of development known as adrenarche, which usually occurs between 6 and 10 years of age. Adrenal androgen production increases during puberty to reach a peak during young adulthood. Levels then reduce due to a process is known as adrenopause, which commences between 30 and 40 years of age. This continues until approximately the age of 70 when DHEAS levels are 5%–10% of the young adult peak [1].

Gonadal sex steroid production

In males, the predominant sex steroid-producing organs are the testes, while in females this role is fulfilled by the ovaries. As is the case in the adrenal cortex, gonadal sex steroid production is under negative feedback control. This feedback loop is known as the hypothalamic-pituitary-gonadal axis. While the upper two elements of this loop are conserved between the sexes, the gonadal elements differ. The relevant hormones and tissues in this pathway are as follows:

- Hypothalamic median eminence—Gonadotropin-releasing hormone (GnRH)
- Anterior pituitary gonadotroph cells—Luteinizing hormone (LH) and follicle-stimulating hormone (FSH)

<u>Males</u>

- Testicular Leydig cells—Testosterone

<u>Females</u>

- Ovarian theca cells—Progesterone and testosterone
- Ovarian granulosa cells—Estradiol

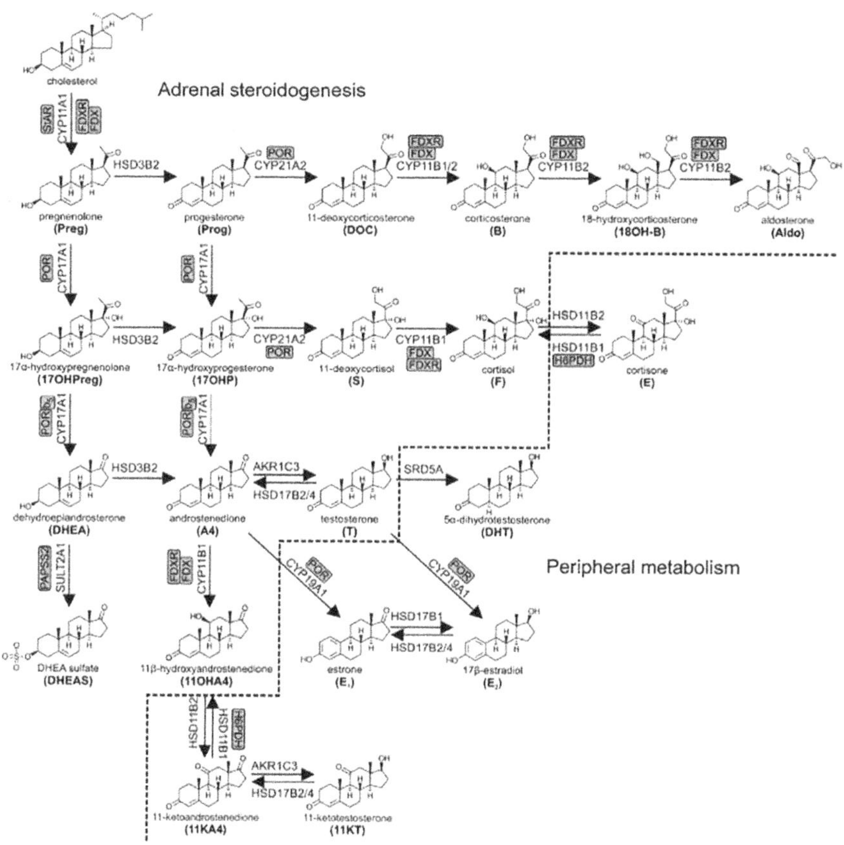

FIG. 1 Steroidogenesis occurs in the adrenal glands *(upper left)* and the peripheries *(bottom right)*. *(Credit: Schiffer L, Barnard L, Baranowski ES, et al. Human steroid biosynthesis, metabolism, and excretion are differentially reflected by serum and urine steroid metabolomes: a comprehensive review. J Steroid Biochem Mol Biol 2019;194:105439. https://doi.org/10.1016/j.jsbmb.2019.105439. Source: https://www.ncbi.nlm.nih.gov/pmc/articles/PMC6857441/.)*

GnRH stimulates LH and FSH. LH stimulates the male testicular Leydig cells and female ovarian theca cells to produce testosterone in both and additionally progesterone in the case of theca cells. FSH stimulates the female ovarian granulosa cells to produce estradiol. In general, gonadal sex steroids exert negative feedback upon GnRH, LH, and FSH. However, the cyclical nature of the feedback loop in females who are menstruating is significantly more complex and such a discussion is beyond the scope of this text.

While testosterone is the major gonadal sex steroid produced in males, estradiol is also found in the male circulation and tissues. Only 20% of circulating estradiol is synthesized directly in the testes. The rest is produced by aromatization of androgens (predominantly testosterone but with some contribution from DHEAS) in bone, adipose, skin, brain, and other tissues, from where it is released back into the circulation [2] (Fig. 2).

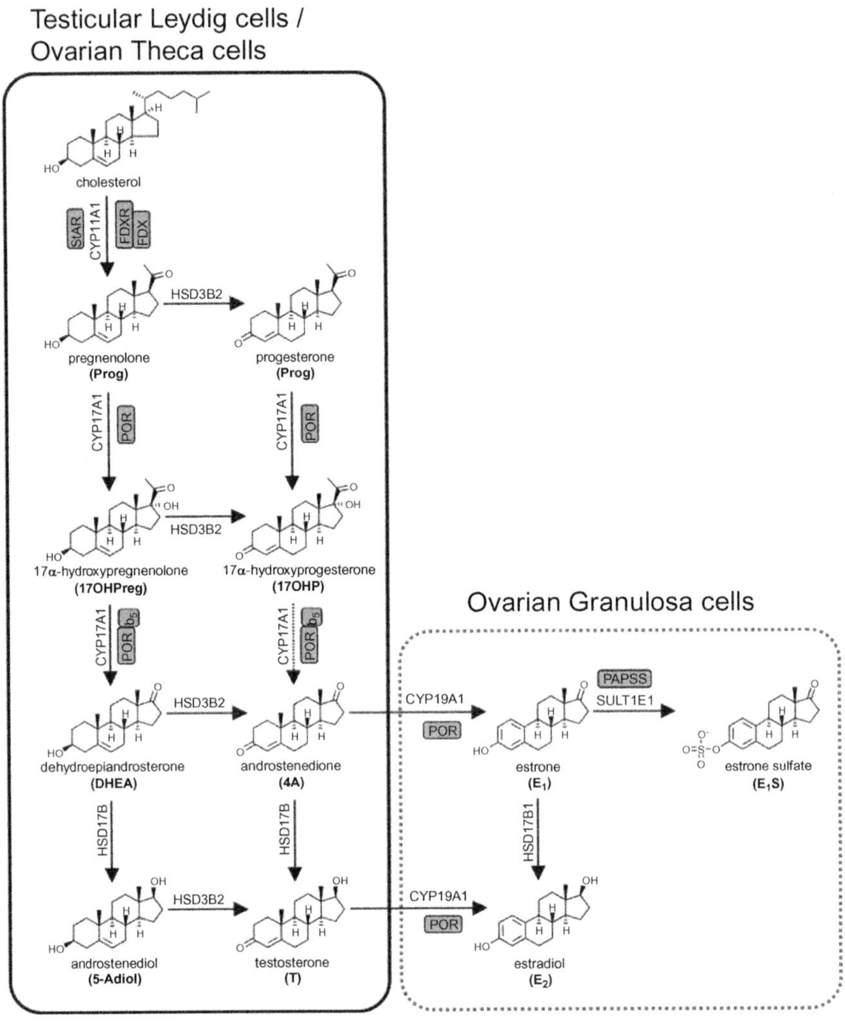

FIG. 2 Steroidogenesis as it occurs in the gonads. *(Credit: Schiffer L, Barnard L, Baranowski ES, et al. Human steroid biosynthesis, metabolism, and excretion are differentially reflected by serum and urine steroid metabolomes: a comprehensive review. J Steroid Biochem Mol Biol 2019;194:105439. https://doi.org/10.1016/j.jsbmb.2019.105439. Source: https://www.ncbi.nlm.nih.gov/pmc/articles/PMC6857441/.)*

Changes across the lifespan—Males

Following infancy, gonadal sex steroid production in males commences at the onset of puberty, LH causes adult Leydig cells to develop and begin producing testosterone. Gonadal sex steroids reach a peak at approximately 20 years of age in males with a gradual decline thereafter. This decline accelerates around the eighth decade of life and is occasionally termed andropause. However, it should be noted that there is disagreement over what constitutes physiologic vs pathologic reductions in androgen levels in males.

Changes across the lifespan—Females

Following infancy, gonadal sex steroid production in females commences at puberty when LH stimulates ovarian theca cells to produce both progesterone and testosterone, while FSH causes granulosa cells to convert thecal androgens to estradiol. Mean levels peak between 16 and 20 years of age and remain stable for the next three decades. Of course, levels of both estradiol and progesterone vary cyclically during the normal menstrual cycle, and change significantly over the course of pregnancy and for the duration of breastfeeding. When menopause occurs, usually between 50 and 55 years of age, there is a rapid and massive reduction in estradiol over no longer than a few years to levels similar to those found in males. Following menopause, most circulating estradiol in females derives from peripheral aromatization of adrenal androgens, primarily in adipose tissue.

Testosterone levels in females, as in males, peak around approximately 20 years of age before rapidly reducing over the next two decades, remaining stable thereafter. Female testosterone is produced exclusively by the ovarian theca cells.

Mechanism of action

In the circulation, steroid hormones are extensively bound to both specific (e.g., sex-hormone-binding globulin) and nonspecific (e.g., albumin) plasma proteins. As lipid-derived hormones, they readily diffuse across the lipid bilayers of cell membranes. However, membrane transporters for steroid hormones do exist and modulate the rate of entry into certain cells. Once inside the cytoplasm of steroid-responsive cells, steroid hormones bind to their specific receptor, activating it. This activated receptor-hormone complex is then able to translocate into the nucleus where it can bind to appropriate deoxyribonucleic acid (DNA) sequences, causing transcription of messenger ribonucleic acid (mRNA) to occur, which is in turn translated into proteins.

The androgen, estrogen, and progesterone receptors have two, two, and three known isoforms, respectively. It is the tissue-specific expression of these isoforms and their respective affinities for various sex steroids that determines some of the tissue-specific heterogeneity in sex steroid effects.

It is typical to differentiate between potent and weak forms of the three types of sex steroids, based on their affinity for their respective receptors. Estradiol is the only potent estrogen while progesterone is the only potent progestogen. Testosterone and its peripheral metabolite dihydrotestosterone (DHT) are both potent androgens.

Sex steroid effects on muscle

Androgens

Testosterone is the major sex steroid that influences skeletal muscle growth with the trophic effects of testosterone on muscle mass and myocyte protein synthesis well-established [3]. Muscle mass is also increased via the growth hormone (GH)/insulin-like growth factor 1 (IGF-1) pathway, with the magnitude of testosterone's effects comparable to this pathway. Testosterone levels correlate with muscle strength independent of muscle mass, suggesting trophic actions on muscle function in addition to tissue volume [4]. While testosterone exerts direct effects upon myocyte-expressed androgen receptors, much of its effects are, in fact, exerted through its metabolite DHT. Myocytes express 5-alpha reductase (5AR), an enzyme that converts testosterone to the much more potent DHT in situ, which binds to androgen receptors with twice the affinity of testosterone while exhibiting a fivefold slower dissociation rate [5].

The direct and independent effects of DHEAS on muscle bulk are less clear with conflicting evidence from related lines of enquiry. While DHEAS levels have been found to correlate with muscle force per cross-sectional area in postmenopausal women in one study, a similar relationship was observed for other sex steroids in the same study [6]. A relatively small, controlled cross-over trial found 6 months of Dehydroepiandrosterone (DHEA) supplementation (functionally similar to DHEAS) to be associated with increased muscle strength in males but not females [7]. A more recent randomized controlled trial found 6 months of DHEA supplementation had no effect on muscle strength in males or females, but in a 4-month extension during which participants engaged in a weight-training program, muscle strength was increased compared with placebo [8].

It has been suggested that the main role of DHEAS in the musculature is to act as a precursor for testosterone and estradiol production since the relevant enzymes in the steroid biosynthesis pathway are expressed by muscle cells. Given the conflicting evidence around its effectiveness, a 2011 review found no benefit of DHEA replacement in postmenopausal women [9].

Estrogens

The evidence for a direct effect of estrogen on skeletal muscle is conflicting. While animal models suggest a clear role of estrogens in contributing to muscle growth, human studies of replacement differ in their conclusions. In a small, controlled cross-over trial, 3 months of hormone replacement therapy (HRT) given to early postmenopausal women resulted in an increase in total body lean mass, presumed to be muscle mass [10]. However, in a similarly-sized prospective cohort trial, 64 weeks of subdermal estradiol implants given to postmenopausal women of similar ages to the previous trial did not result in any significant changes in appendicular skeletal muscle mass [11]. There is some

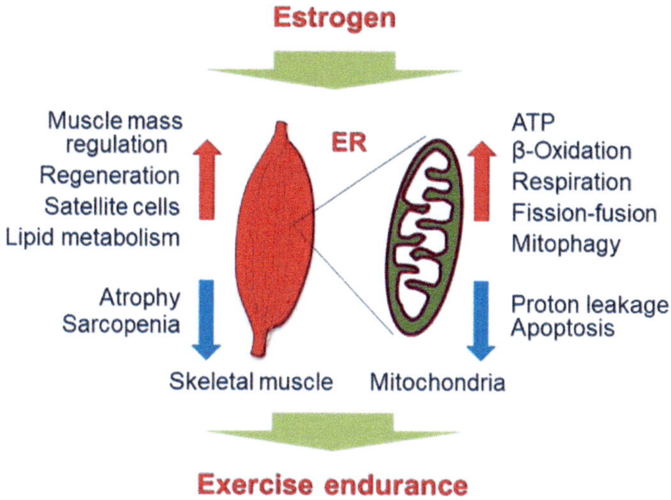

FIG. 3 Putative effects of estrogens on skeletal muscles and myocyte mitochondria. *(Credit: Ikeda K, Horie-Inoue K, Inoue S. Functions of estrogen and estrogen receptor signaling on skeletal muscle. J Steroid Biochem Mol Biol 2019;191:105375. https://doi.org/10.1016/j.jsbmb.2019.105375. Epub 2019 May 5. Source: https://pubmed.ncbi.nlm.nih.gov/31067490/.)*

evidence that estrogens play different and at times opposing roles within the muscle via the alpha and beta isoforms of the estrogen receptor [12].

Estrogens may impact skeletal muscle indirectly through modifying levels of spontaneous activity and resting energy expenditure. It is plausible that declining estrogen levels may contribute to disuse atrophy of muscle through these indirect mechanisms [13] (Fig. 3).

Progestogens

The progesterone receptor is expressed in skeletal muscle cells and progesterone appears to have a direct trophic effect on muscle. In a study of replacing sex steroids in a menstrual cycle-mimicking manner in postmenopausal women, three simulated menstrual cycles of progesterone (three 14-day periods) resulted in increased muscle protein synthesis as measured by mRNA expression [14]. It is unclear whether this translates to increased muscle mass or strength. Progesterone is not currently thought to play a significant role in skeletal muscle growth or strength, but perhaps plays a role in modifying the effects of estradiol on muscle in females.

Male physiology

The rapid increase in testosterone during male puberty is associated with marked gains in muscle mass, with considerable differences between males and females becoming evident over this period. As testosterone decreases following the young adult peak, so does muscle strength and functional performance. It is thought that testosterone explains much of the age-related decline in muscle strength seen in males. This relationship has been explored in numerous cohort studies including the Massachusetts Male Aging Study (muscle strength) and the Framingham Offspring Study (functional performance) [15,16]. Further evidence for this are studies showing an improvement in functional performance with testosterone replacement in older males, most notably the Testosterone in Older Men with Mobility Limitations (TOM) trial, although cardiovascular-related adverse events were also increased [17,18].

However, the relationship between testosterone-related declines in muscle strength and impaired functional performance remains unclear, as does the clinical utility of testosterone supplementation in older males for this purpose [19]. In one 20-week study of healthy men aged 60–75, testosterone supplementation resulted in an increase in both muscle mass and strength but not functional performance [20]. It is also possible that testosterone augments the effects of exercise. In the Testosterone Trials, daily testosterone supplementation for 12 months resulted in improved physical function in those participants with a baseline walk speed of at least 1.2 m/s but not in those with slower walk speeds, suggesting benefit only in those who were likely able to engage in more physical activity and exercise [21]. A recent systematic review and metaanalysis of this question suggest that both testosterone supplementation and exercise have independent beneficial effects upon muscle strength while testosterone alone increases muscle mass [22]. Additionally, the combination of exercise and testosterone supplementation appears to have a greater effect on both parameters than either intervention alone.

While male myocytes express the estrogen and progesterone receptors, the low levels of both of these hormones in circulation mean that serum-derived estrogens and progestogens have minimal effects upon the male musculature. There is also reduced expression of aromatase in muscle compared with other tissues, meaning that there are only low levels of in situ production of estrogen from circulating androgens [23]. What is ultimately clear, however, is that while testosterone levels are related to muscle strength in older males, estradiol is not [4].

Female physiology

As in males, female muscle mass increases during puberty though to a lesser degree, likely explained by the differential testosterone and estrogen levels and effects on muscle. It has long been observed that there is a general decline in female muscle mass from around 30 years of age, which accelerates at the menopausal transition around the age of 50 [24]. It is likely that this acceleration from menopause is related to the precipitous decline in estradiol levels at this time. This is likely largely mediated via a loss of estrogens role in muscle repair leading to accumulation of damage and subsequent atrophy [12]. Androgens likely play a role in the determination of female muscle mass, however, the fact that androgen levels are gradually declining prior to menopause with no precipitous decline at this time (DHEAS often increases around the menopause before continuing its age-related decline [9]), suggests a significant role for estrogens in determining female muscle mass.

Progestogens are thought to play a limited role in determining female muscle strength or mass and are implicated in cyclical changes in muscle protein synthesis over the menstrual cycle as well as during pregnancy and breastfeeding [14]. However, these changes appear not to affect muscle contractile characteristics [25]. The role of progesterone in age-related skeletal muscle changes remains minimally investigated.

Sex steroid effects on bone

Androgens

Androgens appear to have markedly reduced direct effects upon bone compared with estrogens. In both males and females, the androgen receptor does not appear to have a direct regulatory effect upon osteoclasts [26]. However through aromatization of testosterone to estradiol locally within the bone itself, serum testosterone levels do have downstream effects upon bone metabolism, mediated via estradiol. There is some evidence that testosterone has an estradiol-independent role during skeletal growth and maturation preadulthood. Some of this action is mediated via the GH/IGF-1 pathway and appears to contribute to periosteal apposition, which has the net effect of increasing bone size [27]. Testosterone also appears to have greater trophic effects upon cancellous rather than cortical bone. This may relate to differential expression of aromatase between these bone compartments, or an estrogen-independent mechanism.

While there is some evidence that DHEAS and other weak adrenal androgens improve bone mineral density (BMD), evidence is inconsistent [28]. The role of DHEAS in bone metabolism is predominantly to provide a substrate for peripheral aromatization into estradiol. If there is a true independent effect, it is weak compared with estradiol and testosterone and likely does not play a significant role in mediating age-related changes.

Estrogens

In contrast to muscle, the predominant sex steroid influencing bone metabolism is estradiol. The activated estrogen receptor has direct effects upon both osteoblasts and osteoclasts, stimulating bone production by the former and reducing bone resorption by the latter. Preclinical and clinical evidence for this relationship is strong but perhaps nowhere more so than in the Women's Health Initiative trial. In this seminal trial, hormone replacement therapy (HRT) prescribed to postmenopausal and thus estradiol-deficient women resulted in marked improvements in BMD compared with those receiving placebo [29].

Estrogen signaling appears to have greater effects upon cortical bone than cancellous bone, though it is integral to the development of both [26]. This is likely mediated by differential expression of the two estrogen receptor isoforms, alpha, and beta, between the two bone compartments. While both are expressed in cancellous bone, it is predominantly the alpha isoform that is found in cortical bone. Since the beta isoform appears to antagonize the trophic effects of the alpha isoform in bone, this differential receptor expression likely explains these compartment-specific effects [30].

Progestogens

There is some evidence that progesterone may have bone-trophic effects [31]. However, any effect is small compared with other sex steroids and progesterone does not play a role in determining age-related skeletal changes.

Male physiology

Male and female skeletal maturation across puberty is similar, with high levels of sex steroids during this period contributing to longitudinal bone growth, bone mass accrual, and eventually epiphyseal closure to determine the final adult height. Given the low levels of circulating estradiol in males, these effects are predominantly mediated by estradiol produced in situ within bone following aromatization of testosterone. The strongest evidence for this derives from a 3-week trial of pharmacologically suppressing both testosterone and estradiol production in healthy older males, in which the participants were randomized to replacement of none, either, or both of testosterone and estradiol [32]. Comparing bone formation and resorption markers between the groups provided clear evidence that suppressing sex steroid production profoundly increases bone resorption while suppressing its formation. Replacing estradiol alone or both hormones reverses these negative effects. Whereas replacing testosterone, while the body's ability to convert this to estradiol is pharmacologically suppressed, has little to no effect.

Testosterone's estradiol-independent effects upon periosteal apposition and cancellous bone in preference to cortical bone appear to account for some of the gender differences in bone size that become established during puberty. These effects account for the observation that males typically have a greater bone cross-sectional area than females of an equivalent age [17,33].

The gradual reductions in circulating androgens that occur with aging account for much of the age-related decline in BMD. Some of the strongest evidence for this derives from the Testosterone Trials. In these trials of testosterone replacement for 12 months in males at least 65 years of age with low testosterone levels, an improvement in both volumetric BMD and estimated bone strength was observed in the testosterone-treated versus placebo group [34].

Female physiology

As the main circulating sex steroid in females and the predominant effector of bone metabolism within this group, the rapid increase in estradiol during female puberty accounts for much of the skeletal development and maturation during this time. The differential expression of estrogen receptor isoforms between the bone compartments results in a higher cortical: cancellous bone ratio than in males.

Subsequent to puberty there is a small amount of bone loss between early adulthood and menopause. Once the menopausal transition commences, however, there is rapid and marked bone loss, following which the rate of bone loss parallels that in similarly aged males. Postmenopausal female bone density is determined most strongly not by serum estradiol but by serum testosterone [35], consistent with the predominant source of estradiol in the postmenopausal state being local production from androgen aromatization.

In females, there is weak and inconsistent evidence of a direct effect of androgens on bone metabolism [36]. The role of circulating androgens in female bone metabolism is predominantly to act as a substrate for peripheral conversion to estradiol. Strong evidence for this is presented by the accelerated bone lone caused by aromatase inhibitor used for the adjuvant treatment of postmenopausal female breast cancer [37]. This is due to the postmenopausal state being characterized by minimal circulating estradiol such that bone health relies upon local production through aromatization of testosterone and DHEAS (Fig. 4).

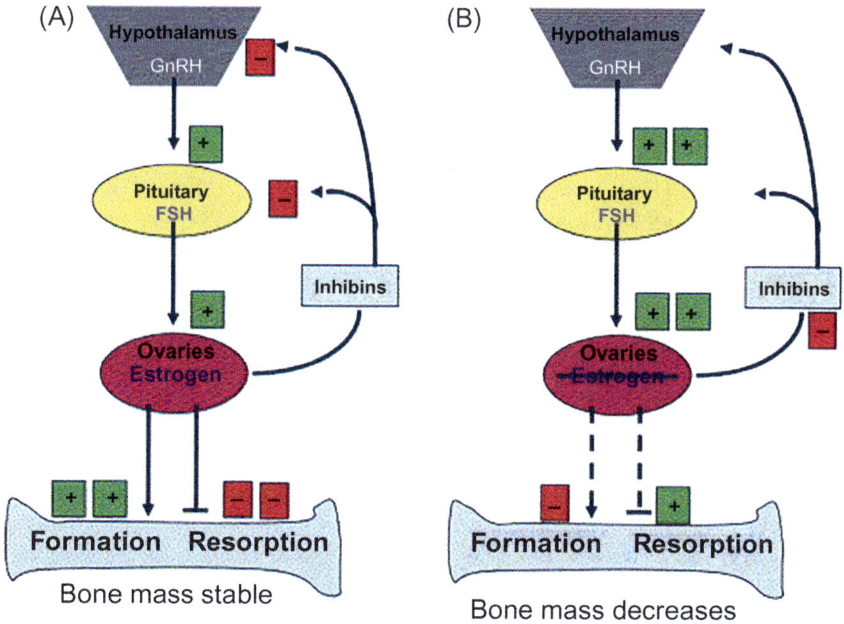

FIG. 4 Classic paradigm of the net contribution of estrogen on bone before (panel A) and after (panel B) menopause. *(Credit: Baron R, FSH versus estrogen: who's guilty of breaking bones? Cell Metab 2006;3(5):302–5. https://doi.org/10.1016/j.cmet.2006.04.007.)*

Sex steroid effects on fat

Androgens

The androgens exhibit a clear lipolytic effect in male adipose tissue. Testosterone has been shown to stimulate lipolysis while inhibiting lipoprotein lipase (LPL) activity and differentiation of adipocyte precursors [38]. The functional effect of these mechanisms is demonstrated in decreased leptin levels, a measure of adipose tissue mass, in males with higher testosterone. While adipose tissue expresses 5AR, it is unclear what role peripheral conversion of testosterone to DHT plays in these mechanisms, since DHT treatment has not been observed to have the same biochemical effects as its precursor [39].

Testosterone's effects in female adipose tissue appear to differ significantly from those in males. The female condition of polycystic ovary syndrome (PCOS) is characterized by elevated levels of androgens, both gonadal and adrenal-derived. In a clinical study comparing nonobese healthy women and women with PCOS matched for body mass index (BMI), and therefore presumably similar levels of other lipolytic and lipogenic hormones, lipolysis was observed to be reduced [40]. In the nondisease state, a positive relationship between serum androgens and BMI in otherwise healthy obese females has been observed [41]. Additionally, though testosterone levels are inversely associated with visceral fat in males, when testosterone is administered in the context of female-to-male gender reassignment therapy there is an increase in visceral fat, suggesting genetically-determined differences in adipose tissue response to androgens [42].

DHEAS does not appear to have significant direct effects upon adipose tissue but has been observed to reduce fat mass. It is most likely that it achieves this through indirect mechanisms. DHEAS stimulates resting metabolic rate and glucose disposal, which has the downstream effect of suppressing insulin release, a potent lipogenic hormone. Thus, DHEAS-mediated insulin suppression is the likely indirect lipolytic mechanism of this hormone [38].

Estrogens

The marked sexual dimorphism seen between males and females in fat volume and distribution is largely attributable to the effects of estrogens. The regulation of fat metabolism by estrogens is complex, fat depot-specific, and involves differences in receptor subtypes as well as tissue concentrations of estrogens. Estradiol is strongly associated with the presence of subcutaneous and lower body fat depots, but a lack of abdominal fat [43]. Given that estradiol appears to inhibit lipogenesis at the molecular level, it is likely that estradiol-signaling preferentially acts at the abdominal fat depots, thus allowing subcutaneous and lower body fat to accumulate uninhibited.

Progestogens

Progesterone has limited effects upon fat, serving primarily to modulate the effects of estradiol during the menstrual cycle. The main effects of progesterone are to increase fat deposition in adipose tissue generally and in breast tissue specifically [44], likely in preparation for a potential pregnancy.

Male physiology

The changes in male fat volume and distribution are largely dictated by changes in androgen levels. Prepubertally there is little difference between the genders, however, once puberty commences the high testosterone levels are seen in males and the resultant increase in muscle mass are accompanied by a similarly rapid decrease in body fat. As testosterone levels fall with age, muscle mass is progressively replaced by fat. Male physiology results in preferential fat accumulation in the visceral and central abdominal fat depots accounting for the so-called "android" body habitus typical of adult males. This progressive replacement of muscle with fat continues throughout life, mirroring the ongoing reduction in the predominant adipocyte-regulating hormone, testosterone. Estrogens and progestogens play a limited role in male fat volume and distribution.

Female physiology

Over the course of puberty, the typical female "gynaecoid" body habitus develops, with fat being deposited preferentially in the gluteal and subcutaneous regions. This fat accumulation appears to be related to increases in both adipocyte number and size. Between puberty and menopause, high levels of estradiol protect against metabolically unhealthy central fat deposition. But at menopause, this protection is lost as estradiol levels fall, and abdominal fat increases. Whole-body fat increases across the menopausal transition as well, however, the magnitude of the increase is not as great as across puberty [43].

The role of progesterone in female fat metabolism is primarily to prepare the female body for potential pregnancy during the menstrual cycle. This is predominantly manifested as increased breast adipose tissue volume toward the end of the menstrual cycle, with significantly greater magnitude effects experienced during pregnancy and breastfeeding. However, the marked reduction in progesterone levels and loss of cycling experienced at menopause is not thought to contribute significantly to postmenopausal changes in female fat mass.

Conclusion

In conclusion, sex steroids play an essential role in muscle, fat, and bone growth and development. Alterations in serum levels or aromatization of those hormones affect bone and muscle mass and function. Although hormone supplementation to correct osteosarcopenia is a subject of another chapter in this book, supplementation of androgens in hypogonadism has not significantly impacted preventing falls and fractures. In contrast, estrogen supplementation in postmenopausal women has demonstrated a beneficial effect on BMD and fracture prevention. However, concerns about safety with estrogen supplementation have prevented their wide use in this condition. In the future, safer and more effective compounds with activity on estrogen or androgen receptors could become a potential alternative to treating osteosarcopenia and preventing its associated outcomes.

References

[1] Papierska L. Adrenopause – does it really exist? Prz Menopauzalny 2017;16(2):57–60.

[2] Finkelstein JS, Lee H, Burnett-Bowie S-AM, Pallais JC, Yu EW, Borges LF, et al. Gonadal steroids and body composition, strength, and sexual function in men. N Engl J Med 2013;369(11):1011–22.

[3] Griggs RC, Kingston W, Jozefowicz RF, Herr BE, Forbes G, Halliday D. Effect of testosterone on muscle mass and muscle protein synthesis. J Appl Physiol 1989;66(1):498–503.

[4] Auyeung TW, Lee JSW, Kwok T, Leung J, Ohlsson C, Vandenput L, et al. Testosterone but not estradiol level is positively related to muscle strength and physical performance independent of muscle mass: a cross-sectional study in 1489 older men. Eur J Endocrinol 2011;164(5):811–7.

[5] Grino PB, Griffin JE, Wilson JD. Testosterone at high concentrations interacts with the human androgen receptor similarly to dihydrotestosterone. Endocrinology 1990;126(2):1165–72.

[6] Pollanen E, Sipila S, Alen M, Ronkainen PHA, Ankarberg-Lindgren C, Puolakka J, et al. Differential influence of peripheral and systemic sex steroids on skeletal muscle quality in pre- and post-menopausal women. Aging Cell 2011;10(4):650–60.

[7] Morales AJ, Haubrich RH, Hwang JY, Asakura H, Yen SS. The effect of six months treatment with a 100 mg daily dose of dehydroepiandrosterone (DHEA) on circulating sex steroids, body composition and muscle strength in age-advanced men and women. Clin Endocrinol 1998;49(4):421–32.

[8] Villareal DT, Holloszy JO. DHEA enhances effects of weight training on muscle mass and strength in elderly women and men. Am J Physiol Endocrinol Metab 2006;291(5):E1003–8.

[9] Davis SR, Panjari M, Stanczyk FZ. Clinical review: DHEA replacement for post-menopausal women. J Clin Endocrinol Metab 2011;96(6):1642–53.

[10] Sorensen MB, Rosenfalck AM, Hojgaard L, Ottesen B. Obesity and sarcopenia after menopause are reversed by sex hormone replacement therapy. Obes Res 2001;9(10):622–6.

[11] Hansen RD, Raja C, Baber RJ, Lieberman D, Allen BJ. Effects of 20-mg oestradiol implant therapy on bone mineral density, fat distribution and muscle mass in post-menopausal women. Acta Diabetol 2003;40(Suppl 1):S191–5.

[12] Ikeda K, Horie-Inoue K, Inoue S. Functions of estrogen and estrogen receptor signaling on skeletal muscle. J Steroid Biochem Mol Biol 2019;191, 105375.

[13] Brown M. Skeletal muscle and bone: effect of sex steroids and aging. Adv Physiol Educ 2008;32(2):120–6.

[14] Smith GI, Yoshino J, Reeds DN, Bradley D, Burrows RE, Heisey HD, et al. Testosterone and progesterone, but not estradiol, stimulate muscle protein synthesis in post-menopausal women. J Clin Endocrinol Metab 2014;99(1):256–65.

[15] O'Donnell AB, Travison TG, Harris SS, Tenover JL, McKinlay JB. Testosterone, dehydroepiandrosterone, and physical performance in older men: results from the Massachusetts male aging study. J Clin Endocrinol Metab 2006;91(2):425–31.

[16] Krasnoff JB, Basaria S, Pencina MJ, Jasuja GK, Vasan RS, Ulloor J, et al. Free testosterone levels are associated with mobility limitation and physical performance in community-dwelling men: the Framingham offspring study. J Clin Endocrinol Metab 2010;95(6):2790–9.
[17] Basaria S, Coviello AD, Travison TG, Storer TW, Farwell WR, Jette AM, et al. Adverse events associated with testosterone administration. N Engl J Med 2010;363(2):109–22.
[18] LeBrasseur NK, Lajevardi N, Miciek R, Mazer N, Storer TW, Bhasin S. Effects of testosterone therapy on muscle performance and physical function in older men with mobility limitations (the TOM trial): design and methods. Contemp Clin Trials 2009;30(2):133–40.
[19] Storer TW, Basaria S, Traustadottir T, Harman SM, Pencina K, Li Z, et al. Effects of testosterone supplementation for 3 years on muscle performance and physical function in older men. J Clin Endocrinol Metab 2017;102(2):583–93.
[20] Storer TW, Woodhouse L, Magliano L, Singh AB, Dzekov C, Dzekov J, et al. Changes in muscle mass, muscle strength, and power but not physical function are related to testosterone dose in healthy older men. J Am Geriatr Soc 2008;56(11):1991–9.
[21] Bhasin S, Ellenberg SS, Storer TW, Basaria S, Pahor M, Stephens-Shields AJ, et al. Effect of testosterone replacement on measures of mobility in older men with mobility limitation and low testosterone concentrations: secondary analyses of the testosterone trials. Lancet Diabetes Endocrinol 2018;6(11):879–90.
[22] Falqueto H, Junior JLR, Silverio MNO, Farias JCH, Schoenfeld BJ, Manfredi LH. Can conditions of skeletal muscle loss be improved by combining exercise with anabolic-androgenic steroids? A systematic review and meta-analysis of testosterone-based interventions. Rev Endocr Metab Disord 2021;22(2):161–78.
[23] Larionov AA, Vasyliev DA, Mason JI, Howie AF, Berstein LM, Miller WR. Aromatase in skeletal muscle. J Steroid Biochem Mol Biol 2003;84(4):485–92.
[24] Aloia JF, McGowan DM, Vaswani AN, Ross P, Cohn SH. Relationship of menopause to skeletal and muscle mass. Am J Clin Nutr 1991;53(6):1378–83.
[25] Janse de Jonge XA, Boot CR, Thom JM, Ruell PA, Thompson MW. The influence of menstrual cycle phase on skeletal muscle contractile characteristics in humans. J Physiol 2001;530(Pt 1):161–6.
[26] Khosla S, Monroe DG. Regulation of bone metabolism by sex steroids. Cold Spring Harb Perspect Med 2018;8(1), a031211.
[27] Almeida M, Laurent MR, Dubois V, Claessens F, O'Brien CA, Bouillon R, et al. Estrogens and androgens in skeletal physiology and pathophysiology. Physiol Rev 2017;97(1):135–87.
[28] Khosla S, Melton 3rd LJ, Atkinson EJ, O'Fallon WM, Klee GG, Riggs BL. Relationship of serum sex steroid levels and bone turnover markers with bone mineral density in men and women: a key role for bioavailable estrogen. J Clin Endocrinol Metab 1998;83(7):2266–74.
[29] Cauley JA, Robbins J, Chen Z, Cummings SR, Jackson RD, LaCroix AZ, et al. Effects of estrogen plus progestin on risk of fracture and bone mineral density: the Women's Health Initiative randomized trial. JAMA 2003;290(13):1729–38.
[30] Nicks KM, Fujita K, Fraser D, McGregor U, Drake MT, McGee-Lawrence ME, et al. Deletion of estrogen receptor beta in osteoprogenitor cells increases trabecular but not cortical bone mass in female mice. J Bone Miner Res 2016;31(3):606–14.
[31] Prior JC. Progesterone as a bone-trophic hormone. Endocr Rev 1990;11(2):386–98.
[32] Falahati-Nini A, Riggs BL, Atkinson EJ, O'Fallon WM, Eastell R, Khosla S. Relative contributions of testosterone and estrogen in regulating bone resorption and formation in normal elderly men. J Clin Invest 2000;106(12):1553–60.
[33] Kanehisa H, Ikegawa S, Fukunaga T. Comparison of muscle cross-sectional area and strength between untrained women and men. Eur J Appl Physiol Occup Physiol 1994;68(2):148–54.

[34] Snyder PJ, Bhasin S, Cunningham GR, Matsumoto AM, Stephens-Shields AJ, Cauley JA, et al. Lessons from the testosterone trials. Endocr Rev 2018;39(3):369–86.
[35] Wu F, Ames R, Clearwater J, Evans MC, Gamble G, Reid IR. Prospective 10-year study of the determinants of bone density and bone loss in normal post-menopausal women, including the effect of hormone replacement therapy. Clin Endocrinol 2002;56(6):703–11.
[36] Raisz LG, Wiita B, Artis A, Bowen A, Schwartz S, Trahiotis M, et al. Comparison of the effects of estrogen alone and estrogen plus androgen on biochemical markers of bone formation and resorption in post-menopausal women. J Clin Endocrinol Metab 1996;81(1):37–43.
[37] Hadji P. Aromatase inhibitor-associated bone loss in breast cancer patients is distinct from post-menopausal osteoporosis. Crit Rev Oncol Hematol 2009;69(1):73–82.
[38] De Pergola G. The adipose tissue metabolism: role of testosterone and dehydroepiandrosterone. Int J Obes Relat Metab Disord 2000;24(Suppl 2):S59–63.
[39] Marin P. Testosterone and regional fat distribution. Obes Res 1995;3(Suppl 4):609S–12S.
[40] Ek I, Arner P, Bergqvist A, Carlstrom K, Wahrenberg H. Impaired adipocyte lipolysis in nonobese women with the polycystic ovary syndrome: a possible link to insulin resistance? J Clin Endocrinol Metab 1997;82(4):1147–53.
[41] Taponen S, Martikainen H, Jarvelin M-R, Laitinen J, Pouta A, Hartikainen A-L, et al. Hormonal profile of women with self-reported symptoms of oligomenorrhea and/or hirsutism: northern Finland birth cohort 1966 study. J Clin Endocrinol Metab 2003;88(1):141–7.
[42] Elbers JM, Asscheman H, Seidell JC, Megens JA, Gooren LJ. Long-term testosterone administration increases visceral fat in female to male transsexuals. J Clin Endocrinol Metab 1997;82(7):2044–7.
[43] Cooke PS, Naaz A. Role of estrogens in adipocyte development and function. Exp Biol Med 2004;229(11):1127–35.
[44] Kalkhoff RK. Metabolic effects of progesterone. Am J Obstet Gynecol 1982;142(6 Pt 2):735–8.

Chapter 8

The role of vitamin D and parathyroid hormone (PTH) in osteosarcopenia

Andrea L. Darling
Department of Nutrition, Food and Exercise Sciences, School of Biosciences and Medicine, Faculty of Health and Medical Sciences, University of Surrey, Guildford, United Kingdom

Introduction

Osteosarcopenia is the combined diagnosis of both osteoporosis and sarcopenia, both of which are conditions associated with aging. Sarcopenia is currently defined by the European Working Group on Sarcopenia in Older People (EWGSOP) (2019) as low muscle strength, quantity, and performance; as defined by performance on specified functional tests [1]. Sarcopenia is known to lead to increased risk of falls, mortality, frailty, and poor function [2]. It is also associated with type 2 diabetes [3], cardiac cachexia [4], and metabolic syndrome [5]. Osteoporosis is a condition of low bone mineral density (BMD), Specifically, it is diagnosed by a dual-X-ray absorptiometry (DXA) T score of less than −2.5. This means that the BMD is 2.5 standard deviations or more below what would be expected at peak bone mineral density (BMD) in young adulthood. Osteoporosis is a condition of reduced bone strength, so it increases the risk of low trauma bone fractures. Hip and vertebral fractures are associated with increased morbidity [6–8] and mortality [9].

With an aging global population, the incidence of osteosarcopenia is increasing, with subsequent large costs to the affected individual and to society. Recent estimates of osteosarcopenia prevalence include 5%–37% of community-dwelling Australian adults over the age of 65 years [10], one-third of older adults in Iran over the age of 60 years [11], and 10%–15% of 75 year old men and women in China [12].

There has been the suggestion that a diagnosis of osteosarcopenia may carry a higher health burden than having either osteoporosis or sarcopenia alone. Persons with both osteoporosis and sarcopenia are likely to be the frailest individuals who are at most risk of fractures, falls, and are most likely to live in a nursing home [13]. For instance, one study found that mortality risk was

Osteosarcopenia. https://doi.org/10.1016/B978-0-12-820088-9.00011-1

1.5 times higher in those with osteosarcopenia, compared with those without either osteoporosis or sarcopenia [14]. However, another study found that those with osteosarcopenia had similar falls and fracture risk with those having osteoporosis or sarcopenia alone [15].

Adequate vitamin D concentration is known to be important for ensuring both bone [16] *and muscle* [17] *health.* Therefore, it is important to establish whether vitamin D deficiency, with concurrent high PTH concentration, is a candidate for influencing the development of osteosarcopenia. Of concern, there is a global epidemic of vitamin D deficiency, with one study finding that less than 50% of the global population in winter are sufficient in 25(OH)D (defined as >50 nmol/L) [18]. Therefore, if vitamin D status does influence the development of osteosarcopenia, it could be an important modifiable factor to address as part of osteosarcopenia treatment and prevention.

Vitamin D

Vitamin D is a prohormone, rather than a vitamin, with clear endocrinological functions in the body. It is ingested from the diet in relatively small amounts, but the main source for most people is dermal production under the action of ultraviolet-B (UVB) radiation on the skin. The active hormone, 1,25-dihydroxy vitamin D ($1,25(OH)_2D$), is produced from the hydroxylation of 25-hydroxyvitamn D (25(OH)D) in the kidney (Fig. 1). There are multiple vitamin D metabolites in the body, but the most measured are 25(OH)D and $1,25(OH)_2D$.

The gold standard marker of vitamin D deficiency is 25(OH)D concentration [19]. This is because the concentration of $1,25(OH)_2D$ is highly regulated in the blood. Conversely, 25(OH)D is not tightly regulated and in serum or plasma it is a proxy estimate of the body's store of vitamin D. However, the level to which it accurately reflects tissue saturation with vitamin D is unclear.

Vitamin D deficiency has been associated with increased risk of a wide range of health conditions, including cancer, heart disease, and osteoporosis; as well as autoimmune conditions and infectious diseases [20]. Vitamin D comes in two forms, vitamin D_2 (from plant and fungal sources) and vitamin D_3 (usually from animal dietary sources, as well as being the form produced dermally). There are few natural rich sources of vitamin D in the diet, the most concentrated ones being oily fish, and to a lesser extent eggs and meat. Vitamin D intake from diet varies by gender, age, and the supplementation and fortification policies of individual countries [21]. Higher intakes are generally seen in countries with high fish or vitamin D supplement consumption, or with mandatory vitamin D food fortification policies [21]. Of concern, *vitamin D deficiency is very common in older people in some parts of the world.* For example, a systematic review and meta analysis reported the following average 25(OH)D concentrations in people aged over 65 years old: Asia/Pacific (66 nmol/L); Europe (52 nmol/L); Middle East (38 nmol/L), and North America (71.7 nmol/L) [22].

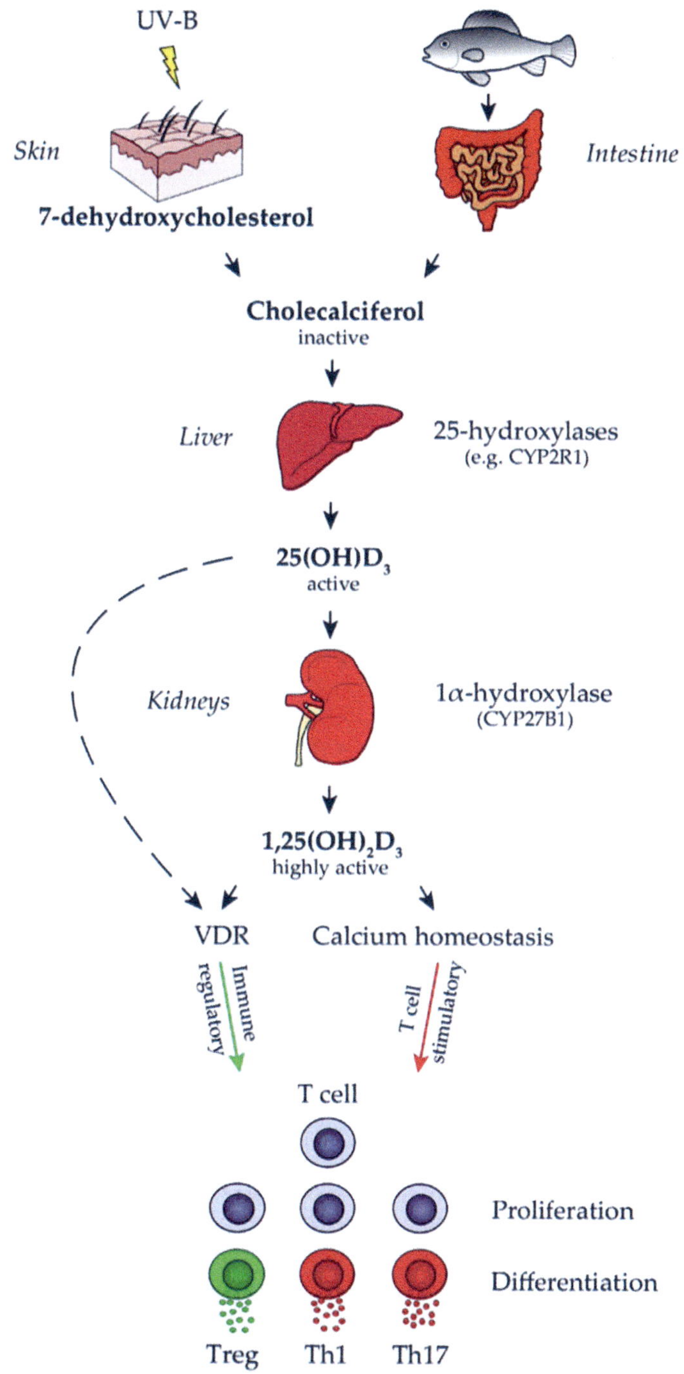

FIG. 1 Vitamin D metabolism. *(Adapted from Hausler D, Weber MS. Vitamin D supplementation in central nervous system demyelinating disease-enough is enough. Int J Mol Sci 2019;20(1):218. https://doi.org/10.3390/ijms20010218; CC-BY 4.0. https://www.mdpi.com/1422-0067/20/1/218/htm.)*

These estimates may contain few frail individuals in nursing homes, so maybe an overestimate. However, they do illustrate that in Europe and the Middle East, a significant number of older individuals have 25(OH)D less than 50 nmol/L (so are deficient using the European Food Safety Agency (EFSA) recommended serum or plasma concentration of >50 nmol/L [23]). Vitamin D deficiency is particularly common in older people in nursing homes or receiving home personal care. For example, a study in Japan found that 15%–20% of older individuals receiving home personal care had vitamin D deficiency in winter (defined as <30 nmol/L) [24]. With aging, there is some evidence of a reduced ability to produce vitamin D in the skin, with production falling by up to 50% between young childhood and age 60 years [25]. Sunlight exposure may also be low for those living in nursing homes, suggested by the fact that a study in the Netherlands (latitude 52.2°N) found low 25(OH)D was low (median of around 15 nmol/L) all year round and did not show the expected seasonal variation [26].

Vitamin D and PTH—Overview of the regulation of calcium metabolism

The physiological regulation of calcium concentration is crucial for life. Serum ionized calcium must be strictly maintained between 2.2 and 2.6 mmol/L. When serum ionized calcium is too low, PTH is released, leading to increased renal reabsorption of calcium. Increased 1,25(OH)$_2$D concentration leads to increased calcium absorption from the gut. Increased PTH leads to loss of calcium from bone by increased osteoclast activity (Fig. 2). These actions lead to a normalization of serum ionized calcium. Conversely, when serum ionized calcium is too high, the hormone calcitonin is released from the thyroid, which stimulates the uptake of calcium into bone tissue by inhibition of osteoclast activity. There is also reduced renal reabsorption of calcium and increased calciuria.

Vitamin D and osteoporosis/osteopenia

Vitamin D has a clear role in bone health. Low 25(OH)D concentration is a known cause of secondary hyperparathyroidism and consequent high bone turnover [27]. For 25(OH)D concentrations, 50 nmol/L has been suggested as the recommended minimum for patients with osteoporosis by the European Society for Clinical and Economic Aspects of Osteoporosis and Osteoarthritis (ESCEO) [28]. They also suggest a minimum of 75 nmol/L for fracture prevention [28].

In addition to its role in regulating calcium metabolism and ensuring adequately mineralized bone, 1,25(OH)$_2$D promotes other aspects of bone health via the vitamin D receptor (VDR). This is a nuclear hormone receptor that is present throughout the body, including in bone tissue [16], and acts as a transcription factor, affecting the expression of multiple genes (Fig. 3). The 1,25(OH)$_2$D ligand binds to the VDR, which heterodimerizes with the retinoid X receptor

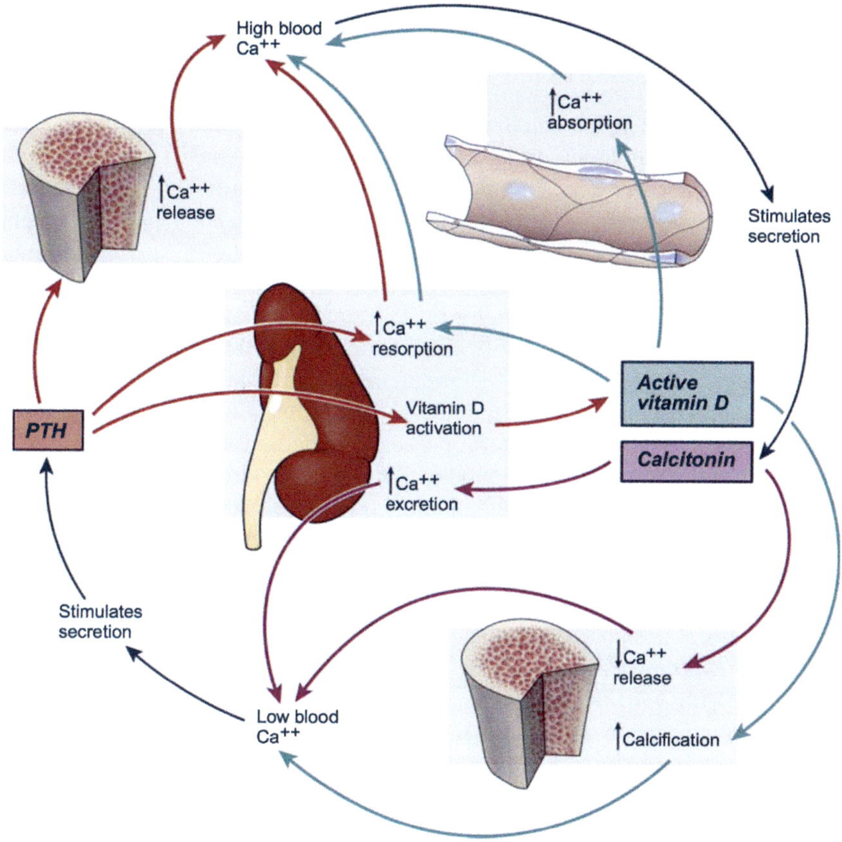

FIG. 2 Calcium metabolism. *(Reprinted from Carlson BM. The endocrine system. In: The human body: linking structure and function. Academic Press Elsevier Science & Technology; 2019. pp. 24-269 [Chapter 9], Copyright (2019), with permission from Elsevier.)*

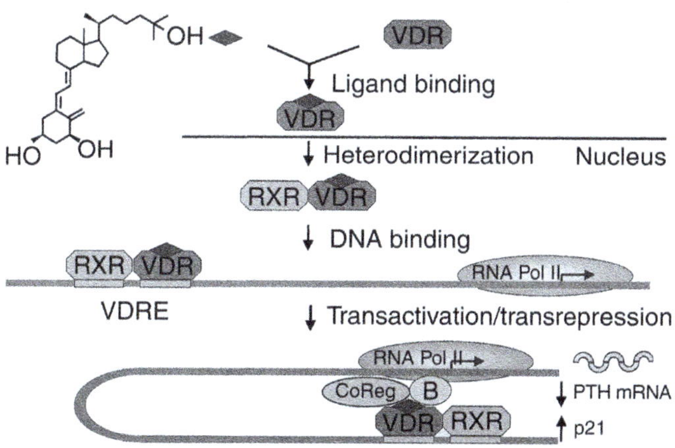

FIG. 3 1,25$(OH)_2D_3$ regulation of gene transcription. *(Reprinted from Dusso AS. Vitamin D receptor: mechanisms for vitamin D resistance in renal failure. Kidney Int 2003;63(Suppl 85):S6–9, Copyright (2003), with permission from Elsevier.)*

(RXR) [29]. It then binds to vitamin D response elements (VDRE), which instigate gene transcription [29]. There are also direct effects of 1,25$(OH)_2$D on the activity of bone cells, which affects calcium transport and signaling of other molecules [16] with knock-on effects on bone tissue function.

There is some evidence that vitamin D supplementation improves bone strength. For example, one peripheral Quantitative Computer Tomography (pQCT) study found that vitamin D supplementation slowed decline in tibial cortical thickness in postmenopausal women [30]. In another pQCT study, there was a benefit of supplementation for bone microarchitectural strength (e.g., trabeculae) but not for overall areal BMD [31]. In terms of DXA studies, one study found that a 1000 IU/d vitamin D supplement attenuated hip bone loss [32], with a secondary analysis of this data showing that vitamin D supplementation only benefited BMD when the participants had a 25(OH)D concentration of $\leq$30 nmol/L [33]. However, another DXA study found a detrimental effect of high dose vitamin D supplementation (4000–10,000 IU/d) on BMD [34]. Moreover, some studies have found no beneficial effect of vitamin D supplementation on BMD [35–39], including two mendelian randomization studies which have found no causal relationship between 25(OH)D concentration and neither femoral neck nor lumbar spine BMD [40] nor total body BMD [41].

For osteoporotic fracture, there has been a relatively large amount of research showing an inverse association between 25(OH)D concentration and fracture prevalence. In observational studies, lower serum 25(OH)D has been associated with higher fracture risk, for hip fracture [42,43], all fractures combined [43] and for faster BMD loss [42]. However, if individuals are calcium deficient then calcium may also need to be supplemented for vitamin D supplements to be able to benefit bone health. A systematic review and meta analysis of randomized controlled trials found that 800 IU of vitamin D and 1200 mg of calcium per day were effective in reducing fracture risk (RR = 0.87 (95% CI 0.77–0.97)) and slowing hip BMD loss in adults aged 50 years or older [44]. Similar results were found in a meta analysis by Avenell et al. (2014) who found a benefit of vitamin D supplementation on fracture prevention in older men and women, but only when calcium was also supplemented [45]. However, some fracture risk systematic reviews and metaanalyses still show no effect of vitamin D supplementation (with or without calcium) on fracture risk in community-dwelling older adults [46] or suggest that only those with specific risk factors should be supplemented [47]. Overall, the situation is complicated in that vitamin D supplements may only reduce fracture risk when calcium is also supplemented [48] and may only benefit certain high-risk groups, such as older people living in institutions [48].

Vitamin D and sarcopenia

Vitamin D, via the VDR, is critical for normal myocyte function [49]. In animals, myocyte-specific vitamin D receptor (mVDR) null mice have been shown to have poor muscle function and sarcopenia [49].

Human studies have assessed whether 25(OH)D concentration is associated with either muscle strength or diagnosed sarcopenia. In observational studies, one study found that in older men, and in both sexes at a very advanced age, low baseline of 25(OH)D may be associated with an increased decline in muscle strength [50]. In sarcopenic older adults, lower overall muscle mass [51] and increased loss of lean mass [52] have been associated with lower 25(OH)D concentration. Two studies found an association between 25(OH)D and sarcopenia or skeletal mass in women only [53,54]. In older adults (60 years or over) 25(OH)D concentrations <40 nmol/L were associated with worse musculoskeletal function than those with 40–94 nmol/L [55]. Another study found increased odds of sarcopenia in middle-aged and older men and women with lower 25(OH)D concentrations [56].

Alternatively, some studies have found that 25(OH)D concentration is only associated with one type of muscle strength. For example, Meng et al. (2017) found no association between 25(OH)D and appendicular muscle mass, but there was a positive association with grip strength [57]. However, one study found an association between low 25(OH)D and reduced muscle mass and poorer physical performance but not frank sarcopenia itself [58]. Finally, a systematic review and meta analysis of observational studies found lower 25(OH)D concentrations in sarcopenic adults than nonsarcopenic controls [59]. Of note, some studies have found no association between 25(OH)D concentration and muscle strength or function. For example, one study found no association between grip strength in men and women over 50 years old [60]. Similarly, in men aged 40–79 years, another study found that 25(OH)D was not associated with the annual change in grip strength, gait speed, or appendicular lean mass or incident sarcopenia [61].

There have been few vitamin D supplementation trials assessing sarcopenia as an outcome, but one trial found that vitamin D supplementation led to improved appendicular muscle mass but there was no increase in grip strength in presarcopenic older men and women [62]. Another trial found improved muscle strength and reduced loss of muscle mass in postmenopausal women [63]. However, one trial in 45–60-year old early postmenopausal women found no effect of vitamin D supplementation on muscle mass or muscle strength [64]. Similarly, another trial in 50–79-year-olds found no effect of vitamin D supplementation of 50,000 IU monthly for 1 year on trunk muscle function [65].

Vitamin D and osteosarcopenia

There are no human observational studies or randomized controlled trials to date assessing the association between vitamin D and osteosarcopenia as a syndrome in itself [66]. There are only separate studies on vitamin D and osteoporosis, or vitamin D and sarcopenia (as discussed above). However, recent research in vitamin D deficient, senescence-accelerated mouse prone 6 (SAMP6)rodents (who have both senile osteoporosis and muscle aging, so are a potential model for osteosarcopenia) has found a higher grip strength and muscle mass in those exposed to UVB radiation than in those not exposed to UVB radiation [67]. This suggests that dermal vitamin D production leads to improved muscle strength in vitamin D deficient aged rodents. However, may have been other biological effects from the radiation itself that are not linked with vitamin D production which may explain the enhanced muscle strength. The authors of the above paper suggest that UVB irradiation may help improve function in those with osteosarcopenia [67]. However, it is unclear as to whether similar observations would be seen in humans, and whether oral dosing of vitamin D would have the same effects.

A recent human study found beneficial effects of resistance training on function in older men with osteosarcopenia, when supplemented with vitamin D and protein [68]. However, as all participants were supplemented with vitamin D it is not possible to show whether the exercise effect was dependent on vitamin D or not. Finally, in kidney transplant patients, vitamin D concentration has not been found to be predictive of having osteosarcopenia or not, once confounders such as age and physical activity levels were controlled for [69]. Therefore, there is only limited literature on the subject and the results are conflicting.

PTH, osteoporosis, sarcopenia and osteosarcopenia

Human parathyroid hormone is an approved treatment for osteoporosis, with a systematic review and meta analysis demonstrating increased BMD at all skeletal sites after administration of PTH treatment, except for the radius [70]. Although long-term high PTH concentrations are detrimental to the bone, intermittent administered PTH actually increases osteoblast activity and number [71]. In terms of endogenous, long-term exposures to high PTH, in older people, increased PTH concentration and lower 25(OH)D have been associated with being sarcopenic [72–74] and longitudinal data shows that lower baseline 25(OH)D in older men is associated with higher sarcopenia incidence over 5 years [75]. Sarcopenic obesity [76] and frailty [77] are associated with higher PTH and lower 25(OH)D. One study found an association between PTH and sarcopenia in men only [53]. However, another study assessing both men and women found no association between PTH and odds of sarcopenia after BMI adjustment [56].

As discussed above, high PTH is associated with osteoporosis and sarcopenia as separate entities. However, it is unclear as to whether PTH is associated with the development of osteosarcopenia [78]. Few research publications have specifically assessed PTH and osteosarcopenia, rather than just osteoporosis and sarcopenia separately. One cross-sectional study found that persons with osteosarcopenia had a higher PTH than those with just sarcopenia, just osteoporosis or neither osteoporosis nor sarcopenia [78]. Similarly, the osteosarcopenia group had higher falls susceptibility than the other groups when PTH was high (>6.8 pmol/L) [78].

Vitamin D, PTH, bone, and muscle interactions

There is much cross-talk between muscle and bone. The muscle provides the mechanical stimulus that regulates bone modeling [79]. There is also non mechanical communication between muscle and bone. For instance, muscle releases a series of mediators such as IGF-1, myostatin, osteoglycin, FAM5C, irisin, osteonectin, FGF2, IL-6, IL-7, IL-15, and MMP-2, which have an effect on bone metabolism [13]. Equally, bone releases mediators such as IGF-1, sclerostin, osteocalcin, MGF, VEGF, and HGF [13]. Both sarcopenia and osteopenia/osteoporosis share common antecedent factors, such as aging, genetics, estrogen, physical activity, 25(OH)D, and anthropometry (Fig. 4) [80]. Moreover, as discussed above, long-term vitamin D deficiency and high PTH concentration negatively affect both muscle and bone health. More research is required into the associations between sarcopenia, osteopenia/osteoporosis, and osteosarcopenia, in order to develop and tailor the correct treatments for the right individuals, and to instigate effective prevention strategies in populations.

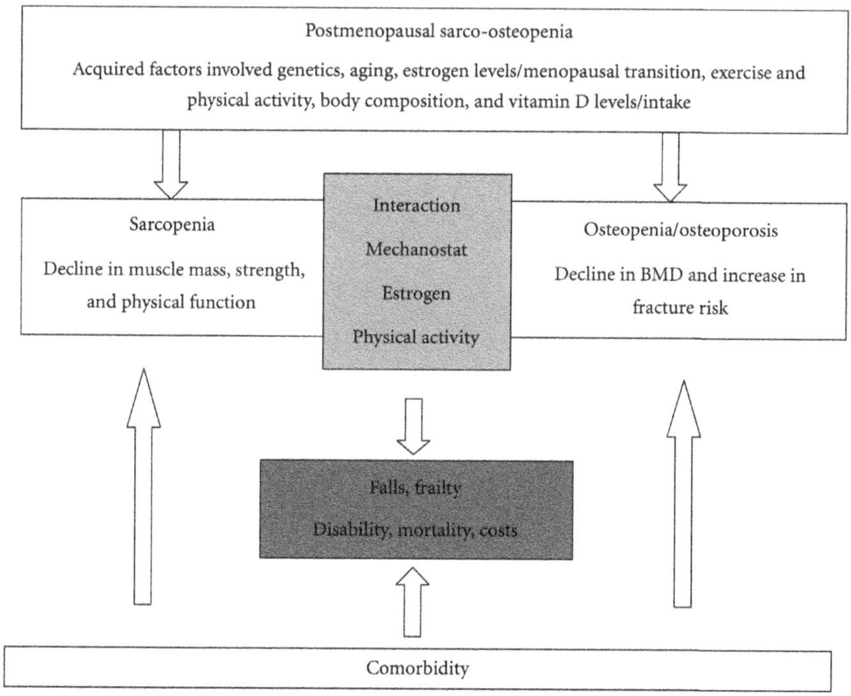

FIG. 4 Sarcopenia, osteoporosis/osteopenia and frailty. *(Reproduced from Sirola J, Kroger H. Similarities in acquired factors related to postmenopausal osteoporosis and sarcopenia. J Osteoporos 2011;2011:536735 under a Creative Commons Attributions License (CC-BY-3.0).)*

Conclusion

PTH and 1,25$(OH)_2$D are key players in the regulation of calcium concentration in the body, with concomitant effects on muscle and bone health. Genomic effects are also exerted widely on muscle and bone by 1,25$(OH)_2$D, via the VDR. Almost all trials of vitamin D supplementation have shown either a beneficial effect or no effect, of vitamin D on indices of bone and muscle health. A high PTH concentration is usually, but not always, associated in research studies with poorer bone and muscle health outcomes. However, intermittent, exogenous PTH treatment is beneficial for bone health. Few studies have assessed the relationship between vitamin D, PTH, and osteosarcopenia as a specific clinical entity. It is therefore unclear as to what extent vitamin D deficiency and high PTH concentration affect the development of osteosarcopenia specifically and more research is urgently needed into this topic.

References

[1] Cruz-Jentoft AJ, Bahat G, Bauer J, et al. Sarcopenia: revised European consensus on definition and diagnosis. Age Ageing 2019;48:601.

[2] Cruz-Jentoft AJ, Sayer AA. Sarcopenia. Lancet 2019;393:2636–46.

[3] Anagnostis P, Gkekas NK, Achilla C, et al. Type 2 diabetes mellitus is associated with increased risk of sarcopenia: a systematic review and meta-analysis. Calcif Tissue Int 2020;107:453–63.

[4] Suzuki T, Palus S, Springer J. Skeletal muscle wasting in chronic heart failure. ESC Heart Fail 2018;5:1099–107.

[5] Kang SY, Lim GE, Kim YK, et al. Association between Sarcopenic obesity and metabolic syndrome in postmenopausal women: a cross-sectional study based on the Korean National Health and nutritional examination surveys from 2008 to 2011. J Bone Metab 2017;24:9–14.

[6] Peeters CM, Visser E, Van de Ree CL, et al. Quality of life after hip fracture in the elderly: a systematic literature review. Injury 2016;47:1369–82.

[7] Ong T, Kantachuvesiri P, Sahota O, et al. Characteristics and outcomes of hospitalised patients with vertebral fragility fractures: a systematic review. Age Ageing 2018;47:17–25.

[8] Veronese N, Maggi S. Epidemiology and social costs of hip fracture. Injury 2018;49:1458–60.

[9] Ercin E, Bilgili MG, Sari C, et al. Risk factors for mortality in geriatric hip fractures: a compressional study of different surgical procedures in 785 consecutive patients. Eur J Orthop Surg Traumatol 2017;27:101–6.

[10] Kirk B, Zanker J, Duque G. Osteosarcopenia: epidemiology, diagnosis, and treatment-facts and numbers. J Cachexia Sarcopenia Muscle 2020;11:609–18.

[11] Fahimfar N, Zahedi Tajrishi F, Gharibzadeh S, et al. Prevalence of osteosarcopenia and its association with cardiovascular risk factors in Iranian older people: Bushehr elderly health (BEH) program. Calcif Tissue Int 2020;106:364–70.

[12] Wang YJ, Wang Y, Zhan JK, et al. Sarco-osteoporosis: prevalence and association with frailty in Chinese community-dwelling older adults. Int J Endocrinol 2015;2015, 482940.

[13] Hirschfeld HP, Kinsella R, Duque G. Osteosarcopenia: where bone, muscle, and fat collide. Osteoporos Int 2017;28:2781–90.

[14] Balogun S, Winzenberg T, Wills K, et al. Prospective associations of osteosarcopenia and osteodynapenia with incident fracture and mortality over 10 years in community-dwelling older adults. Arch Gerontol Geriatr 2019;82:67–73.

[15] Scott D, Seibel M, Cumming R, et al. Does combined osteopenia/osteoporosis and sarcopenia confer greater risk of falls and fracture than either condition alone in older men? The Concord health and ageing in men project. J Gerontol A Biol Sci Med Sci 2019;74:827–34.
[16] Bikle DD. Vitamin D and bone. Curr Osteoporos Rep 2012;10:151–9.
[17] Ceglia L, Harris SS. Vitamin D and its role in skeletal muscle. Calcif Tissue Int 2013;92:151–62.
[18] van Schoor N, Lips P. Global overview of vitamin D status. Endocrinol Metab Clin N Am 2017;46:845–70.
[19] Seamans KM, Cashman KD. Existing and potentially novel functional markers of vitamin D status: a systematic review. Am J Clin Nutr 2009;89:1997S–2008S.
[20] Holick MF. Vitamin D deficiency. N Engl J Med 2007;357:266–81.
[21] Calvo MS, Whiting SJ, Barton CN. Vitamin D intake: a global perspective of current status. J Nutr 2005;135:310–6.
[22] Hilger J, Friedel A, Herr R, et al. A systematic review of vitamin D status in populations worldwide. Br J Nutr 2014;111:23–45.
[23] EFSA. Scientific opinion on dietary reference values for vitamin D., 2016, https://www.efsa.europa.eu/sites/default/files/consultation/160321.pdf. [Accessed 20 August 2017].
[24] Nakamura K, Nishiwaki T, Ueno K, et al. Serum 25-hydroxyvitamin D levels and activities of daily living in noninstitutionalized elderly Japanese requiring care. J Bone Miner Metab 2005;23:488–94.
[25] MacLaughlin J, Holick MF. Aging decreases the capacity of human skin to produce vitamin D3. J Clin Invest 1985;76:1536–8.
[26] Chel VG, Ooms ME, Popp-Snijders C, et al. Ultraviolet irradiation corrects vitamin D deficiency and suppresses secondary hyperparathyroidism in the elderly. J Bone Miner Res 1998;13:1238–42.
[27] Lips P. Vitamin D deficiency and secondary hyperparathyroidism in the elderly: consequences for bone loss and fractures and therapeutic implications. Endocr Rev 2001;22:477–501.
[28] Rizzoli R, Boonen S, Brandi ML, et al. Vitamin D supplementation in elderly or postmenopausal women: a 2013 update of the 2008 recommendations from the European Society for Clinical and Economic Aspects of osteoporosis and osteoarthritis (ESCEO). Curr Med Res Opin 2013;29:305–13.
[29] Dusso AS. Vitamin D receptor: mechanisms for vitamin D resistance in renal failure. Kidney Int 2003;63(Suppl 85):S6–9.
[30] Pop LC, Sukumar D, Schneider SH, et al. Three doses of vitamin D, bone mineral density, and geometry in older women during modest weight control in a 1-year randomized controlled trial. Osteoporos Int 2017;28:377–88.
[31] Bislev LS, Langagergaard Rodbro L, Rolighed L, et al. Bone microstructure in response to vitamin D3 supplementation: a randomized placebo-controlled trial. Calcif Tissue Int 2019;104:160–70.
[32] Macdonald HM, Wood AD, Aucott LS, et al. Hip bone loss is attenuated with 1000 IU but not 400 IU daily vitamin D3: a 1-year double-blind RCT in postmenopausal women. J Bone Miner Res 2013;28:2202–13.
[33] Macdonald HM, Reid IR, Gamble GD, et al. 25-Hydroxyvitamin D threshold for the effects of vitamin D supplements on bone density: secondary analysis of a randomized controlled trial. J Bone Miner Res 2018;33:1464–9.
[34] Burt LA, Billington EO, Rose MS, et al. Effect of high-dose vitamin D supplementation on volumetric bone density and bone strength: a randomized clinical trial. JAMA 2019;322:736–45.
[35] Lerchbaum E, Trummer C, Theiler-Schwetz V, et al. Effects of vitamin D supplementation on bone turnover and bone mineral density in healthy men: a post-hoc analysis of a randomized controlled trial. Nutrients 2019;11:731.

[36] Aloia J, Fazzari M, Islam S, et al. Vitamin D supplementation in elderly black women does not prevent bone loss: a randomized controlled trial. J Bone Miner Res 2018;33:1916–22.
[37] Aspray TJ, Chadwick T, Francis RM, et al. Randomized controlled trial of vitamin D supplementation in older people to optimize bone health. Am J Clin Nutr 2019;109:207–17.
[38] LeBoff MS, Chou SH, Murata EM, et al. Effects of supplemental vitamin D on bone health outcomes in women and men in the VITamin D and OmegA-3 TriaL (VITAL). J Bone Miner Res 2020;35:883–93.
[39] Cooper L, Clifton-Bligh PB, Nery ML, et al. Vitamin D supplementation and bone mineral density in early postmenopausal women. Am J Clin Nutr 2003;77:1324–9.
[40] Larsson SC, Melhus H, Michaelsson K. Circulating serum 25-Hydroxyvitamin D levels and bone mineral density: Mendelian randomization study. J Bone Miner Res 2018;33:840–4.
[41] Sun JY, Zhao M, Hou Y, et al. Circulating serum vitamin D levels and total body bone mineral density: a Mendelian randomization study. J Cell Mol Med 2019;23:2268–71.
[42] Swanson CM, Srikanth P, Lee CG, et al. Associations of 25-hydroxyvitamin D and 1,25-dihydroxyvitamin D with bone mineral density, bone mineral density change, and incident nonvertebral fracture. J Bone Miner Res 2015;30:1403–13.
[43] Feng Y, Cheng G, Wang H, et al. The associations between serum 25-hydroxyvitamin D level and the risk of total fracture and hip fracture. Osteoporos Int 2017;28:1641–52.
[44] Tang BM, Eslick GD, Nowson C, et al. Use of calcium or calcium in combination with vitamin D supplementation to prevent fractures and bone loss in people aged 50 years and older: a meta-analysis. Lancet 2007;370:657–66.
[45] Avenell A, Mak JC, O'Connell D. Vitamin D and vitamin D analogues for preventing fractures in post-menopausal women and older men. Cochrane Database Syst Rev 2014;2014, CD000227.
[46] Zhao JG, Zeng XT, Wang J, et al. Association between calcium or vitamin D supplementation and fracture incidence in community-dwelling older adults: a systematic review and meta-analysis. JAMA 2017;318:2466–82.
[47] Reid IR, Bolland MJ, Grey A. Effects of vitamin D supplements on bone mineral density: a systematic review and meta-analysis. Lancet 2014;383:146–55.
[48] Chung M, Lee J, Terasawa T, et al. Vitamin D with or without calcium supplementation for prevention of cancer and fractures: an updated meta-analysis for the U.S. preventive services task force. Ann Intern Med 2011;155:827–38.
[49] Girgis CM, Cha KM, So B, et al. Mice with myocyte deletion of vitamin D receptor have sarcopenia and impaired muscle function. J Cachexia Sarcopenia Muscle 2019;10:1228–40.
[50] Granic A, Hill TR, Davies K, et al. Vitamin D status, muscle strength and physical performance decline in very old adults: a prospective study. Nutrients 2017;9:379.
[51] Verlaan S, Maier AB, Bauer JM, et al. Sufficient levels of 25-hydroxyvitamin D and protein intake required to increase muscle mass in sarcopenic older adults – the PROVIDE study. Clin Nutr 2018;37:551–7.
[52] Hwang J, Zmuda JM, Kuipers AL, et al. Serum vitamin D and age-related muscle loss in Afro-Caribbean men: the importance of age and diabetic status. J Frailty Aging 2019;8:131–7.
[53] Park S, Ham JO, Lee BK. A positive association of vitamin D deficiency and sarcopenia in 50 year old women, but not men. Clin Nutr 2014;33:900–5.
[54] Iannuzzi-Sucich M, Prestwood KM, Kenny AM. Prevalence of sarcopenia and predictors of skeletal muscle mass in healthy, older men and women. J Gerontol A Biol Sci Med Sci 2002;57:M772–7.
[55] Bischoff-Ferrari HA, Dietrich T, Orav EJ, et al. Higher 25-hydroxyvitamin D concentrations are associated with better lower-extremity function in both active and inactive persons aged > or =60 y. Am J Clin Nutr 2004;80:752–8.

[56] Kim MK, Baek KH, Song KH, et al. Vitamin D deficiency is associated with sarcopenia in older Koreans, regardless of obesity: the fourth Korea National Health and nutrition examination surveys (KNHANES IV) 2009. J Clin Endocrinol Metab 2011;96:3250–6.

[57] Meng L, Man Q, Yuan L, et al. Serum 25-hydroxyvitamin D and elderly skeletal muscle mass and function in urban North China. Asia Pac J Clin Nutr 2017;26:849–55.

[58] Conzade R, Grill E, Bischoff-Ferrari HA, et al. Vitamin D in relation to incident sarcopenia and changes in muscle parameters among older adults: the KORA-age study. Calcif Tissue Int 2019;105:173–82.

[59] Luo J, Quan Z, Lin S, et al. The association between blood concentration of 25- hydroxyvitamin D and sarcopenia: a meta-analysis. Asia Pac J Clin Nutr 2018;27:1258–70.

[60] Kim BJ, Kwak MK, Lee SH, et al. Lack of association between vitamin D and hand grip strength in Asians: a nationwide population-based study. Calcif Tissue Int 2019;104:152–9.

[61] Gielen E, O'Neill TW, Pye SR, et al. Endocrine determinants of incident sarcopenia in middle-aged and elderly European men. J Cachexia Sarcopenia Muscle 2015;6:242–52.

[62] El Hajj C, Fares S, Chardigny JM, et al. Vitamin D supplementation and muscle strength in pre-sarcopenic elderly Lebanese people: a randomized controlled trial. Arch Osteoporos 2018;14:4.

[63] Cangussu LM, Nahas-Neto J, Orsatti CL, et al. Effect of vitamin D supplementation alone on muscle function in postmenopausal women: a randomized, double-blind, placebo-controlled clinical trial. Osteoporos Int 2015;26:2413–21.

[64] Suebthawinkul C, Panyakhamlerd K, Yotnuengnit P, et al. The effect of vitamin D2 supplementation on muscle strength in early postmenopausal women: a randomized, double-blind, placebo-controlled trial. Climacteric 2018;21:491–7.

[65] Cuellar WA, Blizzard L, Hides JA, et al. Vitamin D supplements for trunk muscle morphology in older adults: secondary analysis of a randomized controlled trial. J Cachexia Sarcopenia Muscle 2019;10:177–87.

[66] Bruyere O, Cavalier E, Reginster JY. Vitamin D and osteosarcopenia: an update from epidemiological studies. Curr Opin Clin Nutr Metab Care 2017;20:498–503.

[67] Makida K, Nishida Y, Morita D, et al. Low energy irradiation of narrow-range UV-LED prevents osteosarcopenia associated with vitamin D deficiency in senescence-accelerated mouse prone 6. Sci Rep 2020;10:11892.

[68] Lichtenberg T, von Stengel S, Sieber C, et al. The favorable effects of a high-intensity resistance training on sarcopenia in older community-dwelling men with osteosarcopenia: the randomized controlled FrOST study. Clin Interv Aging 2019;14:2173–86.

[69] Yanishi M, Kinoshita H, Tsukaguchi H, et al. Factors related to Osteosarcopenia in kidney transplant recipients. Transplant Proc 2018;50:3371–5.

[70] Cranney A, Papaioannou A, Zytaruk N, et al. Parathyroid hormone for the treatment of osteoporosis: a systematic review. CMAJ 2006;175:52–9.

[71] Cochenski Borba NZ, Pietszkowski Mañas PC. The use of PTH in the treatment of osteoporosis. Arq Bras Endocrinol Metabol 2010;54(2):213–9.

[72] Chang WT, Wu CH, Hsu LW, et al. Serum vitamin D, intact parathyroid hormone, and Fetuin A concentrations were associated with geriatric sarcopenia and cardiac hypertrophy. Sci Rep 2017;7:40996.

[73] de Souza GP, de Medeiros PM, Szejnfeld VL, et al. Secondary hyperparathyroidism and its relationship with sarcopenia in elderly women. Arch Gerontol Geriatr 2015;60:349–53.

[74] Visser M, Deeg DJ, Lips P, et al. Low vitamin D and high parathyroid hormone levels as determinants of loss of muscle strength and muscle mass (sarcopenia): the longitudinal aging study Amsterdam. J Clin Endocrinol Metab 2003;88:5766–72.

[75] Hirani V, Cumming RG, Naganathan V, et al. Longitudinal associations between vitamin D metabolites and sarcopenia in older Australian men: the Concord health and aging in men project. J Gerontol A Biol Sci Med Sci 2017;73:131–8.
[76] Huo YR, Suriyaarachchi P, Gomez F, et al. Phenotype of sarcopenic obesity in older individuals with a history of falling. Arch Gerontol Geriatr 2016;65:255–9.
[77] Tajar A, Lee DM, Pye SR, et al. The association of frailty with serum 25-hydroxyvitamin D and parathyroid hormone levels in older European men. Age Ageing 2013;42:352–9.
[78] Suriyaarachchi P, Gomez F, Curcio CL, et al. High parathyroid hormone levels are associated with osteosarcopenia in older individuals with a history of falling. Maturitas 2018;113:21–5.
[79] Frost HM. Bone's mechanostat: a 2003 update. Anat Rec A Discov Mol Cell Evol Biol 2003;275:1081–101.
[80] Sirola J, Kroger H. Similarities in acquired factors related to postmenopausal osteoporosis and sarcopenia. J Osteoporos 2011;2011, 536735.

Chapter 9

Falls and fracture risk assessment—The role of osteoporosis, obesity, and sarcopenia

Neema Sharda[a] and Cathleen Colón-Emeric[a,b]

[a]*Geriatrics Division, Department of Medicine, Duke University, Durham, NC, United States,*
[b]*Durham VA Geriatric Research Education and Clinical Center, Durham, NC, United States*

Introduction

As discussed in prior chapters, osteosarcopenia is a geriatric syndrome resulting in falls and fractures as two of its common manifestations. Falls and fractures are consistently among the most frequent reasons for acute care use among older adults, and as a result have a major impact on individuals, families, and society. One out of five falls is injurious, resulting in fracture or head injury [1,2]. Both fractures and head trauma in older adults are associated with increased disability, mortality, and decreased quality of life. In 2010, the medical cost of osteoporotic fractures in Europe was over €37 billion, and this cost is expected to increase by 25% in 2025 [3]. By 2025, the annual medical cost of osteoporotic fractures in the United States is expected to be $25.3 billion [4].

In light of the high burden of falls and fractures, substantial efforts have been made to develop effective screening and prevention strategies. Clinical practice guidelines for treating osteoporosis and preventing falls in older adults have been written and widely disseminated. However, these efforts have largely considered osteoporosis and fall as separate geriatric syndromes in their own right, and have not considered how their overlapping pathogenesis and epidemiology should impact the screening and treatment for the other.

In this chapter, we describe the synergistic contributions of osteoporosis, obesity, and sarcopenia to the epidemiology of falls and fractures in older adults. We define important components of validated risk assessment tools for falls and fractures and point out opportunities to improve their predictive ability

Osteosarcopenia. https://doi.org/10.1016/B978-0-12-820088-9.00004-4

by incorporating markers of both muscle and bone quality. Finally, we highlight the potential of interventions targeting osteosarcopenia to have a pleiotropic impact on falls and fractures in older adults.

Overlapping epidemiology of sarcopenia, osteoporosis, falls, and fractures

Available epidemiology suggests a synergistic and bi-directional relationship between sarcopenia and osteoporosis, falls, and fractures. The association between sarcopenia and subsequent falls has been consistently described, with a recent metaanalysis estimating an 89% higher odds in prospective studies (OR 1.89, 95% CI 1.33–2.68) [5]. Similarly, there is an increased risk of falls among obese individuals in metaanalyses of prospective studies (OR 1.16, 95% CI 1.07–1.26) [6]. Perhaps less well recognized, the odds of fracture are also greater in sarcopenic older adults (OR 1.84, 95% CI 1.30–2.62), even in studies adjusting for bone mineral density (BMD) [5]. This temporal relationship goes both ways. Fractures, especially hip and vertebral, are associated with a subsequent loss in both bone mineral density (BMD) and muscle mass [7]. While the loss of muscle mass and BMD has not been well studied following a fall, activity restriction and declines in physical performance after falls have been well described [8,9], and are likely related in part to the loss of muscle due to deconditioning.

Osteoporosis and falls have an especially important synergistic effect with each other. For example, in a study of more than 2600 women in Europe, women with osteoporosis but without a prior fall had an age- and BMI-adjusted fracture risk that was 2.8 times higher than women with neither. However, women with both osteoporosis and a history of falls had an adjusted fracture risk nearly 25 times higher [10]. The risk of mortality in hip fracture patients is also higher in osteosarcopenic patients compared to those with osteoporosis or sarcopenia alone [11].

Risk assessment: An opportunity for prevention

The underlying common pathophysiology and synergistic, bi-directional relationship between osteoporosis, sarcopenia, falls, and fractures provides an opportunity for streamlined risk assessment and prevention for these conditions simultaneously in clinical care. Fall and fracture risk assessment in older adults should include a medication review and identification of chronic medical conditions that contribute to both osteoporosis and sarcopenia. Body composition measures offer a means of detecting osteosarcopenia, but clinical applications remain limited. Validated clinical tools are available, but have limitations that should be appreciated. Detection of osteosarcopenia is critical to decreasing falls and fractures and subsequently increasing patients' quality of life and ability to age gracefully.

Medications associated with osteosarcopenia, falls, and fractures

Medications are an important target for both screening and prevention of falls and fractures in older adults. While there are several mechanisms by which medications increase the risk of falls and fractures (e.g., sedation, orthostatic hypotension), we will focus on those that directly impact the musculoskeletal system and thus contribute to osteosarcopenia. A summary of these medication classes and how they impact muscle and bone is found in Table 1.

Glucocorticoids are commonly prescribed for prevalent conditions in older adults including rheumatoid arthritis, polymyalgia rheumatica, giant cell arthritis, inflammatory bowel disease, and chronic lung disease. Glucocorticoids negatively impact bone through a multitude of pathways and are the most common cause of secondary osteoporosis [12]. Glucocorticoids directly affect osteoblasts by altering protein synthesis and regulation. Additionally, glucocorticoids reduce the production of growth hormone and insulin-like growth factors, which are osteoblast stimulators. Glucocorticoids enhance bone resorption by increasing the production of receptor activators of nuclear factor kappa-B ligand (RANKL) and decreasing the production of osteoprotegerin. Finally, osteocytes cannot function appropriately and undergo more apoptosis with glucocorticoid treatment. Fractures are the most serious adverse effect related to chronic glucocorticoid use and are associated with an increased fracture risk as quickly as after the first dose [12–14]. Glucocorticoids impact muscle strength and promote skeletal muscle loss, leading to an increased risk of falls and fracture as well. Specifically, glucocorticoids reduce sarcolemmal excitability, decrease serum levels of creatine kinase and myoglobin, and decrease the cross-sectional area and strength of certain myofibers. Additionally, glucocorticoid-induced protein catabolism contributes to muscle atrophy [14,15].

Antidiabetic medications are another class that influences bone, muscle, and fat. Studies have suggested that metformin improves bone quality and decreases the risk of fracture. A key molecule in metformin, AMP-activated protein kinase, is thought to be effective in signaling pathways in bone physiology, having direct osteogenic effects [16–18]. Sulfonylureas increase insulin levels and may positively impact bone metabolism; for example, glimepiride enhances the proliferation of osteoblasts in animal models, though this has not been duplicated in humans. Another study, the ADOPT trial, suggests that patients treated with metformin and sulfonylureas had a similar rate of fracture; these results have been duplicated in other studies as well [16,19]. However, thiazolidinediones influence gene expression for glucose and energy metabolism in adipose tissue, liver, and muscle [16]. They activate peroxisome proliferator-activated receptor γ, suppress insulin-like growth factor, increase osteoclast formation, and decrease osteoblast formation; thus, these have been shown to increase fracture risk and decrease bone mineral density [16–18]. Dipeptidyl peptidase 4 inhibitors may positively influence bone metabolism by reducing osteoclast activity

TABLE 1 Medications and co-morbidities impacting osteosarcopenia, fall, and fracture risk.

Medication/co-morbidity	Proposed mechanism for osteosarcopenia
Medications	
Glucocorticoids	***Detrimental*** • Alters protein synthesis and regulation affecting osteoblasts • Reduces production of growth hormone and insulin-like growth factors, which are osteoblast stimulators • Increases the production of receptor activator of nuclear factor kappa-B ligand (RANKL), which increases bone resorption • Decreases production of osteoprotegerin • Causes osteocytes to function inappropriately and undergo more apoptosis • Reduces sarcolemmal excitability • Decreases serum levels of creatine kinase and myoglobin • Decreases the cross-sectional area and strength of certain myofibers • Induces protein catabolism contributing to muscle atrophy
Metformin	***Protective*** • AMP-activated protein kinase may have direct osteogenic effects
Sulfonylureas	***Protective*** • The proliferation of osteoblasts in animal models
Thiazolidinediones	***Detrimental*** • Activate peroxisome proliferator-activated receptor γ • Suppress insulin-like growth factor • Increase osteoclast formation • Decrease osteoblast formation
Dipeptidyl peptidase 4 inhibitors	***Protective*** • Reducing osteoclast activity • Promoting bone anabolism
Insulin	***Data mixed regarding protective or detrimental*** • Positive anabolic effect on bone metabolism, though clinical data suggest an increased risk of both falls and fracture
Statins	***Data mixed regarding protective or detrimental*** • Unclear mechanism of action; may positively influence bone metabolism, though not reduce fracture risk • Protective against falls but unclear if due to cardioprotective properties

TABLE 1 Medications and co-morbidities impacting osteosarcopenia, fall, and fracture risk—cont'd

Medication/co-morbidity	Proposed mechanism for osteosarcopenia
Co-morbidities	
Type 2 diabetes mellitus	• Advanced glycosylation end-products are toxic to bone tissue • Bone microvascular system is impaired • Hyperglycemia may lead to adipogenic differentiation instead of osteogenesis and enhanced apoptosis of osteoblasts
Chronic liver disease	• Imbalance between RANKL and osteoprotegerin may be related to bone turnover and poor homeostasis maintenance • Higher serum myostatin levels, which in vitro, accelerates RANKL mediated osteoclast formation
Chronic kidney disease	• Renal osteodystrophy
Rheumatoid arthritis	• Systemic inflammation adversely affects cortical and trabecular bone • Sclerostin and dickkopf-1 inhibit signaling pathways leading to reduced bone formation and regeneration • Cytokines and growth factors contribute to muscle wasting
Chronic gastrointestinal disorders (i.e., celiac disease, inflammatory bowel disease)	• Malnutrition due to malabsorption • Inflammatory cytokines such as interleukin 1 and 6 and tumor necrosis factor alfa impact bone metabolism through increasing RANKL

and promoting bone anabolism and subsequent increase in bone mineral density in mice, however human clinical data suggesting this is limited [16]. Finally, though animal studies suggest that insulin has a positive anabolic effect on bone metabolism, clinical data suggest an increased risk of both falls and fracture [20]; it is unclear if this effect in humans is direct or indirect due to hypoglycemia [16]. Insulin therapy is associated with the highest risk of fractures of all antidiabetic medications, although whether this is mediated by the higher risk of hypoglycemia and falls or direct impact on muscle or bone is not clear [21].

Statins have been thought to positively influence bone metabolism, leading to modest increases in BMD. For example, a nationwide retrospective population-based cohort study in Taiwan suggests that long term use of high-potency statins is associated with a decreased risk of osteoporosis [22]. However, other robust studies and reviews, including the JUPITER (Justification for the Use of Statins in Prevention: an Intervention Trial Evaluating Rosuvastatin), suggests that statins do not reduce fracture risk [23,24]. Though statins have been associated with decreased muscle strength and impaired balance, statins have been shown to be protective against falls. However, this may be secondary to its cardioprotective properties [25].

Chronic diseases associated with falls and fractures

The pathophysiology of certain chronic diseases places older adults at risk for changes in bone, muscle, and fat with a resulting increase in the risk of falls and fractures. These are also summarized in Table 1.

Patients with type two diabetes mellitus have an increased fracture risk despite higher BMD, due to obesity, increased risk of falls, sarcopenia, comorbidities, and antidiabetic drugs as noted above [26]. In diabetic patients, advanced glycosylation end-products are toxic to bone tissue, and their bone microvascular system is impaired [17,21,26]. In vitro, hyperglycemia leads to adipogenic differentiation instead of osteogenesis and enhanced apoptosis of osteoblasts [26,27]. Obesity increases the risk and impact of falls, immobility, inflammation, vitamin D insufficiency, and adverse effects of adipose tissue on bone remodeling. Diabetic older adults have reduced muscle strength and impaired gait, independent of peripheral neuropathy or peripheral vascular disease; literature suggests that fat infiltrates muscles, and these patients have lower muscle density [26].

Patients with chronic liver disease are also at increased risk of sarcopenia, osteoporosis, and fracture. One study in Japan revealed an association with body mass index (BMI) in chronic liver disease, and suggest that BMI should be used to predict fracture in these patients [28]. The exact mechanism remains to be elucidated; however, one hypothesis is that the imbalance between RANKL and osteoprotegerin in chronic liver disease and may be related to bone turnover and poor maintenance of bone homeostasis [29,30]. Finally, cirrhotic patients may have higher serum myostatin levels; in vitro, myostatin accelerates RANKL mediated osteoclast formation and may be related to osteoporosis [28]. Sarcopenia has been well-described with chronic liver disease, and is likely related to this increased myostatin, impaired mitochondrial function, and impaired fatty oxidation related to hyperammonemia [31].

It is well known that chronic kidney disease, mainly stages 3–5, is associated with increased fall and fractures in the setting of muscle weakness, neuropathy, polypharmacy, and renal osteodystrophy. The literature and the Kidney Disease: Improving Global Outcomes (KDIGO) guidelines support BMD testing to assess fracture risk in patients with CKD stage 3a to 5 if it will impact treatment decisions [32,33].

Rheumatoid arthritis is also associated with an increased risk of osteoporotic fractures, not only because of treatment with steroids but also due to systemic inflammation. The effects of systemic inflammation adversely affect cortical and trabecular bone [34,35]; sclerostin and dickkopf-1 inhibit signaling pathways leading to reduced bone formation and regeneration [36,37]. Muscle loss and adverse fat distribution also impact BMD in these patients [34,35]. Limited studies suggest that cytokines and growth factors contribute to muscle wasting [38].

Finally, chronic gastrointestinal disorders are associated with osteoporosis and subsequently increased fracture risk. For example, patients with Celiac Disease who have persistent duodenal villous atrophy have increased fracture risk [39]. Inflammatory bowel diseases (IBD) lend to malnutrition, for example, vitamin D and calcium deficiencies, and increase the risk of falling, developing osteoporosis, and sustaining fractures. Additionally, inflammatory cytokines such as interleukin 1 and 6 and tumor necrosis factor α may impact bone metabolism through increasing RANKL, which induces bone resorption [40].

Clinical tools to estimate fall and fracture risk

There are several validated clinical tools that allow the clinician to assess the risk of falls and fracture risks. For example, the FRAX (Fracture Risk Assessment) integrates risks associated with clinical risk factors and medications (including some with overlapping muscle/bone impacts discussed above such as rheumatoid arthritis, glucocorticoids, type 1 diabetes, chronic liver disease, malabsorption, and glucocorticoids) and BMI or BMD at the femoral neck. It is widely generalizable as it was developed from studying population-based cohorts from Europe, North America, Asia, and Australia. The FRAX predicts the 10-year probability of hip fracture and of a major osteoporotic fracture, adjusting for survival probability [41,42]. Notably, FRAX does not include a history of falls which is consistently one of the strongest risk factors for fracture as outlined above and does not provide any assessment of muscle strength or function. The Garvan tool, in contrast, is driven largely by age, BMD, and fall history, and is highly predictive in an Australian cohort. When compared in a separate validation cohort, both calculators have similar, moderate predictive ability with AUCs between 0.60 and 0.70; the 2 tools over- or underestimated fractures variably for different populations, and neither was significantly better than age and BMD alone [43]. The International Osteoporosis Foundation and International Society for Clinical Densitometry have published a position statement suggesting that a history of falls and frailty (which is highly associated with sarcopenia) should ideally be added to FRAX in the future and that in the meantime clinicians should consider these risk factors in addition to the FRAX score [44].

A commonly used tool to evaluate sarcopenia is the SARC-F questionnaire; its components are strength, assistance with walking, rise from a chair, climb stairs, and falls. Scores range from 0 to 10, and a score greater than four is predictive of sarcopenia [45]. This screening tool is useful to prompt the clinician to pursue further diagnostic testing [46]. Validation in some populations has suggested an association with subsequent disability, quality of life, and mortality [47], and the SARC-F score has added predictive value above FRAX for hip fracture risk [48].

The Centers for Disease Control and Prevention developed the "Stopping Elderly Accidents, Deaths and Injuries" (STEADI) initiative for healthcare providers to reduce fall risk. This toolkit has materials to help providers screen to identify older adults at increased fall risk, assess modifiable risk factors, and intervene with effective, evidence-based strategies. While outcome studies of multifactorial interventions have been mixed with regards to fall rates, fall-related injuries, and time of benefit, STEADI has been shown to be feasible and trends toward a decrease in fall-related hospitalizations [49–51]. Notably, the 12-question self-assessment screening tool suggested by STEADI includes only 2 questions related to sarcopenia (difficulty rising from a chair without using arms, difficulty stepping onto a curve), but no questions related to fractures or bone density or the medications/medical conditions related to muscle and bone loss.

Tests to assess muscle quality and quantity exist but are not yet highly utilized clinically. For example, bioelectrical impedance analysis estimates fat-free mass; peripheral quantitative computerized tomography estimates bone structure, muscle cross-sectional area, intramuscular adipose tissue; magnetic resonance imaging measures small muscle volume; and finally, the D3-creatine dilution method measures muscle mass and has shown a strong relationship with falls and fractures in older men [52]. However, these are relatively expensive, may use radiation, and their optimal use in clinical care has not been defined.

In contrast, physical performance tests are a simple, safe indicator of muscle strength and function that are suggested screening tests for older adults. Gait speed has a U-shaped association with falls, such that participants with faster (≥ 1.3 m/s) and slower (<0.6 m/s) gait speeds are at higher risk than those with normal gait speeds [53]. In contrast, gait speed has a linear relationship with hip fracture risk [54], suggesting that the falls in the high gait speed adults may be related to increased physical activity and opportunities for noninjurious falls. The Timed Up and Go (TUG) test is another commonly used screening test that assess hip flexor strength, gait speed, and balance. A metaanalysis suggests that this has poor sensitivity but reasonable specificity in identifying fallers, and its predictive value for future falls is limited [55]. The Short Portable Performance Battery and the Performance-Oriented Mobility Assessment have the modest discriminative ability for fallers vs nonfallers and subsequent falls [56], but their predictive ability for subsequent fracture has not been well defined.

Potential for pleiotropic interventions to reduce both falls and fractures

Because of their clinical overlap, there is a potential for interventions that optimize the interplay between bone, muscle, and fat to subsequently decrease the risk of both falls and fractures. Nutritional interventions are of interest to many older adults. Increased protein consumption not only improves muscle mass but also may protect lumbar spine bone mineral density, especially during weight loss in obese older adults [52,57]. Vitamin D is essential for muscle function and osteoblast activity, and several studies also support calcium and vitamin D supplementation (if meeting dietary recommendations) to reduce fall and fracture risk in the general population [58]. The role of vitamin D in the pathogenesis and treatment of osteosarcopenia is summarized in Chapter 8 of this book.

Resistance and aerobic exercise have the most evidence for a pleiotropic beneficial impact on reducing age-related lean muscle mass and BMD loss. Specifically, resistance exercises stimulate osteoblastogenesis and muscle protein synthesis, which improves bone microarchitecture, muscle mass, strength, and functional capacity. Additionally, physical activity prevents intramuscular adipose tissue increases and its negative impact on muscle quality [52,57]. There is strong evidence from randomized trials linking exercise interventions for both community-dwelling and institutionalized older adults to decrease falls, and at least in some studies, fractures [59–61]. Whole body vibration on portable platforms has been studied as an alternative to weight-bearing exercise in light of the difficulty in sustaining exercise regimens in older populations. Data is mixed and generally low quality but suggests a possible beneficial impact on muscle strength, balance, bone density, and subsequent falls [62] that should be confirmed in well-designed clinical trials. The role of exercise in the treatment of osteosarcopenia is summarized in Chapter 15 of this book.

Treatment of osteoporosis to reduce the risk of fracture is widely available. Pharmacotherapy includes antiresorptive agents (denosumab, bisphosphonates), anabolic agents (teriparatide, abaloparatide), antisclerostin agents (romosozumab), and hormonal agents (hormone replacement therapies, selective estrogen receptor modulators). Generally, these therapies treat bone alone but do not have clinically important impacts on muscle or fat composition. One trial has suggested that denosumab may impact muscle, based on improved handgrip strength and lean body mass [63–65].

No pharmacotherapy options have yet been approved for sarcopenia. However, bimagrumab (a monoclonal antibody that binds to activin type 2 receptors on skeletal muscle fibers), has been shown to induce muscle growth in cell culture and mice. A pilot study suggests that one dose in humans augmented muscle volume and lean body mass. Studies have been mixed regarding improvements in 6-min walking distance. Additionally, no significant changes were seen in quadriceps muscle strength, handgrip and pinch-grip dynamometry, and falls [66].

Conclusions

Falls and fractures are the most important clinical manifestations of osteosarcopenia in older adults, and preventing them is a critical public health goal. Screening and prevention efforts for both should include careful assessment and management of medications and co-morbidities that have a dual impact on muscle, fat, and bone. Current clinical tools do not fully capture the synergistic impact of muscle quality, bone quality, obesity, and prior falls on subsequent fall and fracture risk. We suggest using a combination of validated clinical risk tools, imaging, and brief physical performance testing to optimize management decisions. Exercise and dietary interventions are a key component of fall and fracture prevention; pharmacologic interventions targeting underlying osteosarcopenia are urgently needed.

References

[1] Alexander BH, Rivara FP, Wolf ME. The cost and frequency of hospitalization for fall-related injuries in older adults. Am J Public Health 1992;82(7):1020–3.

[2] Sterling DA, O'Connor JA, Bonadies J. Geriatric falls: injury severity is high and disproportionate to mechanism. J Trauma Acute Care Surg 2001;50(1):116–9.

[3] Hernlund E, Svedbom A, Ivergard M, et al. Osteoporosis in the European Union: medical management, epidemiology and economic burden. A report prepared in collaboration with the International Osteoporosis Foundation (IOF) and the European Federation of Pharmaceutical Industry Associations (EFPIA). Arch Osteoporos 2013;8:136.

[4] Burge R, Dawson-Hughes B, Solomon DH, Wong JB, King A, Tosteson A. Incidence and economic burden of osteoporosis-related fractures in the United States, 2005-2025. J Bone Miner Res 2007;22(3):465–75.

[5] Yeung SSY, Reijnierse EM, Pham VK, et al. Sarcopenia and its association with falls and fractures in older adults: a systematic review and meta-analysis. J Cachexia Sarcopenia Muscle 2019;10(3):485–500.

[6] Neri SGR, Oliveira JS, Dario AB, Lima RM, Tiedemann A. Does obesity increase the risk and severity of falls in people aged 60 years and older? A systematic review and meta-analysis of observational studies. J Gerontol Ser A Biol Sci Med Sci 2020;75(5):952–60.

[7] Fox KM, Magaziner J, Hawkes WG, et al. Loss of bone density and lean body mass after hip fracture. Osteoporos Int 2000;11(1):31–5.

[8] Deshpande N, Metter EJ, Lauretani F, Bandinelli S, Guralnik J, Ferrucci L. Activity restriction induced by fear of falling and objective and subjective measures of physical function: a prospective cohort study. J Am Geriatr Soc 2008;56(4):615–20.

[9] Murphy SL, Williams CS, Gill TM. Characteristics associated with fear of falling and activity restriction in community-living older persons. J Am Geriatr Soc 2002;50(3):516–20.

[10] Geusens P, Autier P, Boonen S, Vanhoof J, Declerck K, Raus J. The relationship among history of falls, osteoporosis, and fractures in postmenopausal women. Arch Phys Med Rehabil 2002;83(7):903–6.

[11] Yoo JI, Kim H, Ha YC, Kwon HB, Koo KH. Osteosarcopenia in patients with hip fracture is related with high mortality. J Korean Med Sci 2018;33(4), e27.

[12] Weinstein RS. Clinical practice. Glucocorticoid-induced bone disease. N Engl J Med 2011;365(1):62–70.

[13] Adami G, Saag KG. Glucocorticoid-induced osteoporosis: 2019 concise clinical review. Osteoporos Int 2019;30(6):1145–56.

[14] Sato AY, Richardson D, Cregor M, et al. Glucocorticoids induce bone and muscle atrophy by tissue-specific mechanisms upstream of E3 ubiquitin ligases. Endocrinology 2017;158(3):664–77.

[15] Schakman O, Gilson H, Thissen JP. Mechanisms of glucocorticoid-induced myopathy. J Endocrinol 2008;197(1):1–10.

[16] Guja C, Guja L, Miulescu RD. Effect of type 2 diabetes medications on fracture risk. Ann Transl Med 2019;7(20):580.

[17] Bahrambeigi S, Yousefi B, Rahimi M, Shafiei-Irannejad V. Metformin; an old antidiabetic drug with new potentials in bone disorders. Biomed Pharmacother 2019;109:1593–601.

[18] Hidayat K, Du X, Wu MJ, Shi BM. The use of metformin, insulin, sulphonylureas, and thiazolidinediones and the risk of fracture: systematic review and meta-analysis of observational studies. Obes Rev 2019;20(10):1494–503.

[19] Kahn SE, Zinman B, Lachin JM, et al. Rosiglitazone-associated fractures in type 2 diabetes: an analysis from a diabetes outcome progression trial (ADOPT). Diabetes Care 2008;31(5):845–51.

[20] Berlie HD, Garwood CL. Diabetes medications related to an increased risk of falls and fall-related morbidity in the elderly. Ann Pharmacother 2010;44(4):712–7.

[21] Lee RH, Sloane R, Pieper C, et al. Glycemic control and insulin treatment alter fracture risk in older men with type 2 diabetes mellitus. J Bone Miner Res 2019;34(11):2045–51.

[22] Lin TK, Chou P, Lin CH, Hung YJ, Jong GP. Long-term effect of statins on the risk of new-onset osteoporosis: a nationwide population-based cohort study. PLoS One 2018;13(5), e0196713.

[23] Pena JM, Aspberg S, MacFadyen J, Glynn RJ, Solomon DH, Ridker PM. Statin therapy and risk of fracture: results from the JUPITER randomized clinical trial. JAMA Intern Med 2015;175(2):171–7.

[24] Shi R, Mei Z, Zhang Z, Zhu Z. Effects of statins on relative risk of fractures for older adults: an updated systematic review with meta-analysis. J Am Med Dir Assoc 2019;20(12):1566–1578.e1563.

[25] de Vries M, Seppala LJ, Daams JG, van de Glind EMM, Masud T, van der Velde N. Fall-risk-increasing drugs: a systematic review and meta-analysis: I. cardiovascular drugs. J Am Med Dir Assoc 2018;19(4):371.e371–9.

[26] Compston J. Type 2 diabetes mellitus and bone. J Intern Med 2018;283(2):140–53.

[27] Wang W, Zhang X, Zheng J, Yang J. High glucose stimulates adipogenic and inhibits osteogenic differentiation in MG-63 cells through cAMP/protein kinase a/extracellular signal-regulated kinase pathway. Mol Cell Biochem 2010;338(1):115–22.

[28] Hayashi M, Abe K, Fujita M, Okai K, Takahashi A, Ohira H. Association between sarcopenia and osteoporosis in chronic liver disease. Hepatol Res 2018;48(11):893–904.

[29] Hegedus D, Ferencz V, Lakatos PL, et al. Decreased bone density, elevated serum osteoprotegerin, and beta-cross-laps in Wilson disease. J Bone Miner Res 2002;17(11):1961–7.

[30] Szalay F, Hegedus D, Lakatos PL, et al. High serum osteoprotegerin and low RANKL in primary biliary cirrhosis. J Hepatol 2003;38(4):395–400.

[31] Dasarathy S. Cause and management of muscle wasting in chronic liver disease. Curr Opin Gastroenterol 2016;32(3):159–65.

[32] Goto NA, Weststrate ACG, Oosterlaan FM, et al. The association between chronic kidney disease, falls, and fractures: a systematic review and meta-analysis. Osteoporos Int 2020;31(1):13–29.

[33] Hall RK, Sloane R, Pieper C, et al. Competing risks of fracture and death in older adults with chronic kidney disease. J Am Geriatr Soc 2018;66(3):532–8.

[34] Baker JF, Long J, Mostoufi-Moab S, et al. Muscle deficits in rheumatoid arthritis contribute to inferior cortical bone structure and trabecular bone mineral density. J Rheumatol 2017;44(12):1777–85.

[35] Carvalho GD, Bonfiglioli K, Caparbo VF, Takayama L, Pereira RMR, Domiciano DS. Changes to body composition in women with long-standing established rheumatoid arthritis: differences by level of disease activity. J Clin Densitom 2020;23(4):639–46.

[36] Ke HZ, Richards WG, Li X, Ominsky MS. Sclerostin and Dickkopf-1 as therapeutic targets in bone diseases. Endocr Rev 2012;33(5):747–83.
[37] Kerschan-Schindl K, Ebenbichler G, Föeger-Samwald U, et al. Rheumatoid arthritis in remission. Wien Klin Wochenschr 2019;131(1):1–7.
[38] Tsai VWW, Husaini Y, Manandhar R, et al. Anorexia/cachexia of chronic diseases: a role for the TGF-β family cytokine MIC-1/GDF15. J Cachexia Sarcopenia Muscle 2012;3(4):239–43.
[39] Lebwohl B, Michaelsson K, Green PH, Ludvigsson JF. Persistent mucosal damage and risk of fracture in celiac disease. J Clin Endocrinol Metab 2014;99(2):609–16.
[40] Piodi LP, Poloni A, Ulivieri FM. Managing osteoporosis in ulcerative colitis: something new? World J Gastroenterol 2014;20(39):14087–98.
[41] FRAX. Fracture risk assessment tool., 2021, https://www.sheffield.ac.uk/FRAX/. [Accessed 25 March 2020].
[42] Edwards MH, Jameson K, Denison H, et al. Clinical risk factors, bone density and fall history in the prediction of incident fracture among men and women. Bone 2013;52(2):541–7.
[43] Bolland MJ, Siu AT, Mason BH, et al. Evaluation of the FRAX and Garvan fracture risk calculators in older women. J Bone Miner Res 2011;26(2):420–7.
[44] Masud T, Binkley N, Boonen S, Hannan MT. Official positions for FRAX® clinical regarding falls and frailty: can falls and frailty be used in FRAX®?: from joint official positions development conference of the International Society for Clinical Densitometry and International Osteoporosis Foundation on FRAX®. J Clin Densitom 2011;14(3):194–204.
[45] Malmstrom TK, Morley JE. SARC-F: a simple questionnaire to rapidly diagnose sarcopenia. J Am Med Dir Assoc 2013;14(8):531–2.
[46] Ida S, Kaneko R, Murata K. SARC-F for screening of sarcopenia among older adults: a meta-analysis of screening test accuracy. J Am Med Dir Assoc 2018;19(8):685–9.
[47] Wu T-Y, Liaw C-K, Chen F-C, Kuo K-L, Chie W-C, Yang R-S. Sarcopenia screened with SARC-F questionnaire is associated with quality of life and 4-year mortality. J Am Med Dir Assoc 2016;17(12):1129–35.
[48] Su Y, Woo JW, Kwok TCY. The added value of SARC-F to prescreening using FRAX for hip fracture prevention in older community adults. J Am Med Dir Assoc 2019;20(1):83–9.
[49] Johnston YA, Bergen G, Bauer M, et al. Implementation of the stopping elderly accidents, deaths, and injuries initiative in primary care: an outcome evaluation. Gerontologist 2018;59(6):1182–91.
[50] Sarmiento K, Lee R. STEADI: CDC's approach to make older adult fall prevention part of every primary care practice. J Saf Res 2017;63:105–9.
[51] Nithman RW, Vincenzo JL. How steady is the STEADI? Inferential analysis of the CDC fall risk toolkit. Arch Gerontol Geriatr 2019;83:185–94.
[52] Kirk B, Zanker J, Duque G. Osteosarcopenia: epidemiology, diagnosis, and treatment-facts and numbers. J Cachexia Sarcopenia Muscle 2020;11(3):609–18.
[53] Quach L, Galica AM, Jones RN, et al. The nonlinear relationship between gait speed and falls: the maintenance of balance, independent living, intellect, and zest in the elderly of Boston study. J Am Geriatr Soc 2011;59(6):1069–73.
[54] Dargent-Molina P, Schott AM, Hans D, et al. Separate and combined value of bone mass and gait speed measurements in screening for hip fracture risk: results from the EPIDOS study. Osteoporos Int 1999;9(2):188–92.
[55] Beauchet O, Fantino B, Allali G, Muir SW, Montero-Odasso M, Annweiler C. Timed up and go test and risk of falls in older adults: a systematic review. J Nutr Health Aging 2011;15(10):933–8.

[56] Lauretani F, Ticinesi A, Gionti L, et al. Short-physical performance battery (SPPB) score is associated with falls in older outpatients. Aging Clin Exp Res 2019;31(10):1435–42.
[57] Colon-Emeric C, Whitson HE, Berry SD, et al. AGS and NIA bench-to bedside conference summary: osteoporosis and soft tissue (muscle and fat) disorders. J Am Geriatr Soc 2020;68(1):31–8.
[58] Cosman F, de Beur SJ, LeBoff MS, et al. Clinician's guide to prevention and treatment of osteoporosis. Osteoporos Int 2014;25(10):2359–81.
[59] Silva RB, Eslick GD, Duque G. Exercise for falls and fracture prevention in long term care facilities: a systematic review and meta-analysis. J Am Med Dir Assoc 2013;14(9):685–689.e682.
[60] El-Khoury F, Cassou B, Charles M-A, Dargent-Molina P. The effect of fall prevention exercise programmes on fall induced injuries in community dwelling older adults: systematic review and meta-analysis of randomised controlled trials. BMJ 2013;347, f6234.
[61] Shea B, Bonaiuti D, Iovine R, et al. Cochrane review on exercise for preventing and treating osteoporosis in postmenopausal women. Eura Medicophys 2004;40(3):199–209.
[62] Jepsen DB, Thomsen K, Hansen S, Jørgensen NR, Masud T, Ryg J. Effect of whole-body vibration exercise in preventing falls and fractures: a systematic review and meta-analysis. BMJ Open 2017;7(12), e018342.
[63] Bonnet N, Bourgoin L, Biver E, Douni E, Ferrari S. RANKL inhibition improves muscle strength and insulin sensitivity and restores bone mass. J Clin Invest 2019;129(8):3214–23. https://doi.org/10.1172/JCI125915. 31120440. PMC6668701.
[64] Phu S, Bani Hassan E, Vogrin S, Kirk B, Duque G. Effect of denosumab on falls, muscle strength, and function in community-dwelling older adults. J Am Geriatr Soc 2019;67(12):2660–1. https://doi.org/10.1111/jgs.16165 [Epub 2019 Sep 4] 31483858.
[65] Chotiyarnwong P, McCloskey E, Eastell R, McClung MR, Gielen E, Gostage J, McDermott M, Chines A, Huang S, Cummings SR. A pooled analysis of fall incidence from placebo-controlled trials of denosumab. J Bone Miner Res 2020;35(6):1014–21. https://doi.org/10.1002/jbmr.3972 [Epub 2020 Apr 2] 31999376.
[66] Hanna MG, Badrising UA, Benveniste O, et al. Safety and efficacy of intravenous bimagrumab in inclusion body myositis (RESILIENT): a randomised, double-blind, placebo-controlled phase 2b trial. Lancet Neurol 2019;18(9):834–44.

Chapter 10

Osteosarcopenic adiposity

Jasminka Z. Ilich[a], Owen J. Kelly[b], Jennifer C. Gilman[c], Selma Cvijetic[d], and Dario Boschiero[e]

[a]*Florida State University, Tallahassee, FL, United States,* [b]*Sam Houston State University College of Osteopathic Medicine, Conroe, TX, United States,* [c]*Independent Writer, Conroe, TX, United States,* [d]*Institute for Medical Research and Occupational Health, Zagreb, Croatia,* [e]*Biotekna®, Marcon-Venice, Venice, Italy*

What is osteosarcopenic adiposity/obesity and what is in its name?

Introduction

Osteosarcopenic adiposity/obesity (OSA/OSO) was officially identified in 2014, when a theoretical concept supported by scientific evidence and research findings, hypothesized its existence and identification as a new condition/syndrome [1]. At that time, it was described as a syndrome in older Caucasian women and subsequently linked to their lower functionality [2]. Since then, OSA has been recognized and studied throughout the world and identified in various populations, age groups, and individuals with different health conditions [3]. The original description of the condition still holds; however, the name was revised from osteosarcopenic obesity (OSO) to osteosarcopenic adiposity (OSA) [4]. The rationale for changing the name is discussed below, but in this paper, the terms (OSA/OSO) are used interchangeably, especially since most of the previous literature refers to the condition as OSO. However, the original working definition did not change: "It is a condition encompassing simultaneous deterioration of bone (osteopenia/osteoporosis) and muscle (sarcopenia/dynapenia), with the increased presence of body fat (adipose tissue), either as an overt overweight/obesity and/or as redistributed fat (particularly in visceral areas) and/or as infiltrated fat (ectopic) into bone and muscle" [1,3,5].

Fig. 1 depicts body composition impairments, where any of the conditions (osteopenic adiposity, osteopenic sarcopenia, sarcopenic adiposity) may result in different stages of body composition derangement, leading ultimately to the most detrimental impairment; the triad of OSA. Also, each of the conditions may arise where the fat infiltration is predominant or where the fat accumulation originated. For example, osteopenic adiposity would be the result of fat infiltrating in bone, due to a multitude of causes, including diet and lifestyle,

Osteosarcopenia. https://doi.org/10.1016/B978-0-12-820088-9.00014-7

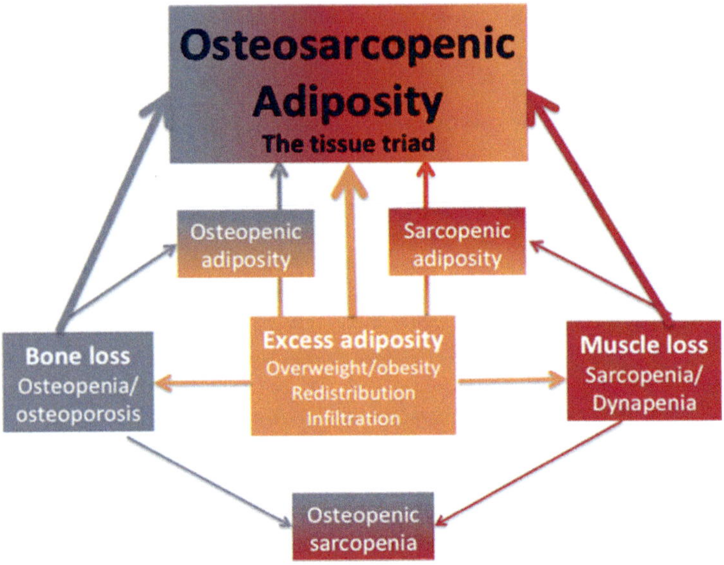

FIG. 1 Osteosarcopenic adiposity as the triad of body composition impairment. *(Credits: Original.)*

aging, inflammation, or other comorbidities, leading to lower bone mass/quality and increased fracture risks. Similar effects may cause fat infiltration into muscle, lowering muscle mass/strength, resulting in sarcopenic adiposity and causing functional disabilities and frailty. In this context, OSA is considered the most advanced impairment in bone, muscle, and body fat [1,6,7]. Actually, there is the possibility that osteoporosis, sarcopenia, osteopenic adiposity, and sarcopenic adiposity are the same disease at different stages of development into OSA. The important point is that the key consequences of OSA are functional disabilities, increased fracture risks, and increased systemic metabolic deregulation leading to various morbidities.

Why the name change?

In the context of this text, and in general terms, body composition includes bone, muscle (or lean tissue as its proxy), and adipose tissues. The criteria to diagnose osteopenia/osteoporosis, based on the dual-energy X-ray absorptiometry (DXA), are well known and widely accepted. To a certain extent, that is also true for sarcopenia, although there are a few working definitions. The most widely accepted one is from the European Working Group on Sarcopenia in Older People [8]. However, there is still no global consensus on cut-offs for obesity or the amount of adipose tissue present in the whole body or its different compartments, as recently addressed [3]. Most of the reasons are due to the high level of heterogeneity of adipose tissue which encompasses visceral, subcutaneous, and ectopic (infiltrated in liver, heart, bone, muscle) fat, as well as white, brown, and beige fat cells, each with different metabolic pathways and molecules secreted. Therefore, the difficulties in identifying either osteopenic/osteoporotic or sarcopenic obesity/adiposity, in addition to reaching the consensus on the cut-off criteria for overall body adiposity become apparent.

Generally, it could be stated that obesity typically refers to overweight, as most often defined by body mass index (BMI) $\geq 30\,kg/m^2$ with all limitations attributed to BMI [3], while body adiposity includes all types of fat discussed above. With that regard, and aligned with our original OSA/OSO definition, some argue that there should be separate terms to include osteosarcopenic subcutaneous obesity and osteosarcopenic visceral obesity [9]. While these terms might provide a clearer picture of the OSA/OSO phenotype, they still do not include ectopic fat infiltrated in bone and muscle, probably the most important aspects in OSA/OSO syndrome, due to their metabolic effects. In view of the heterogeneity of adipose tissue, we believe that the more appropriate term for osteosarcopenic obesity (OSO) should be osteosarcopenic adiposity (OSA), but again, in this text, the terms are used interchangeably.

The proof of concept

In our original concept paper [1], we outlined the cellular, endocrine, and whole-body connections among bone, muscle, and body adiposity. Subsequently, as research in OSA evolved, the possibilities of how each tissue (or in combination with others) may contribute to its development are briefly summarized below [1,4,6,7].

Cellular connections and interactions among three tissues

There is an increasing understanding and appreciation for cellular connections and interactions among bone, muscle, and adipose tissues and the recognition that they should be studied together. With that regard, we summarized some possible pathways for a better understanding of their interactions and connections. For example, as our stem cells age or are exposed to other stressors caused by unfavorable micro or macro environments, they may take different lineage commitments, ultimately producing more adipocytes in bone, muscle, as well as in fat tissue itself [1,4]. In this context, it is particularly important to focus on mesenchymal stem cells (MSC) as precursors for osteoblasts and adipocytes and on myogenic lineage from mesoderm as precursors for myocytes. In short, the stem cells' normal regulatory commitments when affected by adverse metabolic processes in the body, will be disrupted and along the way, both bone and muscle cells may be replaced by fat cells.

As already established, the major osteoblastogenesis and osteoblast maturation and differentiation promoter is runt-related transcription factor 2 (RUNX2) along with the musculoaponeurotic fibrosarcoma oncogene homolog (Maf) [10,11]. In addition, RUNX2 is also essential in shifting the MSC differentiation from adipogenic (slightly favored even under normal conditions) to osteoblastogenic lineage. The key signaling molecules regulating MSC toward myogenesis and promoters of MSC/satellite cells differentiation into myocytes are myogenin and myoD [12,13]. The nuclear peroxisome proliferator-activated receptor gamma (PPAR-gamma) is an ultimate promoter of adipogenesis, adipocyte maturation, and metabolism and it hinders both osteoblastogenesis and myogenesis [14].

Regarding the master cell regulators, transforming growth factor-beta (TGF-beta) is the one that maintains the MSC population and promotes both osteoblastogenesis and myogenesis, but inhibits adipogenesis [15]. Insulin growth factor-1 (IGF-1) exerts similar regulations [16]. On the contrary, tumor necrosis factor-alpha (TNF-alpha), a major proinflammatory cytokine produced by visceral adipocytes, promotes adipogenesis and reduces osteoblastogenesis and myogenesis [17].

Endocrine connections and interactions

Each of the three tissues—bone, muscle, and fat, exerts a specific regulatory action on another one with possible systemic effects. Regarding the crosstalk between bone and muscle, the mechanical loading of muscle exerted on the bone (muscle as a puller, bone as a lever) has been investigated the most and previously believed to be the only connection between two organs. Recently, more insight is gained on bone and particularly on muscle acting as endocrine organs. For example, osteocalcin, a protein secreted by osteoblasts and best known as a bone formation marker, but also coined as the first osteokine [1], is anabolic for muscle and has a role in energy metabolism by regulating insulin sensitivity and glucose utilization, as well as adiponectin secretion by adipocytes [18]. A marker of bone resorption, sclerostin, also causes muscle breakdown, while other molecules, like receptor activator of nuclear factor kappa-B ligand (RANKL) released during bone resorption, has negative effects on both bone and muscle [19,20]. Other bone cells, including osteocytes and their secretory molecules, have been implicated in muscle and other organ regulations, as recently reviewed [19].

Muscle-secreting myokines may influence bone, as well as other organs. For example, myostatin is a major bone and muscle catabolic agent, along with the skeletal muscle-specific troponins (sTnT), the latter including a family of key regulatory contractility proteins which are released only during muscle damage [19]. Interleukin 6 (IL-6) is well known for its strong proinflammatory effects in the systemic circulation, however, when released from the working muscle it exerts antiinflammatory properties and improves glucose utilization and satellite cell proliferation, but also decreases the low-grade chronic inflammation [21] and indirectly bone loss [20]. Other myokines released from the working muscle, interleukins IL-7, and IL-8 mediate fatty acid beta-oxidation, while IL-15, improves glucose utilization, indicating the common link between muscle and fat tissues [22]. Additionally, the irisin-hormonal-system provides probably the best example of muscle-fat axis interaction. Irisin, secreted from the exercising muscle, causes the browning of the white fat cells converting them into the beige fat cells [23], the latter characterized by increased mitochondrial numbers and the expression of uncoupling protein-1, exerting higher thermogenesis. Although irisin effects and pathways are still under investigation, they may explain the higher energy expenditure occurring with exercise, which could not have been expounded by energy expenditure from exercise only [23].

Regarding the endocrine role of adipose tissue, probably the most notable is its endogenous estrogens formation via extra glandular aromatization of androgens. These estrogens are the only ones circulating in postmenopausal women, thus providing beneficial signals to both bone and muscle, and inhibiting adipose tissue accumulation [24]. However, the complex actions of adipose-derived adipokines, namely leptin and adiponectin, are still not quite elucidated. Briefly, leptin and adiponectin have an opposing relationship in circulation, have receptors on both osteoblasts and myocytes, and exert dual effects on bone and muscle, mostly depending on whether their influence is on local or systemic levels [25]. Due to these complexities, it is hard to deduce some general statement about the actions of these two adipokines on bone and muscle, especially in view of their possible involvement in other organ systems and interactions with multiple other molecules.

The adverse influence of the visceral fat and its secretory molecules are widely known and confirmed, not just in bone and muscle deterioration, but also in multiple other organ systems. This is especially important to address in the COVID-19 era (as discussed below). Visceral fat releases multiples of inflammatory cytokines, including tumor necrosis factor (TNF)-alpha, Il-1 and Il-6, C-reactive protein, fibrinogens, and lipoprotein-associated phospholipase, all producing an "inflammatory shift," causing not just the damage to bone and muscle, but to the whole body organ systems [26]. These are some of the same inflammatory cytokines released in a "cytokine storm" that viruses such as COVID-19 trigger, as discussed in the further text.

Whole-body levels

The inevitable changes in body composition occurring with aging, but possibly accelerated by other chronic conditions (e.g., low-grade chronic inflammation, chronic stress, diabetes, some cancers) cause the decrease in bone mass leading to osteopenia/osteoporosis and/or decrease of muscle mass and strength leading to sarcopenia. At the same time, there is an increase in body adiposity, redistribution of fat mass, and its infiltration into bone and muscle. These changes may lead to any of the body composition disturbances and ultimately to osteosarcopenic adiposity (see Fig. 1) with all its detrimental consequences [1].

Fig. 2 depicts the progression of OSA from cellular/endocrine/whole body changes to clinical manifestations.

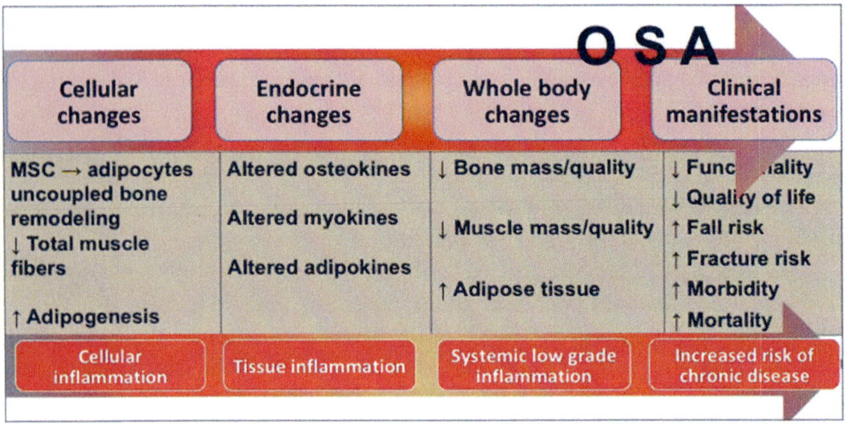

FIG. 2 The connections between three tissues and progression of osteosarcopenic adiposity (OSA) from cellular/endocrine/whole body impairments to clinical manifestations. *(Credits: Original.)*

Identification of OSA and persisting difficulties

The updated diagnostic criteria for both men and women have been recently published [3]. Since OSA is a complex condition involving multiple organs and tissues (each also limited to its own individual diagnosis), it is reasonable to expect that its identification has been difficult and still poses problems. The diagnosis based on deteriorations of body tissue could be performed when clinically relevant stages of bone loss, muscle loss, and fat gain are detected and assessed with some of the available technologies, as discussed below. The tests on functional performance could even precede any of the screening for body composition impairments, as outlined previously [5,7]. When both of these measurements (bone/body composition and functional performance) are available, they can provide a more comprehensive way to grade the extent of the physical and functional deterioration in diagnosing OSA syndrome.

DXA technology has been a gold standard for osteopenia/osteoporosis diagnosis, as well as for the assessment of lean and fat tissue, for many years [27]. However, the limitations of DXA for bone assessment are well recognized; it yields only areal bone mineral density (BMD), does not distinguish between trabecular and cortical bone (except the rough assumptions based on which parts of the skeleton are analyzed), and provides no information about bone structure/quality, thus limiting predictability for fracture risks. Additionally, utilizing DXA to assess lean (often used as a proxy for muscle) and fat tissue, each has its own limitations when considering mass screening and remains dependent on its availability, costs, and radiation exposure. Therefore, using some alternative technologies to measure body composition have been explored, including the bioelectrical impedance analysis (BIA). Most of the BIA devices assess total lean mass (muscle, organs, and body water) as a proxy for muscle. This limitation is offset in some devices by measuring only the appendicular tissue, mostly comprising muscle [28]. However, the presence of ectopic fat complicates this approach. Additionally, most of these devices do not detect bone, thus cannot be utilized for OSA identification.

New technologies

Bone and muscle

Recently, a new device, BIA-ACC (BioTekna, Marcon-Venice, Italy), based on multi-frequency bioelectrical impedance and able to assess quantitative and qualitative body composition parameters, has been introduced. It was validated against DXA [29] and was used to detect OSO in young men and women [30]. This instrument detects total bone mass in the body (kg), along with minerals, calcium, magnesium, and phosphorus, but cannot distinguish among different skeletal sites or types of bone. The bone status is determined based on a normal reference population (which may be instrument-specific); therefore, a T-score of ≤ -1 SD would indicate osteopenia/osteoporosis. This technology does not assess the ectopic fat in bone or changes in bone marrow fat; in other words, it does not address the quality of bone. However, BIA-ACC provides the information on skeletal muscle mass (kg and % fat-free mass) and S-score for muscle (analog to T-scores for bone), as well as intramuscular adipose tissue (IMAT). It also yields the amount of fat mass (kg and % body weight), total body water, and extracellular and intracellular water. The BIA-ACC may be complemented by another device, the PPG-StressFlow (BioTekna, Marcon-Venice, Italy), which assesses the biofeedback of the autonomic nervous system including heart rate, and provides information on chronic stress, systemic inflammation, oxidative stress, and insulin resistance [31,32]. Therefore, in addition to their portability and ease of use, the synergy of BIA-ACC and PPG-StressFlow provides body composition assessment enabling the diagnosis of OSA, and at the same time shows underlying metabolic derangements such as low-grade chronic inflammation and stress, offering a more comprehensive assessment about overall health.

The unique material properties of bone regarding its strength and quality could not be measured in vivo (other than with some invasive technologies, like computerized tomography or expensive MRI) until recently. However, the introduction of impact micro-indentation (IMI) technology lent the evaluation of in vivo tissue-level properties of bone in humans. The metaanalysis evaluating studies using this technology, focusing on the OsteoProbe (ActiveLife Scientific Inc., Santa Barbara, California, United States), has been recently published [33]. Briefly, the IMI measures the reference point micro-indentation and bone's ability to resist the separation of mineralized collagen fibrils after the probe insertion. The final output is a calculated bone material strength index (BMSi), a ratio of the indentation distance in bone versus a reference material; the compromised bone strength allows the deeper probe indentation resulting in the lower BMSi. However, the OsteoProbe technology is invasive as it requires the application of a local anesthetic at a mid-shaft tibia where the probe is inserted through the skin. Nevertheless, this is a promising technology for the in vivo bone material properties and bone quality and fragility evaluation, especially when complemented with other technologies (e.g., DXA) [33].

Regarding the muscle quality assessment, the easiest way would be to calculate the phase angle from the BIA data by finding the arc-tangent of the reactance/resistance ratio [34]. Although this does not directly measure the infiltrated fat in muscle, it could serve as a proxy for muscle tissue quality. Similarly, some researchers are using the knee extension measurements to assess muscle quality, as well as the lower body strength, where one repetition maximum in kg from the knee extension is divided by the leg lean mass in kg (most measured by DXA or BIA) [35]. The BIA-ACC conveniently provides the analysis of phase angle, in addition to other muscle and body composition properties mentioned above (e.g., IMAT). Recent attention has been given to the advanced assessment of muscle tissue via ultrasound technology, particularly regarding its ability to distinguish different properties of the muscle. For example, the high-frequency ultrasound can evaluate the quality of skeletal muscle (e.g., quadriceps) by finding the echo intensity and using grayscale analysis with software such as Adobe Photoshop that can identify myosteatosis (infiltrated fat), otherwise negatively correlated with muscle strength and thickness, as well as age.

Adipose tissue

In order to offset the lack of consensus for overall obesity cut-offs, as well as a technological limitation for detection of ectopic/infiltrated fat, we recently proposed some alternatives for body fat assessment to help in OSA diagnosis [3]. For example, instead of using the total percent of body fat, fat mass index (FMI) can be used, with the proposed cut-offs for men and women of ≥ 9 and $\geq 13\,kg/m^2$, respectively [36]. Regarding visceral fat, several criteria could be used including the ratio of visceral to subcutaneous fat or ratio of android to gynoid fat (when DXA measurements are available). In other words, several options are available, however, there is a need to establish the scientific group on osteosarcopenic adiposity to guide researchers in its diagnosis and identification, as is currently established for sarcopenia [8].

Serum biomarkers for bone, muscle, fat, inflammation, and stress—Developing the omics for OSA

Research within OSA identification is needed in the development of serum biomarkers, to eventually develop the omics for body composition and complement them with physical and functional measurements. The markers of bone turnover are well developed and have been used extensively in clinical and research settings with various successes for their predictability of bone status or fractures. The biomarkers for muscle breakdown/turnover are being investigated with heightened interest. We recently reported that sclerostin and skeletal muscle-specific troponin (sTnT), the markers of bone and muscle breakdown, respectively, were more sensitive in identifying OSA in overweight/obese older women than some other serum indicators [37]. Serum sTnT has been previously associated with the onset of sarcopenia in older adults, and it decreased during their strength training, particularly in those who showed improvement in handgrip strength [38]. The search for biomarkers may be accelerated by using and developing both female and male animal models, as it has been introduced for the former [39].

The circulating levels of inflammatory cytokines such as TNF-α, IL-1, and IL-6 and C-reactive protein increase with increased adiposity, particularly visceral [40], and cause low-grade chronic inflammation perpetuating obesity and damaging both muscle and bone [41,42]. Additionally, it is of crucial importance to account for chronic stress that could affect a multitude of organs, including body composition via immune system modulation, all contributing to MSC lineage shift toward adipogenesis. In this context, the Western-type proinflammatory diet, altered lifestyle with reduced physical activity, and misaligned circadian rhythm, all create a vicious cycle contributing to compromised body composition and health [4].

The bottom line

While all mentioned instruments and technologies could be used in research and special circumstances, the mainstay technologies (although not available for a mass use or routine measurements) include MRI or EchoMRI and computed tomography (CT) that give the most comprehensive picture about any of the tissues discussed. The development of new technologies and easier use of the existing ones will enable a more universal identification of OSA and any of its components. Overall, while further studies are needed to determine the exact cut-offs and validation for various instruments, it is important to keep assessing body composition components with whatever tools are available and contribute them to the OSA diagnostic criteria. With such an approach, it will be possible to eventually assess all other ethnic and age groups of the population, as well as the individuals of various body composition categories and health conditions, and develop diagnostic cut-offs for each, and ultimately, gain better insights into the OSA syndrome.

What has the research on OSA/OSO showed so far?

Since its identification in 2014, the published research on OSA/OSO has grown rapidly, either based on retrospective and epidemiological studies, prospective analyses, or clinical interventions in different age and ethnic groups and populations across the world. Even more important is the fact that numerous published studies have accumulated data from which OSA/OSO could be retrospectively identified and related to various conditions, although at the time the condition was not reported as such. The problems for determining the overall prevalence of OSA/OSO in men and women still exist, due to the different ethnic groups and populations in which it has been studied and to the lack of uniformly accepted diagnostic criteria (as discussed above). In addition to the recently published review [3], the newest brief appraisal is captured in the following few paragraphs.

Several published studies originated from the Korean National Health and Nutrition Examination Surveys (mostly data from 2008 to 2009 and/or 2010 to 2011) and showed that individuals with OSO (≥50 years) had lower serum vitamin D levels [43], poorer diet quality [44], higher dietary inflammatory index [45] and consumed a diet lower in fruit [46] compared to their counterparts without OSO, but with some other of its components. Similarly, another cross-sectional study in individuals with OSO, showed that they had a less favorable body composition, fat distribution, and vitamin D levels, compared with only obese individuals in both sexes [47]. Based on fracture site, OSO prevalence was more common in men with vertebral, hip, and ankle fracture while among women, only those with ankle fracture had higher OSO prevalence [48]. However, another recent study showed no stronger correlation with insulin resistance in individuals with OSO compared to those with any other co-existing components or obesity alone [49], indicating greater fat mass is the strongest contributor to insulin resistance.

Researchers from other Asian countries reported various findings as well. For example, Chinese older women with OSO had significantly poorer blood lipid profiles compared to their counterparts without OSO [50]. Another Chinese study conducted in four minority populations reported that those with OSO had a higher prevalence of hypertension [51]. A Japanese study investigating the body composition impairments in patients with cardiovascular disease (CVD) and comparing them with community-dwelling controls, showed that the prevalence of sarcopenia, osteosarcopenia, and osteosarcopenic obesity was higher in the CVD patients than in the controls (16.9% vs 4.4%, $P<.001$; 8.8% vs 2.6%, $P=.009$; and 4.4% vs 0.9%, $P=.036$, respectively) [52] indicating that CVD may aggravate body composition, or vice versa, creating a vicious cycle. Another Japanese study (only the abstract is in English) reported that the prevalence of sarcopenic obesity was 16% among older Japanese women (mean age 72.5 years), however, over half of them also had osteopenia, identifying them as actually having OSO [53].

Our previous study in Caucasian, overweight/obese postmenopausal women showed that those with OSO had lower handgrip strength, poorer balance, and inferior walking abilities compared to women with obesity-only [2]. This lower functionality may emphasize even more the intrinsic complex nature of the OSO syndrome and the increased risk for falls. For example, in the study with 543 Mexican middle-aged and older males and females, OSO (16.6%of study population) was independently associated with frailty (as measured by the Frailty Phenotype and FRAIL scale) and a lower Short Physical Performance battery score [54].

There were also a few interventional studies with resistance training examining its effect on various OSO markers. A Brazilian study in older women with OSO showed that a 12-week resistance training improved some of their functionalities, even in a dose-response, where three sets induced more benefits than one set [55]. Another study in older Brazilian women who were followed for 24 months with regard to their functionality and habitual physical activity, showed that regardless of whether they had OSO or not, the physical activity was inversely related to their functionality. However, those who had OSO were less active and presented with higher functional disabilities [56]. The intervention with elastic band resistance training for 12 weeks (three times/week) was conducted as a randomized controlled trial in Iranian older women with OSO. The results showed that women who received training improved in some of the functionality measures (e.g., handgrip strength, 30-s chair test), but not in others (e.g., gait speed) or any of the body composition parameters (BMI, BMD, or body fat). Likewise, there was no improvement in the serum sclerostin and skeletal troponin [57], the markers shown previously as sensitive indicators for bone and muscle loss, respectively [37].

In the Australian Busselton Healthy Aging Study, higher body fat was associated with a lower bone mineral density in females but not in males; however, the highest body fat groups also had the lowest lean mass index (kg/m^2) in both males and females [58], indicating the presence of OSO. The Louisiana Osteoporosis Study, a large cross-sectional study of $\geq$18 years individuals, showed the prevalence of sarcopenic obesity of 7% in males and 2.5% in females, with the older age groups contributing the most [59]. This is another important study as it also collected bone density measurements, making it an ideal database to estimate the prevalence of OSO in that wide age-range population. However, the most striking report was the presence of OSO in apparently healthy young overweight/obese Greek males and females compared to their normal-weight counterparts [30] as the OSO phenotype was not anticipated in young, healthy individuals. Another striking result is a recent finding of high prevalence of OSA in Croatian nursing home residents (Keser et al., abstract in press). In that study, $n=84$ nursing home residents (82.1% females, 81.2 ± 6.8 years old with BMI of $29.2 \pm 5.0\,kg/m^2$), were analyzed by bioimpedance devices, BIA-ACC and PPG-Stress Flow (BioTekna, Marcon-Venice, Italy). The prevalence of OSA was 66.7% in women and 40.0% in men, with a very low phase angle and a high percentage of extracellular water indicating poor health. These findings indicate the urgency of evaluating body composition and OSA in that population (Keser et al., abstract in press), particularly during COVID-19, as addressed below.

To our knowledge, there were no explicit longitudinal or other studies investigating various diseased states and how they might influence OSA/OSO or vice versa. However, there are some correlational studies, worth mentioning. For example, Carsote and colleagues reported that malignancy might lead to OSO and that malignancy of all causes in the presence of OSO would result in a worse prognosis [60]. In another study investigating males with or without HIV, all three components of OSO, osteoporosis, sarcopenia, and obesity (visceral adipose tissue area), were associated with frailty, although BMI or subcutaneous fat were not associated with similar relationships [61]. The authors emphasized that interventions for all three conditions (OSO) would help to treat and reduce the risk for frailty in this population. In a sample of 40 women (mean age of 40.7 years) with rheumatoid arthritis, 42.5% were diagnosed with OSO [62], suggesting rheumatoid arthritis may promote its development or vice versa. A case study in male identical twins 76 years of age suggested that the twin undergoing androgen deprivation therapy for prostate cancer was at higher risk for OSO and frailty due to the overt worsening in body composition, namely increase in visceral adiposity and muscle weakening [63]. It is known that both estrogen and androgen deprivation therapies in breast and prostate cancers respectively, result in hypogonadism and altered bone and body composition. Therefore, it was recently suggested that when evaluating fracture risk in those patients, it might not be enough to just evaluate BMD and Fracture Risk Assessment Tool (FRAX) scores, but also overall body composition (often underestimated in cancer patients), indicating the need for comprehensive analysis for the presence of OSA syndrome [64]. A recent study in a group of patients with Cushing's disease identified significantly lower irisin levels compared to controls, and irisin's independent relationship with osteosarcopenic obesity, suggesting irisin could serve as a possible marker for OSO in Cushing's Disease [65].

While low-grade chronic inflammation has been linked earlier to the development of osteoporosis, obesity, and subsequently to OSA [41], recent reviews show the association of chronic stress, including dehydration, with OSA [31], as well as the immune system modulating stress and body composition [4]. This insight gives rise to yet another component; chronic stress affects body composition via immune system and opens up the less explored area where nutritional and lifestyle measures could be implemented for the improvement of body composition, inflammation, and stress.

Overall, there is a growing body of evidence supporting the existence of OSA/OSO as a separate entity in populations of different ethnicities and backgrounds, not limited just to aging or to women (as initially identified) and indicating that its consequences are larger than the sum of each condition alone, as discussed below.

OSA health consequences

It is reasonable to hypothesize that due to fat infiltration, inflammation and metabolic and functional dysfunction in three tissues, the health consequences of OSA with comorbidities are greater than the sum of its individual components, despite some doubts [66]. For example, when examining each of the individual conditions, osteopenia/osteoporosis with its diminished BMD leads to increased risk of fractures, which will be aggravated by impaired mobility and increased falls secondary to sarcopenia. The weakened muscle might weaken the bone even more, or vice versa. The distorted and redistributed adipose tissue with its infiltration in bone and muscle will weaken each, as well as cause low-grade chronic inflammation resulting in multiple ill consequences to all other organs and tissues, including susceptibility to and poor outcomes in COVID-19 infection, as discussed below. In other words, although each individual condition has its associated comorbidities, health outcomes are compounded when all three are present (osteopenia/osteoporosis + sarcopenia + adiposity) and their outcomes are worse than just a sum of three. Crosstalk occurs between all three tissues, therefore in the OSA syndrome, each tissue may worsen another, multiplying the overall ill effects and resulting in heightened vulnerability to chronic poor health, risk of falls and bone fractures, disability, and frailty. Such conditions lead to low quality of life, nursing home placement, and morbidity, as well as premature death—definitely more than just the sum of each of OSA components alone.

Since a progressive loss of bone and muscle and increase in adipose tissue is inevitable with normal aging (and even more so in some chronic conditions), identification of the epidemiological overlap of osteoporosis, sarcopenia, and increased adiposity is crucial, especially given the common risk factors and cellular origins. Evidence for the pathophysiological overlap of these conditions is expanding, particularly with more understanding about the interplay of inflammatory and hormonal mechanisms. However, a causal relationship among osteosarcopenic adiposity components is not clearly identified, although some origins were pointed out in the text above. Obviously, more comprehensive research to understand the underlying biological phenomena linking the three conditions are needed. In other words, the OSA model is ideal for studying, monitoring, and possibly managing and treating changes after any internal or external insults (including age) affect body composition, especially considering that those tissues originate from the same stem cell lineage.

OSA in the time of COVID-19

The COVID-19 pandemic has brought much-deserved attention to the importance of the immune system and the fact that underlying conditions worsen the outcomes from COVID-19, especially in obesity [67]. The OSA syndrome emphasizes the interconnected nature of the human body and the postulate that having one condition may result in the development of others with the resulting ill condition being greater than the sum of its parts. The evidence for crosstalk between bone, muscle, and adipose tissues [1,68] and the connection between the immune system and inflammation [69], the common traits in OSA, are well known. The cytokine storm described in COVID-19 [70] may be rooted in the low-grade chronic inflammation present before contracting COVID-19.

All tissues may have resident immune cells and the immune system involvement in bone resorption/formation is known as osteoimmunology [71,72]. Skeletal muscle is no different; for example, there is a distinct type of regulatory T-cells present in the muscle of mice [73]. Some of the myokines released from working muscles may be part of the crosstalk with the immune system and the absence of these (e.g., in sedentary muscle), may result in some immune dysfunction in muscle tissue [74]. Muscle goes through a regulated cycle of events when undergoing repair; injury—inflammation—repair initiated—resolved, and a disruption of this can result in fat infiltration [75]. Other acute or chronic muscle diseases as well as aging may disrupt the immune-cell-muscle balance [76]. Compared to the role of the immune system in bone and muscle metabolism, the immune system's role in excess adiposity is better known. Low-grade inflammation due to the increasing number and size of adipocytes is at the heart of the systemic metabolic disorders associated with obesity [77,78]. In fact, it is possible that crosstalk between the immune system and adipose tissue regulates adipose tissue homeostasis [79].

For OSA specifically, no direct data on its relationship with COVID-19 are available (both conditions are new and the latter one has taken us by storm). That obesity increases the risk for contracting COVID-19 and worsen the outcomes has been shown recently [67]. Regarding bone health and COVID-19, a small study ($n = 10$) from China showed that patients with fractures and limited mobility had a higher mortality rate compared to those without fractures [80]. Data from the New York City hospital showed an increased need for oxygen in patients with hip fracture after surgery, but those with asymptomatic or mild COVID-19 infection had only a 10% mortality rate (compared to more than 40% in other countries) [81]. Regarding sarcopenia and COVID-19, no data are available to distinguish the outcomes for those with or without sarcopenia. However, COVID-19 probably results in muscle loss in patients who are symptomatic, even just considering the reduced food intake and lack of activity, with even more detrimental muscle loss in those who are severely affected or who drastically change their lifestyle during social isolation (sedentary, poor diet, depression, etc.) [82,83].

Our recommendations within the auspices of personalized nutrition/medicine

We have already published comprehensive nutritional and physical activity recommendations for OSA [84–87] and we recently provided a preliminary algorithm for its treatment and management [3]. Briefly, after a global medical, nutritional, and functional assessment has been performed, the strategies to maintain or treat OSA would depend on each individual's status and may be considered within the auspices of personalized nutrition/medicine. Additionally, the steps to reduce low-grade chronic inflammation, chronic stress, and the importance of maintaining a healthy microbiome with nutrition, exercise, or even pharmacological agents, should be considered [4]. No less important is the robust circadian rhythm for the proper functioning and synchronization of all body processes. Unfortunately, modern humans' lifestyle does not always translate to the optimal chrono-biology leading to increased risks for metabolic disturbances and diseases of modern time, including altered body composition [4].

Below are general suggestions that could be individually adapted and fine-tuned for each patient. The target for energy intake would depend on the need for weight loss or maintenance, but in general should be 25–30 kcal/kg/day, with about 1–1.2 g/kg/day of good quality protein (possibly ~25% of overall energy intake). The remaining energy intake should be balanced between carbohydrate and fat, to include: ~40% from nonprocessed carbohydrates with very limited simple sugars and ~35% from fat with $<10\%$ saturated fatty acids and no or very limited trans fatty acids. A focus should be to increase omega-3 polyunsaturated fatty acids, including more than 1 g/day (combination of eicosapentaenoic acid [EPA], docosahexaenoic acid [DHA], and the essential, alpha-linolenic acid). Fiber in the amount of 25–30 g/day is recommended, but it is usually harder to achieve. Some pre or pro-biotic foods or supplements may be recommended instead.

The micronutrients should include balanced minerals and vitamins intake, mostly at or above the Dietary Reference Intakes (DRI). That includes calcium, magnesium, and potassium (with about 1200 mg/day, 320 mg/day, and 4500 mg/day, respectively), but also adequate intake of zinc, selenium, manganese, and copper (deficiencies implicated in depression). All of them also improve the antioxidative capacity of mitochondria in repairing DNA damage and reducing inflammation and stress. On the other hand, among other minerals, sodium and phosphorus (except in severely sick patients) should be reduced and kept in check, along with too much iron [4].

Among vitamins, vitamin D has been studied most extensively and as of now, the intake of about 800 IU/day is recommended to keep the serum levels ≥ 20 ng/mL in older or otherwise compromised individuals. Besides its undisputed involvement in bone metabolism/calcium absorption, it also has a role in preventing falls and increasing muscle performance and its deficiency is associated with sarcopenia. Other antioxidant vitamins, like vitamin A, C, E, and carotenoids, along with vitamins from the B group are all involved in multiple metabolic processes regulating body composition, inflammation, and related chronic stress. In this respect, B_1 (thiamine), B_3 (niacin), and B_6 (pyridoxine) have been implicated in impaired neurotransmitter synthesis, while B_9 (folic acid) and B_{12} (cyanocobalamin), both involved in the recycling of homocysteine (toxic to mitochondria and cardiovascular system) into methionine, have been implicated not just in somebody composition regulation but also in stress-related mitochondrial damage and impaired neurotransmitter signaling [4].

Regarding the exercise program, we also suggest that activities be developed on an individual basis and centered on preference and abilities. While following the official exercise regimens (e.g., for weight loss, muscle strength or balance improvement, or overall well-being) could serve as some general guideline, it depends on each individual's condition, abilities, and state of the mind. Therefore, in the personalized-physical activity approach, the exercise or the amount and kind of physical activity should be addressed individually and recommended depending on the overall assessment. However, based on the evidence we have so far on OSA, we do recommend a comprehensive exercise program, depending on needs, but mostly on preferences, as the latter ensures adherence and regularity. The program could include all or some of the following varieties and options: aerobic, resistance, endurance, weight-bearing, strength, flexibility, and balance in the duration and frequency found most achievable by each individual. The official recommendations are 60 min of some exercise 5 days/week. However, performing each kind or amount according to the abilities and preferences makes each one easier to achieve and eventually leads to the overall goals; benefits to weight, body fat, bone, and muscle, improvements in balance, flexibility, cognition, and decrease in proinflammatory cytokines. Additionally, exercises like yoga, pilates, and tai chi have shown similar benefits but perhaps to a milder degree, especially considering body composition outcomes [84,87]. However, more studies in these exercise forms will provide evidence regarding their benefits for the prevention and treatment of OSA.

Conclusions

The evidence presented highlights the interconnectedness between bone, muscle, and adipose tissues and the central role of the immune system in their homeostasis. OSA is a multifactorial syndrome with its adverse health consequences larger than the sum of its parts (osteoporosis, sarcopenia, and obesity) alone. Crosstalk occurs between all three tissues, therefore within the OSA syndrome, each tissue may worsen another, multiplying the overall ill effects and resulting in heightened vulnerability to chronic poor health, risk of falls and bone fractures, disability and frailty, leading to low quality of life, nursing home placement, and morbidity, as well as premature death. All these effects are heightened and magnified in the COVID-19 pandemic. Optimizing the nutritional and lifestyle habits may contribute to better bone, muscle, and adipose tissues health as well as prevent/treat underlying conditions, including inflammation, and at the same time increase resilience.

In view that a progressive loss of bone and muscle and increase in adipose tissue is inevitable with aging and even more so in the presence of other comorbidities, identification of the epidemiological overlap of osteoporosis, sarcopenia, and adiposity is crucial. However, a causal relationship among osteosarcopenic adiposity components is not clearly identified although some common risk factors and cellular origins are outlined in the text. More comprehensive research to understand the underlying biological phenomena linking the three conditions and the inescapable impact of the immune system is needed.

References

[1] Ilich JZ, et al. Interrelationship among muscle, fat, and bone: connecting the dots on cellular, hormonal, and whole body levels. Ageing Res Rev 2014;15:51–60.
[2] Ilich JZ, et al. Osteosarcopenic obesity is associated with reduced handgrip strength, walking abilities, and balance in postmenopausal women. Osteoporos Int 2015;26(11):2587–95.
[3] Kelly OJ, et al. Osteosarcopenic obesity: current knowledge, revised identification criteria and treatment principles. Nutrients 2019;11(4):747.
[4] Ilich JZ, et al. Chronic stress contributes to osteosarcopenic adiposity via inflammation and immune modulation: the case for more precise nutritional investigation. Nutrients 2020;12(4):989.
[5] Ilich JZ, Kelly OJ, Inglis JE. Osteosarcopenic obesity syndrome: what is it and how can it be identified and diagnosed? Curr Gerontol Geriatr Res 2016;2016:7325973.
[6] Ilich JZ. Another impairment in older age: what does osteosarcopenic obesity syndrome mean for middle-aged and older women? J Am Med Dir Assoc 2017;18(8):648–50.
[7] JafariNasabian P, et al. Aging human body: changes in bone, muscle and body fat with consequent changes in nutrient intake. J Endocrinol 2017;234(1):R37–51.
[8] Cruz-Jentoft AJ, et al. Sarcopenia: revised European consensus on definition and diagnosis. Age Ageing 2018;48(1):16–31.
[9] Perna S, et al. Osteosarcopenic visceral obesity and osteosarcopenic subcutaneous obesity, two new phenotypes of sarcopenia: prevalence, metabolic profile, and risk factors. J Aging Res 2018;2018:6147426.
[10] Nishikawa K, et al. Maf promotes osteoblast differentiation in mice by mediating the age-related switch in mesenchymal cell differentiation. J Clin Invest 2010;120(10):3455–65.
[11] Zaidi SK, et al. Runx2 deficiency and defective subnuclear targeting bypass senescence to promote immortalization and tumorigenic potential. Proc Natl Acad Sci USA 2007;104(50):19861–6.
[12] Chen SE, Jin B, Li YP. TNF-alpha regulates myogenesis and muscle regeneration by activating p38 MAPK. Am J Phys Cell Phys 2007;292(5):C1660–71.
[13] Langen RC, et al. Tumor necrosis factor-alpha inhibits myogenic differentiation through MyoD protein destabilization. FASEB J 2004;18(2):227–37.
[14] Lecka-Czernik B, Suva LJ. Resolving the two "bony" faces of PPAR-gamma. PPAR Res 2006;2006:27489.
[15] Clarke DC, Liu X. Decoding the quantitative nature of TGF-beta/Smad signaling. Trends Cell Biol 2008;18(9):430–42.
[16] Sandhu MS, et al. Association between insulin-like growth factor-I: insulin-like growth factor-binding protein-1 ratio and metabolic and anthropometric factors in men and women. Cancer Epidemiol Biomark Prev 2004;13(1):166–70.
[17] Cawthorn WP, Sethi JK. TNF-alpha and adipocyte biology. FEBS Lett 2008;582(1):117–31.
[18] Karsenty G, Ferron M. The contribution of bone to whole-organism physiology. Nature 2012;481(7381):314–20.
[19] Bonewald L. Use it or lose it to age: a review of bone and muscle communication. Bone 2019;120:212–8.
[20] Gomarasca M, Banfi G, Lombardi G. Myokines: the endocrine coupling of skeletal muscle and bone. Adv Clin Chem 2020;94:155–218.
[21] Serrano AL, et al. Interleukin-6 is an essential regulator of satellite cell-mediated skeletal muscle hypertrophy. Cell Metab 2008;7(1):33–44.
[22] Pedersen BK. Muscles and their myokines. J Exp Biol 2011;214(Pt 2):337–46.

[23] Bostrom P, et al. A PGC1-alpha-dependent myokine that drives brown-fat-like development of white fat and thermogenesis. Nature 2012;481(7382):463–8.
[24] Reid IR. Relationships between fat and bone. Osteoporos Int 2008;19(5):595–606.
[25] Lecke SB, Morsch DM, Spritzer PM. Leptin and adiponectin in the female life course. Braz J Med Biol Res 2011;44:381–7.
[26] Ryan PM, Caplice NM. Is adipose tissue a reservoir for viral spread, immune activation, and cytokine amplification in coronavirus disease 2019? Obesity 2020;28(7):1191–4.
[27] Cosman F, et al. Clinician's guide to prevention and treatment of osteoporosis. Osteoporos Int 2014;25(10):2359–81.
[28] Shepherd JA, et al. Body composition by DXA. Bone 2017;104:101–5.
[29] Peppa M, et al. Bioimpedance analysis vs. DEXA as a screening tool for osteosarcopenia in lean, overweight and obese caucasian postmenopausal females. Hormones 2017;16(2):181–93.
[30] Stefanaki C, et al. Healthy overweight/obese youth: early osteosarcopenic obesity features. Eur J Clin Investig 2016;46(9):767–78.
[31] Stefanaki C, et al. Chronic stress and body composition disorders: implications for health and disease. Hormones 2018;17(1):33–43.
[32] Tsigos C, et al. Stress and inflammatory biomarkers and symptoms are associated with bioimpedance measures. Eur J Clin Investig 2015;45(2):126–34.
[33] Schoeb M, et al. Added value of impact microindentation in the evaluation of bone fragility: a systematic review of the literature. Front Endocrinol 2020;11:15.
[34] Barbosa-Silva MC, et al. Bioelectrical impedance analysis: population reference values for phase angle by age and sex. Am J Clin Nutr 2005;82(1):49–52.
[35] Brooks N, et al. Strength training improves muscle quality and insulin sensitivity in hispanic older adults with type 2 diabetes. Int J Med Sci 2006;4(1):19–27.
[36] Kelly TL, Wilson KE, Heymsfield SB. Dual energy X-ray absorptiometry body composition reference values from NHANES. PLoS One 2009;4(9):e7038.
[37] JafariNasabian P, et al. Metabolic profile of osteosarcopenic obesity syndrome: identifying biomarkers for diagnostic criteria. FASEB J 2017;31(1 Suppl):151.5.
[38] Abreu EL, et al. Skeletal muscle troponin as a novel biomarker to enhance assessment of the impact of strength training on fall prevention in the older adults. Nurs Res 2014;63(2):75–82.
[39] Ezzat-Zadeh Z, et al. The cooccurrence of obesity, osteoporosis, and sarcopenia in the ovariectomized rat: a study for modeling osteosarcopenic obesity in rodents. J Aging Res 2017;2017:1454103.
[40] Liu P-Y, et al. Evidence for the association between abdominal fat and cardiovascular risk factors in overweight and obese African American women. J Am Coll Nutr 2012;31(2):126–32.
[41] Ilich JZ, et al. Low-grade chronic inflammation perpetuated by modern diet as a promoter of obesity and osteoporosis. Arh Hig Rada Toksikol 2014;65(2):139–48.
[42] Schaap LA, et al. Higher inflammatory marker levels in older persons: associations with 5-year change in muscle mass and muscle strength. J Gerontol A Biol Sci Med Sci 2009;64(11):1183–9.
[43] Kim J, et al. Association of serum vitamin D with osteosarcopenic obesity: Korea National Health and Nutrition Examination Survey 2008-2010. J Cachexia Sarcopenia Muscle 2017;8(2):259–66.
[44] Kim J, et al. Diet quality and osteosarcopenic obesity in community-dwelling adults 50 years and older. Maturitas 2017;104:73–9.
[45] Park S, Na W, Sohn C. Relationship between osteosarcopenic obesity and dietary inflammatory index in postmenopausal Korean women: 2009 to 2011 Korea National Health and Nutrition Examination Surveys. J Clin Biochem Nutr 2018;63(3):211–6.

[46] Bae YJ. Fruit intake and osteosarcopenic obesity in Korean postmenopausal women aged 50-64 years. Maturitas 2020;134:41–6.
[47] Kim YM, et al. Clinical manifestations and factors associated with osteosarcopenic obesity syndrome: a cross-sectional study in Koreans with obesity. Calcif Tissue Int 2019;105(1):77–88.
[48] Hong W, et al. Prevalence of sarcopenia and its relationship with sites of fragility fractures in elderly Chinese men and women. PLoS One 2015;10(9):e0138102.
[49] Lee K. Association of osteosarcopenic obesity and its components: osteoporosis, sarcopenia and obesity with insulin resistance. J Bone Miner Metab 2020;38(5):695–701.
[50] Mo D, et al. Osteosarcopenic obesity and its relationship with dyslipidemia in women from different ethnic groups of China. Arch Osteoporos 2018;13(1):65.
[51] Chen X, et al. Association between osteosarcopenic obesity and hypertension among four minority populations in China: a cross-sectional study. BMJ Open 2019;9(7):e026818.
[52] Sasaki KI, et al. The prevalence of sarcopenia and subtypes in cardiovascular diseases, and a new diagnostic approach. J Cardiol 2020;76(3):266–72.
[53] Takayama M, et al. Sarcopenic obesity is associated with osteopenia among Japanese elderly women: a cross-sectional study from comprehensive health checkups. Health Eval Promot 2018;45(4):573–8.
[54] Szlejf C, Parra-Rodriguez L, Rosas-Carrasco O. Osteosarcopenic obesity: prevalence and relation with frailty and physical performance in middle-aged and older women. J Am Med Dir Assoc 2017;18(8):733 e1–5.
[55] Cunha PM, et al. The effects of resistance training volume on osteosarcopenic obesity in older women. J Sports Sci 2018;36(14):1564–71.
[56] Dos Santos VR, Gobbo LA. Physical activity is associated with functional capacity of older women with osteosarcopenic obesity: 24-month prospective study. Eur J Clin Nutr 2020;74(6):912–9.
[57] Banitalebi E, et al. Osteosarcopenic obesity markers following elastic band resistance training: a randomized controlled trial. Exp Gerontol 2020;135:110884.
[58] Zhu K, et al. Discordance between fat mass index and body mass index is associated with reduced bone mineral density in women but not in men: the Busselton Healthy Ageing Study. Osteoporos Int 2017;28(1):259–68.
[59] Jeng C, et al. Race and socioeconomic effect on sarcopenia and sarcopenic obesity in the Louisiana Osteoporosis Study (LOS). JCSM Clin Rep 2018;3(2):e00027.
[60] Carsote M, et al. Particular types of non-age related sarcopenia: osteosarcopenic obesity and malignancy-associated muscle waste. Arch Balk Med Union 2016;51(3):369–72.
[61] Hawkins KL, et al. Abdominal obesity, sarcopenia, and osteoporosis are associated with frailty in men living with and without HIV. AIDS 2018;32(10):1257–66.
[62] Yatsyshyn R, Stoika I. AB0358 phenotypes of secondary sarcopenia in patients with rheumatoid arthritis. Ann Rheum Dis 2018;77(Suppl. 2):1351.
[63] Fui MNT, Grossmann M. Hypogonadism from androgen deprivation therapy in identical twins. Lancet 2016;388(10060):2653.
[64] Dalla Volta A, et al. Bone mineral density and FRAX score may not predict fracture risk in patients with cancer undergoing hormone deprivation therapies. J Clin Oncol 2020;JCO2000434.
[65] Guarnotta V, et al. Circulating Irisin levels as a marker of osteosarcopenic-obesity in Cushing's disease. Diab Metab Syndr Obes 2020;13:1565–74.
[66] Bauer JM, et al. Is there enough evidence for osteosarcopenic obesity as a distinct entity? A critical literature review. Calcif Tissue Int 2019;105(2):109–24.
[67] Kassir R. Risk of COVID-19 for patients with obesity. Obes Rev 2020;21(6):e13034.

[68] Kirk B, et al. Muscle, bone, and fat crosstalk: the biological role of myokines, osteokines, and adipokines. Curr Osteoporos Rep 2020;18(4):388–400.
[69] Serhan CN, Chiang N, Van Dyke TE. Resolving inflammation: dual anti-inflammatory and pro-resolution lipid mediators. Nat Rev Immunol 2008;8(5):349–61.
[70] Konig MF, et al. Preventing cytokine storm syndrome in COVID-19 using alpha-1 adrenergic receptor antagonists. J Clin Invest 2020;130(7):3345–7.
[71] Weitzmann MN. T-cells and B-cells in osteoporosis. Curr Opin Endocrinol Diabetes Obes 2014;21(6):461–7.
[72] Weitzmann MN, Ofotokun I. Physiological and pathophysiological bone turnover—role of the immune system. Nat Rev Endocrinol 2016;12(9):518–32.
[73] Wang K, et al. Neuronal, stromal, and T-regulatory cell crosstalk in murine skeletal muscle. Proc Natl Acad Sci USA 2020;117(10):5402–8.
[74] Pedersen BK. Exercise-induced myokines and their role in chronic diseases. Brain Behav Immun 2011;25(5):811–6.
[75] Gharaibeh B, et al. Biological approaches to improve skeletal muscle healing after injury and disease. Birth Defects Res C Embryo Today 2012;96(1):82–94.
[76] Tidball JG. Regulation of muscle growth and regeneration by the immune system. Nat Rev Immunol 2017;17(3):165–78.
[77] Seijkens T, et al. Immune cell crosstalk in obesity: a key role for costimulation? Diabetes 2014;63(12):3982–91.
[78] Maurizi G, et al. Adipocytes properties and crosstalk with immune system in obesity-related inflammation. J Cell Physiol 2018;233(1):88–97.
[79] DiSpirito JR, Mathis D. Immunological contributions to adipose tissue homeostasis. Semin Immunol 2015;27(5):315–21.
[80] Mi B, et al. Characteristics and early prognosis of COVID-19 infection in fracture patients. J Bone Joint Surg Am 2020;102(9):750–8.
[81] Cheung ZB, Forsh DA. Early outcomes after hip fracture surgery in COVID-19 patients in New York City. J Orthop 2020;21:291–6.
[82] Boreskie KF, Hay JL, Duhamel TA. Preventing frailty progression during the COVID-19 pandemic. J Frailty Aging 2020;9(3):130–1.
[83] Morley JE, Kalantar-Zadeh K, Anker SD. COVID-19: a major cause of cachexia and sarcopenia? J Cachexia Sarcopenia Muscle 2020;11(4):863–5.
[84] Kelly OJ, Gilman JC. Can unconventional exercise be helpful in the treatment, management and prevention of osteosarcopenic obesity? Curr Aging Sci 2017;10(2):106–21.
[85] Kelly OJ, et al. Micronutrient intake in the etiology, prevention and treatment of osteosarcopenic obesity. Curr Aging Sci 2016;9(4):260–78.
[86] Kelly OJ, et al. Macronutrient intake and distribution in the etiology, prevention and treatment of osteosarcopenic obesity. Curr Aging Sci 2017;10(2):83–105.
[87] JafariNasabian P, et al. Osteosarcopenic obesity in women: impact, prevalence, and management challenges. Int J Women's Health 2017;9:33–42.

Chapter 11

Diagnosis of osteosarcopenia—Clinical

Ahmed M. Negm[a,b] and Alexandra Papaioannou[a,c]
[a]*GERAS Centre for Aging Research, St Peter's Hospital, Hamilton, ON, Canada,* [b]*Department of Surgery, University of Calgary, Calgary, AB, Canada,* [c]*Division of Geriatric Medicine, McMaster University, Hamilton, ON, Canada*

Overview

Osteosarcopenia is an age-related syndrome characterized by a low mass of the musculoskeletal unit composed of muscles and bones [1–3]. Osteosarcopenia was first described in 2009 as the coexistence of osteoporosis/osteopenia [4] (characterized by low bone mass and microarchitectural deterioration of bone tissue [5]) and sarcopenia (age-related loss of muscle mass, strength, and physical performance [6]). During the past decade, the negative impact of osteosarcopenia was proven to be more than only the cumulative effect of osteoporosis and sarcopenia (known as a hazardous duet) due to the interaction of their risk factors (including hormonal, nutritional, genetic, and lifestyle factors) [3,7]. The general consensus on the interaction between sarcopenia and osteoporosis/osteopenia is that it is first the loss of muscle that reduces bone mineral density (BMD) via a reduction in mechanical loading by gravitational forces, which usually stimulate bone formation [8,9].

The prevalence of osteosarcopenia

Epidemiological studies examining the prevalence of osteosarcopenia are fairly limited due to the recent origin of this syndrome [10]. The prevalence of osteosarcopenia was estimated to be between 5% and 40% [11]. The varied prevalence is likely due to a non-unified diagnostic criterion for this syndrome, with various screening tools being utilized for low muscle mass and function (sarcopenia), a key component of osteosarcopenia [12]. A recent study compared the performance of five screening tools for identifying older adults at risk of sarcopenia against five diagnostic definitions [13–17]. They found the prevalence of sarcopenia varied from 5.7% to 16.7%, depending on the definition. This study suggested using one of these clinical criteria to identify individuals with sarcopenia [18]. The prevalence of osteosarcopenia

Osteosarcopenia. https://doi.org/10.1016/B978-0-12-820088-9.00009-3

varies in epidemiological studies due to including heterogeneous populations. For example, the prevalence of osteosarcopenia in people with hip fracture was 27.2% [19]; however, the prevalence in community-dwelling older adults ranged from 4% to 15.1% [20,21]. Also, the prevalence of osteosarcopenia appear to vary in different countries; community-dwelling older adults range from 4.7% in Japan [22] to 13% in China [20], and 28% in Germany [23], with the highest rates observed in Australia (40%) [2] and Iran (34%) [24]. Despite the differences in reported prevalence of osteosarcopenia in previous studies, osteosarcopenia is a global health concern and a serious problem in the elderly due to its increasing incidence and the associated unfavorable outcomes [19].

Impact of osteosarcopenia

With aging of the global population, the impact of osteosarcopenia is increasing [19]. One-year mortality of older adults with osteosarcopenia (15.1%) was higher than people with osteoporosis (4.9%) or sarcopenia only (9.1%) [19]. After adjusting for covariates, osteosarcopenia had a 1.8 times higher mortality rate than nonosteosarcopenia (hazard ratio, 1.84; 95% confidence interval, 0.69–4.92) [19]. People with osteosarcopenia are at a higher risk of falls and fractures [1,25–28]. In addition, fracture risk in older men with osteosarcopenia is 3.5-fold higher than having only sarcopenia or osteopenia alone [26]. Compared with the nonosteosarcopenic group, those with osteosarcopenia had greater impairment in physical performance and balance (measured by short physical performance battery and timed-up and go) [25]. With physical performance impairment, osteosarcopenia is associated with a significant physical disability, representing a substantial threat to loss of independence later in life [29,30]. Indeed, the osteosarcopenic population is at higher risk not only for fractures but also for institutionalization, depression, and impaired mobility and quality of life [2,3].

Osteosarcopenia complications are associated with substantially increased morbidity and mortality, placing a significant economic burden on healthcare services [2,3]. An American study estimated the lifetime attributable cost of hip fracture in an 80 years old community dweller person to be $81,300, and the total yearly cost of all hip fractures in the United States of more than $20 billion [31]. Also, in the United States, another study calculated the direct cost of sarcopenia to be $18.5 billion in 2000, represented by hospitalization, nursing home admissions, and home healthcare expenditure [32]. In Europe, an estimate in 2010 calculated the direct cost of all osteoporotic fractures at €29 billion in the five largest EU countries (France, Germany, Italy, Spain, and the United Kingdom) and €38.7 billion in 27 EU countries [33,34]. Given the clinical outcomes associated with osteosarcopenia, the diagnosis of osteosarcopenia is imperative to enable clinical care [35]. The diagnosis and screening for osteosarcopenia and hence implementing different prevention and treatment strategies will improve health outcomes and quality of life of older adults.

Osteosarcopenia diagnostic algorithm

There are several diagnostic and screening tools to identify people with osteosarcopenia; specifically, the sarcopenia component of osteosarcopenia. In this chapter, we are presenting an algorithm to screen and diagnose people at risk of osteosarcopenia. The algorithm is shown in Fig. 1. We are also describing a number of validated tools to be used in each stage of the algorithm.

Case finding

Early identification of older adults with osteosarcopenia will allow clinicians to implement preventative or intervention strategies and avoid complications. Patients with one or more of the following osteosarcopenia risk factors need to be further screened and tested.

Clinical risk factors

Personal

Age

Sarcopenia and osteoporosis are age-related diseases by definition [25,36]. The mean age of the subjects with osteosarcopenia is close to 80 years (79–82 years), as observed in most studies. People in this age group have a significant increase in the incidence of fractures. This significant increase is caused by the greater physical functional loss resulting from sarcopenia, and the lower BMD observed in osteosarcopenic patients as compared to older persons with sarcopenia or osteoporosis only [3,24].

Sex

Osteosarcopenia occurs more frequently in women than in men. Studies have shown variation between 55% and 65% of prevalence in women [2,19,20]. The association with the female is mainly due to the estrogenic deprivation of menopause, which causes a marked decrease in muscle strength in women [37,38]. The lower muscle strength promotes less mechanostatic action, decreasing the stimulus on bone growth and, consequently, more significant loss of BMD, contributing to the incidence of osteosarcopenia.

Body composition

Obesity

Obesity, i.e., excess body fat, usually defined as body mass index (BMI) $\geqslant 30\,kg/m^2$, is a major public health problem and is well recognized as a risk factor for morbidity and mortality in older adults [39]. Aging is associated with significant changes in body composition with a substantial reduction in

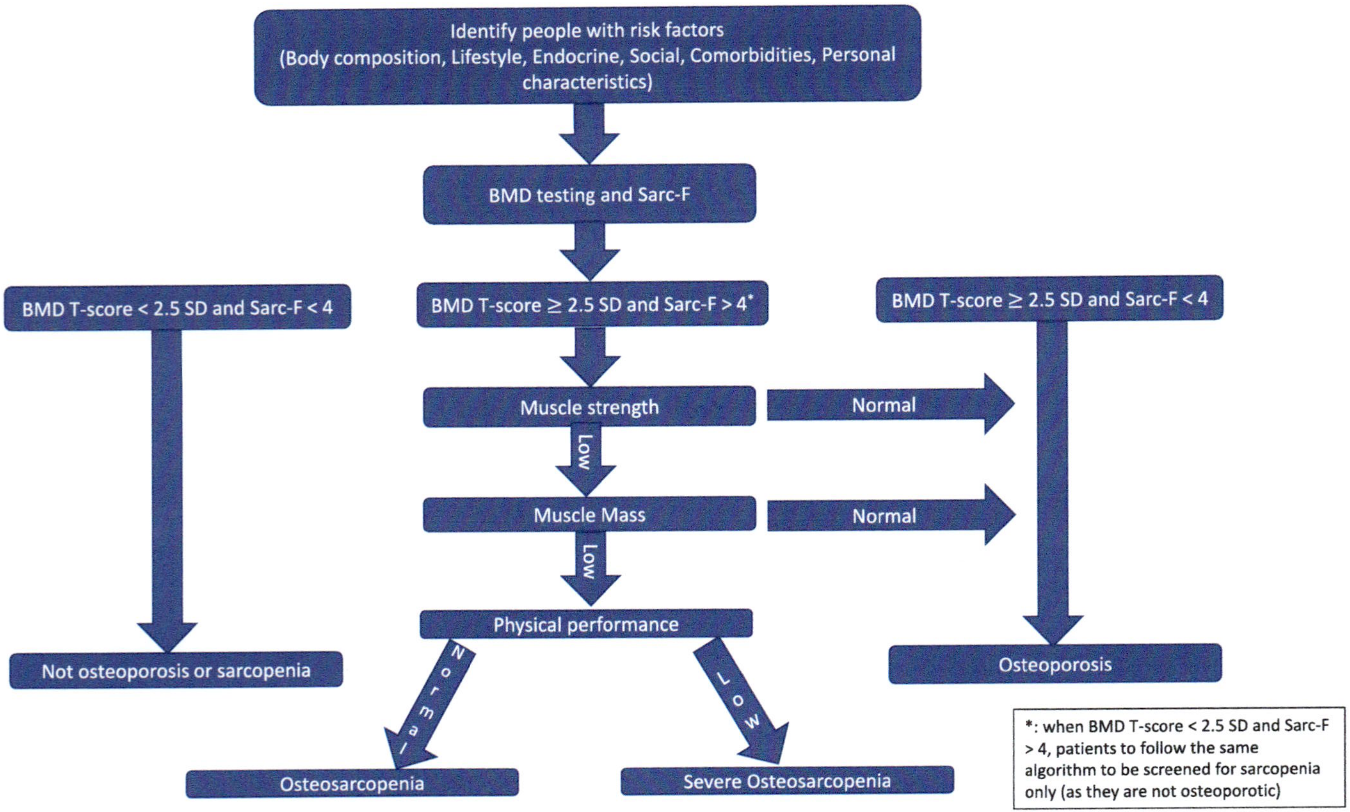

FIG. 1 Osteosarcopenia diagnostic algorithm.

fat-free mass and muscle mass and an increase in visceral fat [40–42]. Given the age-related changes in body composition, sarcopenia often coexists with an increase in fat mass. Visceral fat and muscle mass are known to be interrelated from a pathogenic point of view and are reported to share common inflammatory pathways [42]. In addition, sarcopenia reduces physical activity, resulting in decreased energy expenditure, leading to an increased risk of obesity [42]. Alternatively, visceral fat induces inflammation, contributing to osteoporosis and sarcopenia [43]. The interplay between sarcopenia and rising trends in obesity in an aging population is emerging as a paramount public health concern in the older population. The term sarcopenic obesity was first introduced by Baumgartner [41] and is defined by the combination of sarcopenia and obesity. Obesity and sarcopenia may act synergistically; sarcopenic obesity may have a greater effect on metabolic disorders and mortality, disability, or physical function as outcomes than either obesity or sarcopenia alone [42,44,45]. Therefore, screening people with obesity for osteosarcopenia is indicated to prevent unfavorable outcomes of older adults.

Fat infiltration

Since BMI does not distinguish between fat mass and fat-free mass, which have opposing effects on the risk of morbidity and mortality, the use of BMI in older persons may have limitations [46]. Therefore, to fully understand the impact of obesity on older persons, it is essential also to take both fat mass and lean mass into account. Several studies have observed that osteosarcopenic individuals present a high percentage of fat independent of BMI [2]. There is still no consensus as to the percentage of better specificity and sensitivity for these patients. At present, high fat is present when it is above 30% or 40% [47] or the percentage body fat percentage by the squared height is equal to or above the upper quintile of the sample.

Low body weight

Low body weight, defined by low BMI, is associated with sarcopenia [48]. The few studies that evaluated the BMI of older subjects with osteosarcopenia showed that the mean BMI of these individuals is lower when compared to individuals with sarcopenia and osteoporosis only. However, due to the ethnic and gender variety of study populations, there is some discrepancy as to the mean that can best characterize osteosarcopenia, since they ranged from 20.7 (3.5) kg/m^2 in Asian elderly with hip fracture to 27.2 (6.2) kg/m^2 in a population of community-dwelling older persons with a high prevalence of obesity [2,19].

Lifestyle

Sedentary lifestyle/poor mobility

Both bone and muscle are adaptive, modifying their mass and strength in response to mechanical loading. Therefore, mechanical stimulus is essential for the health of both tissues, and thus, decreased levels of physical activity may shift the delicate balance in favor of muscle degradation and bone resorption [3]. Physical activity diminishes with aging, with up to 80% of waking hours spent sedentary in older adults [49], leading to a loss of mechanical loading and associated bone and muscle loss [50]. Low mobility is a prevalent and specific clinical feature among the osteosarcopenic population. The risk of loss of mobility was about three times higher among osteosarcopenic patients than the control group, whereas people with sarcopenia had no significant association with loss of mobility [2,23,51].

Malnutrition

Caloric intake diminishes by around 25% between the ages of 40 and 70 [52], with reduced vitamin D levels and protein intake correlated with declining muscle strength [53]. Vitamin D deficiency also increases the risk of falls and fractures through its multiple effects on muscle and bone [54]. Malnutrition was described in a study with the Mini-Nutritional Assessment (MNA) tool. In this study, osteosarcopenic individuals present a twofold higher risk for malnutrition (MNA < 12) than individuals in the control group [2,55].

Smoking

Smoking may have detrimental effects on the skeletal system. Recent evidence demonstrates tobacco smoking causes an imbalance in the mechanisms of bone turnover, leading to lower bone BMD making bone vulnerable to osteoporosis and fracture [56–63]. Similarly, components of cigarette smoke enter the bloodstream and reach the skeletal muscles of smokers and accelerate muscle wasting [64–66]. A metaanalysis of 12 studies (22,515 participants) indicated that cigarette smoking as an isolated factor might contribute to the development of sarcopenia. Therefore, cigarette smoking should be counted among the risk factors of osteosarcopenia [67–69].

Alcohol consumption

Alcohol is a significant risk factor for osteoporosis, with an intake of ≥ 3 units of alcohol/day increasing fracture risk in a dose-dependent fashion [70].

Endocrine

Glucocorticoids

The increased incidence of various diseased states during aging is associated with the hypersecretion of glucocorticoids [71–73]. Glucocorticoid-associated atrophy appears to be specific to type II or phasic muscle fibers. In a study of controlled hypercortisolemia in healthy men [74], experimental inactivity increased the catabolic effect of glucocorticoids, suggesting that an absence of mechanical signals potentiates the impact. The mechanism of glucocorticoid-induced atrophy may involve an upregulated expression of myostatin and glutamine synthetase, the latter via the glucocorticoid receptor's interaction with the glutamine synthetase promoter [75]. Glucocorticoids inhibit the physiological secretion of growth hormone and appear to induce IGF-I activity in target organs [76]. Also, prolonged use of systemic glucocorticoids (i.e., at least three months cumulative use during the preceding year at a prednisone-equivalent dose ≥7.5 mg daily) increases the risk of fracture independent of BMD [77].

Low vitamin D

Vitamin D has been considered a key regulator of bone metabolism and calcium and phosphorus homeostasis through negative feedback with the parathyroid hormone [78,79]. It is also well established that vitamin D deficiency is a risk factor for osteoporosis in older adults. A large and growing body of evidence suggests that vitamin D is necessary for bone tissue and calcium metabolism [78,80]. Approximately 1 billion, mostly older persons, worldwide have vitamin D deficiency [81–83]. The prevalence of low vitamin D concentrations in subjects older than 65 years of age has been estimated at approximately 50% [81–83]. Similarly, there is an age-dependent reduction in vitamin D receptor expression in skeletal muscle [84]. Prolonged vitamin D deficiency has been associated with severe muscle weakness, which improves with vitamin D supplementation [85]. Interestingly, muscle biopsies performed before and after vitamin D supplementation have documented an increased number and sectional area of type II (or fast) muscle fibers [84,86]. More comprehensive knowledge of vitamin D-related mechanisms may provide a helpful tool for preventing muscle atrophy in older persons (sarcopenia).

Hypogonadism (male)

In males, levels of testosterone decrease by 1% per year, and those of bioavailable testosterone by 2% per year from age 30 [87–89]. In women, testosterone levels drop rapidly from 20 to 45 years of age [90]. Testosterone increases muscle protein synthesis [91], and its effects on muscle are modulated by several factors, including genetic background, nutrition, and exercise [92]. Numerous studies of treatment with testosterone in older persons have been performed over the past few years [93–96]. In 1999, Snyder et al. [96] suggested that increasing the level of testosterone in older men to that seen in young men increased muscle mass but did not result in functional gains in strength. Systemic reviews of the literature [97] have concluded that testosterone supplementation attenuates several sarcopenic symptoms, including decreases in muscle mass [94–96] and grip strength [93]. For instance, a recent study of 6 months of supraphysiological dosage of testosterone in a randomized placebo-controlled trial reported increased leg lean body mass and leg and arm strength [98]. Although there are significant increases in strength among older males given high doses of testosterone, the potential risks may outweigh the benefits. Risks associated with testosterone therapy in older men include sleep apnea, thrombotic complications, and the increased risk of prostate cancer [99].

Menopause (female)

Menopause is a natural part of aging, and it encompasses the loss of ovarian reproductive function. Osteoporosis is a common, asymptomatic postmenopausal disease that substantially impacts the quality of life of older women. Osteoporosis-related fractures are one of the causes of disability among the older population [100]. One in two postmenopausal women will have an osteoporotic fracture in their lifetime [101].

It has been hypothesized that menopause transition and the subsequent decline in estrogen may play a role in muscle mass loss [102,103]. Van Geel et al. [104] reported a positive relationship between lean body mass and estrogen levels. Similarly, Iannuzzi-Sucich et al. [105] observed that muscle mass is correlated significantly with plasma estrone and estradiol levels in women. The mechanisms by which a decrease in estrogen levels may have a negative effect on muscle mass are not well understood but may be associated with an increase in proinflammatory cytokines, such as TNF-α and IL-6, which might be implicated in the apparition of sarcopenia [106]. Furthermore, estrogen could directly affect muscle mass since it has been shown that skeletal muscle has estrogen beta-receptors on the cell membrane [107]. Therefore, a direct potential mechanistic link could exist between low estrogen levels and a decrease in protein synthesis.

Low growth hormone

Growth hormone (GH) is a single-chain peptide of 191 amino acids produced and secreted mainly by the somatotrophs of the anterior pituitary gland. GH coordinates the postnatal growth of multiple target tissues, including skeletal muscle [108]. Indeed, circulating GH levels decline progressively after 30 years of age at a rate of $\sim 1\%$ per year [109]. In aged men, daily GH secretion is 5- to 20-fold lower than in young adults [110]. The age-dependent decline in GH secretion is secondary to a decrease in GHRH and an increase in somatostatin secretion [111]. There is evidence that the age-associated decline in GH levels in combination with lower IGF-I levels contributes to the development of sarcopenia [112,113]. The effects of GH administration on muscle mass, strength, and physical performance are still under debate [114]. In animal models, GH treatment effectively inhibits sarcopenic symptoms such as muscle atrophy and decreases in protein synthesis, particularly in combination with exercise training [115]. The effect of GH treatment on older subjects is controversial. Some groups demonstrated an improvement in strength after long-term administration (3–11 months) of GH [116]. In contrast, many researchers have found that muscle strength or muscle mass did not improve on supplementation with GH [114,116].

Hyperparathyroidism

Hyperparathyroidism is due to increased parathyroid gland activity, which leads to osteoporosis with related fractures [117]. Proximal muscle weakness due to type II muscle fiber atrophy can be seen in association with severe bone disease (such as osteoporosis) [118]. High serum levels of parathyroid hormone have been recently associated with osteosarcopenia independently of serum vitamin D or renal function (summarized in Chapter 8).

Social

Living in a residential care facility

Dependent older adults pose a particular challenge for researchers because advanced functional and cognitive impairment may limit their capacity to perform tests, especially for speed and strength. As the population ages, a greater number of older adults will need residential support such as residential care facility (RACF). RACF residents are often frail since their multiple physical and cognitive deficits place them at high risk of falls, disability, and death [119–121]. The fracture rate for adults living in RACF is two to four times that of adults of a similar age living in the community, and one-third of older adults who experience hip fracture are residents in RACF [122].

A systematic review and metaanalysis published in 2017 by Shafiee et al. [123] addressed the worldwide prevalence of sarcopenia but excluded studies carried out in hospitals or nursing homes for older adults. The prevalence of sarcopenia was shown to be higher in RACF residents. A review followed the consensus of the European Working Group on Sarcopenia in Older People (EWGSOP) [13], described prevalence values of 1%–29% among older adults living at home, 14%–68% among those in RACF, and 10% among people hospitalized in acute care [13]. Another review included studies that evaluated the prevalence of sarcopenia among older adults (aged ≥60 years) living in RACF. Forty-four studies were identified, of which 21 studies were included after applying eligibility criteria. The reported prevalence of sarcopenia ranged widely between 17.7% and 73.3% in RACF and between 22% and 87% in assisted-living facilities [124]. Therefore, it is critical to identify RACF residents with osteosarcopenia.

Comorbidities

A large proportion is of older adults are suffering from chronic comorbidities such as cardiovascular failure, renal failure, or cancer [125]. These comorbidities are associated with a decline of skeletal muscle and bone mass, potentially leading to osteosarcopenia [126–128].

Previous fragility fracture

History of fragility fracture is associated with osteoporosis and sarcopenia. In a recent study, 70 out of 139 hip fracture patients (50.36%) were diagnosed with sarcopenia. Hip fracture patients with sarcopenia also have insufficient activity of daily living and a lower quality of life than patients without sarcopenia before the injury and 6 months after the operation [129]. Clinicians should examine people with a history of fragility fracture for sarcopenia and osteoporosis (if not diagnosed already).

Frailty

The odds of frailty are significantly higher in osteosarcopenic patients than those with osteoporosis or sarcopenia alone [20]. Bone and muscle loss also may be tightly linked to the risk of frailty as shown in a 2015 study conducted in China in which osteosarcopenia was found in 26.3% of men and 38.5% of women with frailty and only in 1.6% and 1.9% of nonfrail men and women, respectively [20].

Sarc-F and BMD

People with one or more osteosarcopenia risk factors need to be screened using the Sarc-F questionnaires, as well as BMD measurement to determine whether a patient is at risk of osteosarcopenia, sarcopenia, or osteoporosis alone.

Sarc-F

To identify candidates for sarcopenia assessment, the Sarc-F questionnaire will be used. Sarc-F comprises five components: strength, assistance with walking, rise from a chair, stair climbing, and falls. The scores range from 0 to 10, with 0 to 2 points for each component. A score equal to or greater than four is predictive of sarcopenia [130]. SARC-F was valid and consistent for identifying people at risk of sarcopenia-associated adverse outcomes. SARC-F has a low-to-moderate sensitivity and a very high specificity to predict low muscle strength [131]. As such, SARC-F primarily detects severe cases. As an inexpensive and convenient method for sarcopenia risk screening, SARC-F is recommended as a way to introduce assessment and treatment of sarcopenia into clinical practice.

BMD

The World Health Organization (WHO) established diagnostic criteria for osteoporosis based on BMD T scores [132]. The T score describes the patient's BMD in terms of the number of SDs by which it differs from the mean peak value in young, healthy persons of the same sex [133]. The WHO uses a threshold of 2.5 SDs below the mean of young adult women as the criterion for a diagnosis of osteoporosis [132]. The criterion for diagnosing osteopenia (low bone mass) is more than 1.0 SD, but less than 2.5 SDs below the reference mean [132]. However, T scores were developed to estimate the prevalence of osteoporosis across populations, not for the assessment of osteoporosis in specific patients

[134]. Moreover, although T scores originally were based on the BMD of the hip measured by dual-energy X-ray absorptiometry (DXA), the scores are now applied to BMD at other skeletal sites and/or measured by different methods [135]. Currently, the National Osteoporosis Foundation and the International Society for Clinical Densitometry consider central DXA of the hip and/or spine as the preferred measurement for a diagnosis of osteoporosis [136,137]. In this chapter, radiologic diagnostic measures of osteoporosis will be discussed in more detail.

Muscle strength

In patients with osteosarcopenia risk factors who scored 4 or more on Sarc-F, muscle strength needs to be measured. There are several clinical measures of muscle strength.

Grip strength

Grip strength is a simple method to measure muscle strength. Low grip strength is associated with poor patient outcomes such as disability, longer hospital stays, increased functional limitations, poor health-related quality of life, morbidity, and mortality [138–140]. Measurements of grip strength taken with the Jamar dynamometer have evidence for good to excellent ($r > 0.80$) test-retest reliability [141] and excellent ($r = 0.98$) interrater reliability [142]. High test-retest reliability has been shown among older American community-dwelling volunteers (mean age 75 years) repeatedly tested over 12 weeks [143]. Grip strength correlates moderately with strength in other body compartments, so it serves as a reliable surrogate for more complicated measures of arm and leg strength [36]. Because of its ease of use, grip strength is advised for routine use in hospital practice, specialty clinical settings, and community healthcare [138,139,144–146].

Accurate measurement of grip strength requires using a calibrated handheld dynamometer under well-defined test conditions with measurement protocol to improve the validity of assessment [147,148]. It was demonstrated that the choice of equipment and measurement protocol for assessing grip strength varies widely between studies. The Jamar hand dynamometer is the most widely cited instrument in the literature and appears to be a generally accepted gold standard with the most normative data [147].

Measurement protocol

The American Society of Hand Therapists (ASHT) recommends standardized positioning: patient seated, shoulders adducted and neutrally rotated, elbow flexed at 90°, forearm in neutral, and wrist between 0° and 30° of dorsiflexion [147]. Different methods of instruction and/or verbal encouragement can affect the patients' performance [149] and thus introduce measurement error [150].

Mathiowetz et al. [141] have a set of standardized instructions: "I want you to hold the handle like this and squeeze as hard as you can." The examiner demonstrates and then gives the dynamometer to the subject. After the subject is positioned appropriately, the examiner says, "Are you ready? Squeeze as hard as you can." As the subject begins to squeeze, the examiner says, "Harder!... Harder!... Relax" [141].

Sarcopenia cut-off points for grip strength vary according to the sarcopenia definition used. Table 1 summarizes the cut-off points for EWGSOP2, Asian Working Group for Sarcopenia, and The Foundation for the National Institutes of Health (FNIH) [16,17,36].

Chair stand

The chair stand test can be used as a proxy for the strength of leg muscles (quadriceps muscle group). The chair stand test measures the amount of time needed for a patient to rise five times from a seated position without using their arms; the timed chair stand test is a variation that counts how many times a patient can rise and sit in the chair over a 30-s interval [145,151,152]. Since the chair stand test requires both strength and endurance, this test is a qualified but convenient measure of strength.

In the chair stand test, participants are asked to stand up five times in a row as quickly as possible from a chair without stopping, keeping arms folded across the chest. Participants have to come to a full standing position each time they stood up and to sit all the way down each time. Timing starts when the examiner says "Go!" and stops when the participant sits down for the fifth time. Time (in seconds) or inability to perform the test is used as a result of the test [151]. According to EWGSOP2, older adults who complete 5 rises in more than 15 s are considered sarcopenic [13].

TABLE 1 Sarcopenia cut-off points of grip strength using 3 different definitions.

Sarcopenia definition	Measurement modality (cut-off points)
EWGSOP2	(Men <27 kg; women <16 kg)
SDOC	Handgrip strength (men <35.5 kg; women <20 kg)
	Handgrip strength:BMI (men ≪1.05 kg/kg/m^2; women <0.79 kg/kg/m^2)
Asian Working Group for Sarcopenia	Handgrip strength (men <26 kg; women <18 kg)

EWGSOP2, the European Working Group on Sarcopenia in Older People; *SDOC*, Sarcopenia Definitions and Outcomes Consortium.

Lower limb strength

When measurement of grip is not possible due to hand disability (e.g., with advanced arthritis or stroke), isometric torque methods can be used to measure lower limb strength (most frequently of the quadriceps) [153]. Commercial dynamometers can enable isometric and/or isokinetic measurements of strength [145]. Even if these measurements are feasible in frail people [154,155], they are often limited in clinical practice by their relative expense, the need to purchase dedicated equipment, the lack of trained staff, and limited data in older populations. Harbo et al. described a lower limb strength measurement protocol for research purposes [156].

Muscle mass

If a participant has low muscle strength, muscle mass needs to be measured to confirm the diagnosis of sarcopenia. Muscle mass can be estimated using different techniques, and there are multiple methods of adjusting the result for height or BMI [157–159]. Muscle (lean)mass can be reported as total body Skeletal Muscle Mass (SMM), as Appendicular Skeletal Muscle Mass (ASM), or as cross-sectional muscle area of specific muscle groups or body locations. The diagnostic measures of muscle mass include DXA (the most commonly used diagnostic measure [160]), Computed Tomography (CT)/Magnetic Resonance Imaging (MRI) (considered the gold standard), ultrasound, or bioimpedance analysis (BIA). In this chapter, the radiological and nonradiological diagnostic measures of muscle mass will be discussed in detail.

Physical performance

Physical performance is a multidimensional concept that involves not only muscles but also central and peripheral nervous functions, including balance [145]. Measuring physical performance aims to determine the severity of osteosarcopenia. Physical performance can be measured by gait speed, Short Physical Performance Battery (SPPB), Timed-Up and Go test (TUG), or 400-m walk test, among other tests.

Gait speed

The most widely used tool in clinical practice for assessing physical performance is the gait speed measurement. The test is highly acceptable for participants and health professionals in clinical settings [161]. No special equipment is required as it only needs a flat floor devoid of obstacles with a straight, clearly marked course. A trained operator with a stopwatch is also needed as an evaluator [162]. Patients are instructed to walk at their usual pace from a still-standing position behind the starting line. Timing starts at the first foot movement and ends when a foot completely crossed the finish line. Canes and walkers are allowed if a patient normally used this equipment in their daily life. In the 4-m gait speed test, which the EWGSOP2 recommends for assessing sarcopenia, men and women with a gait speed <0.8 m/s are described as having poor physical performance [36].

400-m walk test

The 400-m walk test assesses walking ability and endurance. For this test, patients are asked to complete 20 laps of 20 m, each lap as fast as possible, and are allowed up to two rest stops during the test. Measurement protocol and equipment are similar to the gait speed test [36].

Short physical performance battery

The Short Performance Physical Battery (SPPB) is an objective physical performance measure focused on lower extremity physical function and measures balance, strength, and coordination [51], which are important contributors to mobility and independence [51]. In older adults with a high degree of frailty and impairment, age- and gender-adjusted SPPB is associated with increased emergency room visits and hospitalizations [163]. The SPPB is a composite test that includes an assessment of gait speed, a balance test, and a chair stand test, and each component is scored between 0 and 4 [51]. This performance-based tool is a continuous measure with total scores ranging from 0 to 12. From previous validation [164,165], scores of 0–4, 5–8, and 9–12 indicate poor, intermediate, and good lower extremity function, respectively. For the assessment of sarcopenia, a score of ≤8 points indicates poor physical performance [13,145].

Timed-up and go test

The Timed-Up and Go test (TU & Go) is the most used test worldwide [166]. This test measures the dynamic balance and functional mobility in older adults, as well as in the neurological population [167–169]. The TU & Go is a simple test that can be performed anywhere and consists of a patient getting up from a chair from the sitting to the bipedal position, walking three meters, turning, returning, and sitting on the chair again. The variable measured is the total time taken by the test, and then the score assigned in seconds is observed, which is correlated with the risk of falls [167,170]. Some of the advantages of the TU & Go test are the simplicity in its application and its short duration. In addition, it requires little equipment and allows the possibility that people with a functional impairment can perform the test [166]. The EWGSOP2 suggested that patients with a TU & Go of 20 s or more are described as having poor physical performance [36].

TABLE 2 Sarcopenia cut-off points of physical performance using 3 different definitions.

Sarcopenia definition	Measurement modality (cut-off points)
EWGSOP2	Gait speed: ≤0.8 m/s SPPB: ≤8-point score TUG: ≥20 s 400 m walk test: noncompletion or ≥6 min for completion
FNIH	Gait speed: ≤0.8 m/s
Asian Working Group for Sarcopenia	Gait speed: <0.8 m/s

EWGSOP2, the European Working Group on Sarcopenia in Older People; *SDOC*, Sarcopenia Definitions and Outcomes Consortium.

Table 2 summarizes the sarcopenia cut points of sarcopenia cut-off points of physical performance measures for EWGSOP2, Asian Working Group for Sarcopenia, and the FNIH [16,17,36].

Summary

Osteosarcopenia syndrome is the age-related process of musculoskeletal tissue degeneration with impaired physical and functional performance. Osteosarcopenia leads to a greater risk of disability, frailty, morbidity, and mortality predominantly among our older population. Osteosarcopenia is characterized by low muscle mass and BMD, muscle weakness, and lower physical function. The proposed osteosarcopenia identification algorithm in this chapter is fundamental for screening at-risk older adults in various settings. Early identification and diagnosis of people with osteosarcopenia could be followed by interventions and prevention strategies tailored to improve older adults' musculoskeletal health and prevent potential complications.

References

[1] Huo YR, Suriyaarachchi P, Gomez F, Curcio CL, Boersma D, Gunawardene P, et al. Comprehensive nutritional status in sarco-osteoporotic older fallers. J Nutr Health Aging 2015;19(4):474–80.

[2] Huo YR, Suriyaarachchi P, Gomez F, Curcio CL, Boersma D, Muir SW, et al. Phenotype of osteosarcopenia in older individuals with a history of falling. J Am Med Dir Assoc 2015;16(4):290–5.

[3] Hirschfeld HP, Kinsella R, Duque G. Osteosarcopenia: where bone, muscle, and fat collide. Osteoporos Int 2017;28(10):2781–90.

[4] Binkley N, Buehring B. Beyond FRAX: it's time to consider "sarco-osteopenia". J Clin Densitom 2009;12(4):413–6.

[5] Edwards MH, Dennison EM, Aihie Sayer A, Fielding R, Cooper C. Osteoporosis and sarcopenia in older age. Bone 2015;80:126–30.
[6] Fuggle N, Shaw S, Dennison E, Cooper C. Sarcopenia. Best Pract Res Clin Rheumatol 2017;31(2):218–42.
[7] Zanker J, Duque G. Osteosarcopenia: the path beyond controversy. Curr Osteoporos Rep 2020;18(2):81–4.
[8] Park JH, Song YM, Sung J, Lee K, Kim YS, Kim T, et al. The association between fat and lean mass and bone mineral density: the Healthy Twin Study. Bone 2012;50(4):1006–11.
[9] Verschueren S, Gielen E, O'Neill TW, Pye SR, Adams JE, Ward KA, et al. Sarcopenia and its relationship with bone mineral density in middle-aged and elderly European men. Osteoporos Int 2013;24(1):87–98.
[10] Paintin J, Cooper C, Dennison E. Osteosarcopenia. Br J Hosp Med (Lond) 2018;79(5):253–8.
[11] Nielsen BR, Abdulla J, Andersen HE, Schwarz P, Suetta C. Sarcopenia and osteoporosis in older people: a systematic review and meta-analysis. Eur Geriatr Med 2018;9(4):419–34.
[12] Kirk B, Al Saedi A, Duque G. Osteosarcopenia: a case of geroscience. Aging Med (Milton) 2019;2(3):147–56.
[13] Cruz-Jentoft AJ, Baeyens JP, Bauer JM, Boirie Y, Cederholm T, Landi F, et al. Sarcopenia: European consensus on definition and diagnosis: report of the European Working Group on Sarcopenia in Older People. Age Ageing 2010;39(4):412–23.
[14] Fielding RA, Vellas B, Evans WJ, Bhasin S, Morley JE, Newman AB, et al. Sarcopenia: an undiagnosed condition in older adults. Current consensus definition: prevalence, etiology, and consequences. International working group on sarcopenia. J Am Med Dir Assoc 2011;12(4):249–56.
[15] Morley JE, Abbatecola AM, Argiles JM, Baracos V, Bauer J, Bhasin S, et al. Sarcopenia with limited mobility: an international consensus. J Am Med Dir Assoc 2011;12(6):403–9.
[16] Chen LK, Liu LK, Woo J, Assantachai P, Auyeung TW, Bahyah KS, et al. Sarcopenia in Asia: consensus report of the Asian Working Group for Sarcopenia. J Am Med Dir Assoc 2014;15(2):95–101.
[17] Studenski SA, Peters KW, Alley DE, Cawthon PM, McLean RR, Harris TB, et al. The FNIH sarcopenia project: rationale, study description, conference recommendations, and final estimates. J Gerontol A Biol Sci Med Sci 2014;69(5):547–58.
[18] Locquet M, Beaudart C, Reginster JY, Petermans J, Bruyère O. Comparison of the performance of five screening methods for sarcopenia. Clin Epidemiol 2018;10:71–82.
[19] Yoo JI, Kim H, Ha YC, Kwon HB, Koo KH. Osteosarcopenia in patients with hip fracture is related with high mortality. J Korean Med Sci 2018;33(4):e27.
[20] Wang YJ, Wang Y, Zhan JK, Tang ZY, He JY, Tan P, et al. Sarco-osteoporosis: prevalence and association with frailty in chinese community-dwelling older adults. Int J Endocrinol 2015;2015:482940.
[21] Kobayashi K, Imagama S, Ando K, Machino M, Ota K, Tanaka S, et al. Epidemiology and effect on physical function of osteosarcopenia in community-dwelling elderly people in Japan. Mod Rheumatol 2019;1–6.
[22] Yoshimura N, Muraki S, Oka H, Iidaka T, Kodama R, Kawaguchi H, et al. Is osteoporosis a predictor for future sarcopenia or vice versa? Four-year observations between the second and third ROAD study surveys. Osteoporos Int 2017;28(1):189–99.
[23] Drey M, Sieber CC, Bertsch T, Bauer JM, Schmidmaier R, FiAT Intervention Group. Osteosarcopenia is more than sarcopenia and osteopenia alone. Aging Clin Exp Res 2016;28(5):895–9.

[24] Fahimfar N, Zahedi Tajrishi F, Gharibzadeh S, Shafiee G, Tanha K, Heshmat R, et al. Prevalence of osteosarcopenia and its association with cardiovascular risk factors in iranian older people: bushehr elderly health (BEH) program. Calcif Tissue Int 2020;106(4):364–70.
[25] Sepulveda-Loyola W, Phu S, Bani Hassan E, Brennan-Olsen SL, Zanker J, Vogrin S, et al. The joint occurrence of osteoporosis and sarcopenia (osteosarcopenia): definitions and characteristics. J Am Med Dir Assoc 2020;21:220–5.
[26] Yu R, Leung J, Woo J. Incremental predictive value of sarcopenia for incident fracture in an elderly Chinese cohort: results from the Osteoporotic Fractures in Men (MrOs) Study. J Am Med Dir Assoc 2014;15(8):551–8.
[27] Chalhoub D, Cawthon PM, Ensrud KE, Stefanick ML, Kado DM, Boudreau R, et al. Risk of nonspine fractures in older adults with sarcopenia, low bone mass, or both. J Am Geriatr Soc 2015;63(9):1733–40.
[28] Lexell J. Human aging, muscle mass, and fiber type composition. J Gerontol A Biol Sci Med Sci 1995. 50 Spec No:11-6.
[29] Curtis E, Litwic A, Cooper C, Dennison E. Determinants of muscle and bone aging. J Cell Physiol 2015;230(11):2618–25.
[30] Ha YC, Kim TY, Lee A, Lee YK, Kim HY, Kim JH, et al. Current trends and future projections of hip fracture in South Korea using nationwide claims data. Osteoporos Int 2016;27(8):2603–9.
[31] Braithwaite RS, Col NF, Wong JB. Estimating hip fracture morbidity, mortality and costs. J Am Geriatr Soc 2003;51(3):364–70.
[32] Janssen I, Shepard DS, Katzmarzyk PT, Roubenoff R. The healthcare costs of sarcopenia in the United States. J Am Geriatr Soc 2004;52(1):80–5.
[33] Ström O, Borgström F, Kanis JA, Compston J, Cooper C, McCloskey EV, et al. Osteoporosis: burden, health care provision and opportunities in the EU: a report prepared in collaboration with the International Osteoporosis Foundation (IOF) and the European Federation of Pharmaceutical Industry Associations (EFPIA). Arch Osteoporos 2011;6:59–155.
[34] Kanis JA, McCloskey EV, Johansson H, Cooper C, Rizzoli R, Reginster JY, et al. European guidance for the diagnosis and management of osteoporosis in postmenopausal women. Osteoporos Int 2013;24(1):23–57.
[35] Turkmen I, Ozcan C. Osteosarcopenia increases hip fracture risk: a case-controlled study in the elderly. J Back Musculoskelet Rehabil 2019;32(4):613–8.
[36] Cruz-Jentoft AJ, Bahat G, Bauer J, Boirie Y, Bruyère O, Cederholm T, et al. Sarcopenia: revised European consensus on definition and diagnosis. Age Ageing 2019;48(1):16–31.
[37] Phillips SK, Rook KM, Siddle NC, Bruce SA, Woledge RC. Muscle weakness in women occurs at an earlier age than in men, but strength is preserved by hormone replacement therapy. Clin Sci (Lond) 1993;84(1):95–8.
[38] Greeves JP, Cable NT, Reilly T, Kingsland C. Changes in muscle strength in women following the menopause: a longitudinal assessment of the efficacy of hormone replacement therapy. Clin Sci (Lond) 1999;97(1):79–84.
[39] Mathus-Vliegen EM. Obesity and the elderly. J Clin Gastroenterol 2012;46(7):533–44.
[40] Zamboni M, Mazzali G, Zoico E, Harris TB, Meigs JB, Di Francesco V, et al. Health consequences of obesity in the elderly: a review of four unresolved questions. Int J Obes (Lond) 2005;29(9):1011–29.
[41] Baumgartner RN. Body composition in healthy aging. Ann N Y Acad Sci 2000;904:437–48.
[42] Zamboni M, Mazzali G, Fantin F, Rossi A, Di Francesco V. Sarcopenic obesity: a new category of obesity in the elderly. Nutr Metab Cardiovasc Dis 2008;18(5):388–95.

[43] Gregor MF, Hotamisligil GS. Inflammatory mechanisms in obesity. Annu Rev Immunol 2011;29:415–45.
[44] Waters DL, Baumgartner RN. Sarcopenia and obesity. Clin Geriatr Med 2011;27(3):401–21.
[45] Dominguez LJ, Barbagallo M. The cardiometabolic syndrome and sarcopenic obesity in older persons. J Cardiometab Syndr 2007;2(3):183–9.
[46] Wannamethee SG, Atkins JL. Muscle loss and obesity: the health implications of sarcopenia and sarcopenic obesity. Proc Nutr Soc 2015;74(4):405–12.
[47] Hassan EB, Duque G. Osteosarcopenia: a new geriatric syndrome. Aust Fam Physician 2017;46(11):849–53.
[48] Nasimi N, Dabbaghmanesh MH, Sohrabi Z. Nutritional status and body fat mass: determinants of sarcopenia in community-dwelling older adults. Exp Gerontol 2019;122:67–73.
[49] Harvey JA, Chastin SF, Skelton DA. How sedentary are older people? A systematic review of the amount of sedentary behavior. J Aging Phys Act 2015;23(3):471–87.
[50] Frost HM. Bone's mechanostat: a 2003 update. Anat Rec A Discov Mol Cell Evol Biol 2003;275(2):1081–101.
[51] Guralnik JM, Simonsick EM, Ferrucci L, Glynn RJ, Berkman LF, Blazer DG, et al. A short physical performance battery assessing lower extremity function: association with self-reported disability and prediction of mortality and nursing home admission. J Gerontol 1994;49(2):M85–94.
[52] Nieuwenhuizen WF, Weenen H, Rigby P, Hetherington MM. Older adults and patients in need of nutritional support: review of current treatment options and factors influencing nutritional intake. Clin Nutr 2010;29(2):160–9.
[53] Marty E, Liu Y, Samuel A, Or O, Lane J. A review of sarcopenia: enhancing awareness of an increasingly prevalent disease. Bone 2017;105:276–86.
[54] Kaji H. Interaction between muscle and bone. J Bone Metab 2014;21(1):29–40.
[55] Hou L, Lei Y, Li X, Huo C, Jia X, Yang J, et al. Effect of protein supplementation combined with resistance training on muscle mass, strength and function in the elderly: a systematic review and meta-analysis. J Nutr Health Aging 2019;23(5):451–8.
[56] Cusano NE. Skeletal effects of smoking. Curr Osteoporos Rep 2015;13(5):302–9.
[57] Wong PK, Christie JJ, Wark JD. The effects of smoking on bone health. Clin Sci (Lond) 2007;113(5):233–41.
[58] Ward KD, Klesges RC. A meta-analysis of the effects of cigarette smoking on bone mineral density. Calcif Tissue Int 2001;68(5):259–70.
[59] Law MR, Hackshaw AK. A meta-analysis of cigarette smoking, bone mineral density and risk of hip fracture: recognition of a major effect. BMJ 1997;315(7112):841–6.
[60] Al-Bashaireh AM, Haddad LG, Weaver M, Kelly DL, Chengguo X, Yoon S. The effect of tobacco smoking on musculoskeletal health: a systematic review. J Environ Public Health 2018;2018:4184190.
[61] Kanis JA, Johnell O, Oden A, Johansson H, De Laet C, Eisman JA, et al. Smoking and fracture risk: a meta-analysis. Osteoporos Int 2005;16(2):155–62.
[62] Vestergaard P, Mosekilde L. Fracture risk associated with smoking: a meta-analysis. J Intern Med 2003;254(6):572–83.
[63] De Laet C, Kanis JA, Odén A, Johanson H, Johnell O, Delmas P, et al. Body mass index as a predictor of fracture risk: a meta-analysis. Osteoporos Int 2005;16(11):1330–8.
[64] Rom O, Kaisari S, Aizenbud D, Reznick AZ. Sarcopenia and smoking: a possible cellular model of cigarette smoke effects on muscle protein breakdown. Ann NY Acad Sci 2012;1259:47–53.
[65] Rom O, Kaisari S, Aizenbud D, Reznick AZ. The effects of acetaldehyde and acrolein on muscle catabolism in C2 myotubes. Free Radic Biol Med 2013;65:190–200.

[66] Al-Bashaireh AM, Haddad LG, Weaver M, Chengguo X, Kelly DL, Yoon S. The effect of tobacco smoking on bone mass: an overview of pathophysiologic mechanisms. J Osteoporos 2018;2018:1206235.

[67] Lee JS, Auyeung TW, Kwok T, Lau EM, Leung PC, Woo J. Associated factors and health impact of sarcopenia in older chinese men and women: a cross-sectional study. Gerontology 2007;53(6):404–10.

[68] Landi F, Liperoti R, Fusco D, Mastropaolo S, Quattrociocchi D, Proia A, et al. Prevalence and risk factors of sarcopenia among nursing home older residents. J Gerontol A Biol Sci Med Sci 2012;67(1):48–55.

[69] Steffl M, Bohannon RW, Petr M, Kohlikova E, Holmerova I. Relation between cigarette smoking and sarcopenia: meta-analysis. Physiol Res 2015;64(3):419–26.

[70] Compston J, Cooper A, Cooper C, Gittoes N, Gregson C, Harvey N, et al. UK clinical guideline for the prevention and treatment of osteoporosis. Arch Osteoporos 2017;12(1):43.

[71] Dardevet D, Sornet C, Taillandier D, Savary I, Attaix D, Grizard J. Sensitivity and protein turnover response to glucocorticoids are different in skeletal muscle from adult and old rats. Lack of regulation of the ubiquitin-proteasome proteolytic pathway in aging. J Clin Invest 1995;96(5):2113–9.

[72] Savary I, Debras E, Dardevet D, Sornet C, Capitan P, Prugnaud J, et al. Effect of glucocorticoid excess on skeletal muscle and heart protein synthesis in adult and old rats. Br J Nutr 1998;79(3):297–304.

[73] Sakuma K, Yamaguchi A. Sarcopenia and age-related endocrine function. Int J Endocrinol 2012;2012:127362.

[74] Ferrando AA, Stuart CA, Sheffield-Moore M, Wolfe RR. Inactivity amplifies the catabolic response of skeletal muscle to cortisol. J Clin Endocrinol Metab 1999;84(10):3515–21.

[75] Carballo-Jane E, Pandit S, Santoro JC, Freund C, Luell S, Harris G, et al. Skeletal muscle: a dual system to measure glucocorticoid-dependent transactivation and transrepression of gene regulation. J Steroid Biochem Mol Biol 2004;88(2):191–201.

[76] Sacheck JM, Ohtsuka A, McLary SC, Goldberg AL. IGF-I stimulates muscle growth by suppressing protein breakdown and expression of atrophy-related ubiquitin ligases, atrogin-1 and MuRF1. Am J Physiol Endocrinol Metab 2004;287(4):E591–601.

[77] Kanis JA, Johansson H, Oden A, Johnell O, de Laet C, Melton III LJ, et al. A meta-analysis of prior corticosteroid use and fracture risk. J Bone Miner Res 2004;19(6):893–9.

[78] Holick MF. Vitamin D deficiency. N Engl J Med 2007;357(3):266–81.

[79] DeLuca HF. Overview of general physiologic features and functions of vitamin D. Am J Clin Nutr 2004;80(6 Suppl):1689S–96S.

[80] Gloth FM, Gundberg CM, Hollis BW, Haddad JG, Tobin JD. Vitamin D deficiency in homebound elderly persons. JAMA 1995;274(21):1683–6.

[81] Goldray D, Mizrahi-Sasson E, Merdler C, Edelstein-Singer M, Algoetti A, Eisenberg Z, et al. Vitamin D deficiency in elderly patients in a general hospital. J Am Geriatr Soc 1989;37(7):589–92.

[82] Wicherts IS, van Schoor NM, Boeke AJ, Visser M, Deeg DJ, Smit J, et al. Vitamin D status predicts physical performance and its decline in older persons. J Clin Endocrinol Metab 2007;92(6):2058–65.

[83] Bischoff-Ferrari HA, Borchers M, Gudat F, Dürmüller U, Stähelin HB, Dick W. Vitamin D receptor expression in human muscle tissue decreases with age. J Bone Miner Res 2004;19(2):265–9.

[84] Sato Y, Iwamoto J, Kanoko T, Satoh K. Low-dose vitamin D prevents muscular atrophy and reduces falls and hip fractures in women after stroke: a randomized controlled trial. Cerebrovasc Dis 2005;20(3):187–92.

[85] Montero-Odasso M, Duque G. Vitamin D in the aging musculoskeletal system: an authentic strength preserving hormone. Mol Aspects Med 2005;26(3):203–19.
[86] Sørensen OH, Lund B, Saltin B, Andersen RB, Hjorth L, Melsen F, et al. Myopathy in bone loss of ageing: improvement by treatment with 1 alpha-hydroxycholecalciferol and calcium. Clin Sci (Lond) 1979;56(2):157–61.
[87] Sakuma K, Yamaguchi A. Sarcopenia and cachexia: the adaptations of negative regulators of skeletal muscle mass. J Cachexia Sarcopenia Muscle 2012;3(2):77–94.
[88] Feldman HA, Longcope C, Derby CA, Johannes CB, Araujo AB, Coviello AD, et al. Age trends in the level of serum testosterone and other hormones in middle-aged men: longitudinal results from the Massachusetts male aging study. J Clin Endocrinol Metab 2002;87(2):589–98.
[89] Morley JE, Kaiser FE, Perry HM, Patrick P, Morley PM, Stauber PM, et al. Longitudinal changes in testosterone, luteinizing hormone, and follicle-stimulating hormone in healthy older men. Metabolism 1997;46(4):410–3.
[90] Morley JE, Perry HM. Androgens and women at the menopause and beyond. J Gerontol A Biol Sci Med Sci 2003;58(5):M409–16.
[91] Urban RJ, Bodenburg YH, Gilkison C, Foxworth J, Coggan AR, Wolfe RR, et al. Testosterone administration to elderly men increases skeletal muscle strength and protein synthesis. Am J Physiol 1995;269(5 Pt. 1):E820–6.
[92] Bhasin S, Woodhouse L, Storer TW. Proof of the effect of testosterone on skeletal muscle. J Endocrinol 2001;170(1):27–38.
[93] Bakhshi V, Elliott M, Gentili A, Godschalk M, Mulligan T. Testosterone improves rehabilitation outcomes in ill older men. J Am Geriatr Soc 2000;48(5):550–3.
[94] Ferrando AA, Sheffield-Moore M, Yeckel CW, Gilkison C, Jiang J, Achacosa A, et al. Testosterone administration to older men improves muscle function: molecular and physiological mechanisms. Am J Physiol Endocrinol Metab 2002;282(3):E601–7.
[95] Morley JE, Perry HM. Androgen deficiency in aging men: role of testosterone replacement therapy. J Lab Clin Med 2000;135(5):370–8.
[96] Snyder PJ, Peachey H, Hannoush P, Berlin JA, Loh L, Lenrow DA, et al. Effect of testosterone treatment on body composition and muscle strength in men over 65 years of age. J Clin Endocrinol Metab 1999;84(8):2647–53.
[97] Bhasin S, Calof OM, Storer TW, Lee ML, Mazer NA, Jasuja R, et al. Drug insight: testosterone and selective androgen receptor modulators as anabolic therapies for chronic illness and aging. Nat Clin Pract Endocrinol Metab 2006;2(3):146–59.
[98] Sinha-Hikim I, Cornford M, Gaytan H, Lee ML, Bhasin S. Effects of testosterone supplementation on skeletal muscle fiber hypertrophy and satellite cells in community-dwelling older men. J Clin Endocrinol Metab 2006;91(8):3024–33.
[99] Mudali S, Dobs AS. Effects of testosterone on body composition of the aging male. Mech Ageing Dev 2004;125(4):297–304.
[100] Dempster DW. Osteoporosis and the burden of osteoporosis-related fractures. Am J Manag Care 2011;17(Suppl. 6):S164–9.
[101] Eastell R, Rosen CJ, Black DM, Cheung AM, Murad MH, Shoback D. Pharmacological management of osteoporosis in postmenopausal women: an endocrine society clinical practice guideline. J Clin Endocrinol Metab 2019;104(5):1595–622.
[102] Roubenoff R, Hughes VA. Sarcopenia: current concepts. J Gerontol A Biol Sci Med Sci 2000;55(12):M716–24.
[103] Thomas DR. Loss of skeletal muscle mass in aging: examining the relationship of starvation, sarcopenia and cachexia. Clin Nutr 2007;26(4):389–99.

[104] van Geel TA, Geusens PP, Winkens B, Sels JP, Dinant GJ. Measures of bioavailable serum testosterone and estradiol and their relationships with muscle mass, muscle strength and bone mineral density in postmenopausal women: a cross-sectional study. Eur J Endocrinol 2009;160(4):681–7.
[105] Iannuzzi-Sucich M, Prestwood KM, Kenny AM. Prevalence of sarcopenia and predictors of skeletal muscle mass in healthy, older men and women. J Gerontol A Biol Sci Med Sci 2002;57(12):M772–7.
[106] Roubenoff R. Catabolism of aging: is it an inflammatory process? Curr Opin Clin Nutr Metab Care 2003;6(3):295–9.
[107] Brown M. Skeletal muscle and bone: effect of sex steroids and aging. Adv Physiol Educ 2008;32(2):120–6.
[108] Florini JR, Ewton DZ, Coolican SA. Growth hormone and the insulin-like growth factor system in myogenesis. Endocr Rev 1996;17(5):481–517.
[109] Hermann M, Berger P. Hormonal changes in aging men: a therapeutic indication? Exp Gerontol 2001;36(7):1075–82.
[110] Ryall JG, Schertzer JD, Lynch GS. Cellular and molecular mechanisms underlying age-related skeletal muscle wasting and weakness. Biogerontology 2008;9(4):213–28.
[111] Veldhuis JD, Iranmanesh A. Physiological regulation of the human growth hormone (GH)-insulin-like growth factor type I (IGF-I) axis: predominant impact of age, obesity, gonadal function, and sleep. Sleep 1996;19(10 Suppl):S221–4.
[112] Ferrucci L, Penninx BW, Volpato S, Harris TB, Bandeen-Roche K, Balfour J, et al. Change in muscle strength explains accelerated decline of physical function in older women with high interleukin-6 serum levels. J Am Geriatr Soc 2002;50(12):1947–54.
[113] Philippou A, Maridaki M, Halapas A, Koutsilieris M. The role of the insulin-like growth factor 1 (IGF-1) in skeletal muscle physiology. In Vivo 2007;21(1):45–54.
[114] Giovannini S, Marzetti E, Borst SE, Leeuwenburgh C. Modulation of GH/IGF-1 axis: potential strategies to counteract sarcopenia in older adults. Mech Ageing Dev 2008;129(10):593–601.
[115] Andersen NB, Andreassen TT, Orskov H, Oxlund H. Growth hormone and mild exercise in combination increases markedly muscle mass and tetanic tension in old rats. Eur J Endocrinol 2000;143(3):409–18.
[116] Blackman MR, Sorkin JD, Münzer T, Bellantoni MF, Busby-Whitehead J, Stevens TE, et al. Growth hormone and sex steroid administration in healthy aged women and men: a randomized controlled trial. JAMA 2002;288(18):2282–92.
[117] Mazzaglia PJ, Berber E, Kovach A, Milas M, Esselstyn C, Siperstein AE. The changing presentation of hyperparathyroidism over 3 decades. Arch Surg 2008;143(3):260–6.
[118] Fraser WD. Hyperparathyroidism. Lancet 2009;374:145–58.
[119] Abellan van Kan G, Rolland Y, Houles M, Gillette-Guyonnet S, Soto M, Vellas B. The assessment of frailty in older adults. Clin Geriatr Med 2010;26(2):275–86.
[120] Negm AM, Ioannidis G, Jantzi M, Bucek J, Giangregorio L, Pickard L, et al. Validation of a one year fracture prediction tool for absolute hip fracture risk in long term care residents. BMC Geriatr 2018;18(1):1–10.
[121] Bergman H, Ferrucci L, Guralnik J, Hogan DB, Hummel S, Karunananthan S, et al. Frailty: an emerging research and clinical paradigm—issues and controversies. J Gerontol A Biol Sci Med Sci 2007;62(7):731–7.
[122] Crilly RG, Tanner DA, Kloseck M, Chesworth BM. Hip fractures in long-term care: is the excess explained by the age and gender distribution of the residents? J Aging Res 2010;2010:291258.

[123] Shafiee G, Keshtkar A, Soltani A, Ahadi Z, Larijani B, Heshmat R. Prevalence of sarcopenia in the world: a systematic review and meta- analysis of general population studies. J Diabetes Metab Disord 2017;16:21.
[124] Rodríguez-Rejón AI, Ruiz-López MD, Wanden-Berghe C, Artacho R. Prevalence and diagnosis of sarcopenia in residential facilities: a systematic review. Adv Nutr 2019;10(1):51–8.
[125] Shibahashi K, Sugiyama K, Kashiura M, Hamabe Y. Decreasing skeletal muscle as a risk factor for mortality in elderly patients with sepsis: a retrospective cohort study. J Intensive Care 2017;5:8.
[126] Mak RH, Ikizler AT, Kovesdy CP, Raj DS, Stenvinkel P, Kalantar-Zadeh K. Wasting in chronic kidney disease. J Cachexia Sarcopenia Muscle 2011;2(1):9–25.
[127] Suzuki T, Palus S, Springer J. Skeletal muscle wasting in chronic heart failure. ESC Heart Fail 2018;5(6):1099–107.
[128] Burckart K, Beca S, Urban RJ, Sheffield-Moore M. Pathogenesis of muscle wasting in cancer cachexia: targeted anabolic and anticatabolic therapies. Curr Opin Clin Nutr Metab Care 2010;13(4):410–6.
[129] Chen YP, Wong PK, Tsai MJ, Chang WC, Hsieh TS, Leu TH, et al. The high prevalence of sarcopenia and its associated outcomes following hip surgery in Taiwanese geriatric patients with a hip fracture. J Formos Med Assoc 2020;119(12):1807–16.
[130] Malmstrom TK, Morley JE. SARC-F: a simple questionnaire to rapidly diagnose sarcopenia. J Am Med Dir Assoc 2013;14(8):531–2.
[131] Bahat G, Yilmaz O, Kılıç C, Oren MM, Karan MA. Performance of SARC-F in regard to sarcopenia definitions, muscle mass and functional measures. J Nutr Health Aging 2018;22(8):898–903.
[132] Kanis JA. Assessment of fracture risk and its application to screening for postmenopausal osteoporosis. Report of a WHO Study Group. World Health Organ Tech Rep Ser 1994;843:1–129.
[133] Brunader R, Shelton DK. Radiologic bone assessment in the evaluation of osteoporosis. Am Fam Physician 2002;65(7):1357–64.
[134] Faulkner KG, von Stetten E, Miller P. Discordance in patient classification using T-scores. J Clin Densitom 1999;2(3):343–50.
[135] NIH Consensus Development Panel on Osteoporosis Prevention Da, and Therapy. Osteoporosis prevention, diagnosis, and therapy. JAMA 2001;285(6):785–95.
[136] Leib ES, Lewiecki EM, Binkley N, Hamdy RC. Official positions of the international society for clinical densitometry. J Clin Densitom 2004;7:1–6.
[137] Lane NE. Epidemiology, etiology, and diagnosis of osteoporosis. Am J Obstet Gynecol 2006;194:S3–11.
[138] Ibrahim K, May C, Patel HP, Baxter M, Sayer AA, Roberts H. A feasibility study of implementing grip strength measurement into routine hospital practice (GRImP): study protocol. Pilot Feasibility Stud 2016;2:27.
[139] Leong DP, Teo KK, Rangarajan S, Lopez-Jaramillo P, Avezum A, Orlandini A, et al. Prognostic value of grip strength: findings from the Prospective Urban Rural Epidemiology (PURE) study. Lancet 2015;386(9990):266–73.
[140] Dodds RM, Syddall HE, Cooper R, Benzeval M, Deary IJ, Dennison EM, et al. Grip strength across the life course: normative data from twelve British studies. PLoS One 2014;9(12):e113637.
[141] Mathiowetz V, Weber K, Volland G, Kashman N. Reliability and validity of grip and pinch strength evaluations. J Hand Surg Am 1984;9(2):222–6.
[142] Peolsson A, Hedlund R, Oberg B. Intra- and inter-tester reliability and reference values for hand strength. J Rehabil Med 2001;33(1):36–41.

[143] Bohannon RW, Schaubert KL. Test-retest reliability of grip-strength measures obtained over a 12-week interval from community-dwelling elders. J Hand Ther 2005;18(4):426–7.
[144] Steiber N. Strong or weak handgrip? Normative reference values for the german population across the life course stratified by sex, age, and body height. PLoS One 2016;11(10):e0163917.
[145] Beaudart C, McCloskey E, Bruyère O, Cesari M, Rolland Y, Rizzoli R, et al. Sarcopenia in daily practice: assessment and management. BMC Geriatr 2016;16(1):170.
[146] Rossi AP, Fantin F, Micciolo R, Bertocchi M, Bertassello P, Zanandrea V, et al. Identifying sarcopenia in acute care setting patients. J Am Med Dir Assoc 2014;15(4). 303.e7–12.
[147] Roberts HC, Denison HJ, Martin HJ, Patel HP, Syddall H, Cooper C, et al. A review of the measurement of grip strength in clinical and epidemiological studies: towards a standardized approach. Age Ageing 2011;40(4):423–9.
[148] Spijkerman DC, Snijders CJ, Stijnen T, Lankhorst GJ. Standardization of grip strength measurements. Effects on repeatability and peak force. Scand J Rehabil Med 1991;23(4):203–6.
[149] Rendos NK, Harriell K, Qazi S, Regis RC, Alipio TC, Signorile JF. Variations in verbal encouragement modify isokinetic performance. J Strength Cond Res 2019;33(3):708–16.
[150] Johansson CA, Kent BE, Shepard KF. Relationship between verbal command volume and magnitude of muscle contraction. Phys Ther 1983;63(8):1260–5.
[151] Cesari M, Kritchevsky SB, Newman AB, Simonsick EM, Harris TB, Penninx BW, et al. Added value of physical performance measures in predicting adverse health-related events: results from the Health, Aging And Body Composition Study. J Am Geriatr Soc 2009;57(2):251–9.
[152] Jones CJ, Rikli RE, Beam WC. A 30-s chair-stand test as a measure of lower body strength in community-residing older adults. Res Q Exerc Sport 1999;70(2):113–9.
[153] Francis P, Toomey C, Mc Cormack W, Lyons M, Jakeman P. Measurement of maximal isometric torque and muscle quality of the knee extensors and flexors in healthy 50- to 70-year-old women. Clin Physiol Funct Imaging 2017;37(4):448–55.
[154] Brown M, Sinacore DR, Binder EF, Kohrt WM. Physical and performance measures for the identification of mild to moderate frailty. J Gerontol A Biol Sci Med Sci 2000;55(6):M350–5.
[155] Callahan D, Phillips E, Carabello R, Frontera WR, Fielding RA. Assessment of lower extremity muscle power in functionally-limited elders. Aging Clin Exp Res 2007;19(3):194–9.
[156] Harbo T, Brincks J, Andersen H. Maximal isokinetic and isometric muscle strength of major muscle groups related to age, body mass, height, and sex in 178 healthy subjects. Eur J Appl Physiol 2012;112(1):267–75.
[157] Maden-Wilkinson TM, Degens H, Jones DA, McPhee JS. Comparison of MRI and DXA to measure muscle size and age-related atrophy in thigh muscles. J Musculoskelet Neuronal Interact 2013;13(3):320–8.
[158] Cooper C, Fielding R, Visser M, van Loon LJ, Rolland Y, Orwoll E, et al. Tools in the assessment of sarcopenia. Calcif Tissue Int 2013;93(3):201–10.
[159] Cawthon PM, Peters KW, Shardell MD, McLean RR, Dam TT, Kenny AM, et al. Cutpoints for low appendicular lean mass that identify older adults with clinically significant weakness. J Gerontol A Biol Sci Med Sci 2014;69(5):567–75.
[160] Guerri S, Mercatelli D, Aparisi Gómez MP, Napoli A, Battista G, Guglielmi G, et al. Quantitative imaging techniques for the assessment of osteoporosis and sarcopenia. Quant Imaging Med Surg 2018;8(1):60–85.
[161] Karpman C, Lebrasseur NK, Depew ZS, Novotny PJ, Benzo RP. Measuring gait speed in the out-patient clinic: methodology and feasibility. Respir Care 2014;59(4):531–7.
[162] Maggio M, Ceda GP, Ticinesi A, De Vita F, Gelmini G, Costantino C, et al. Instrumental and non-instrumental evaluation of 4-meter walking speed in older individuals. PLoS One 2016;11(4):e0153583.

[163] Negm AM, Kennedy CC, Pritchard JM, Ioannidis G, Vastis V, Marr S, et al. The short performance physical battery is associated with one-year emergency department visits and hospitalization. Can J Aging 2019;38:507–11.

[164] Bandinelli S, Lauretani F, Boscherini V, Gandi F, Pozzi M, Corsi AM, et al. A randomized, controlled trial of disability prevention in frail older patients screened in primary care: the FRASI study. Design and baseline evaluation. Aging Clin Exp Res 2006;18(5):359–66.

[165] Subra J, Gillette-Guyonnet S, Cesari M, Oustric S, Vellas B, Platform T. The integration of frailty into clinical practice: preliminary results from the Gerontopole. J Nutr Health Aging 2012;16(8):714–20.

[166] Ortega-Bastidas P, Aqueveque P, Gómez B, Saavedra F, Cano-de-la-Cuerda R. Use of a single wireless IMU for the segmentation and automatic analysis of activities performed in the 3-m timed up & go test. Sensors (Basel) 2019;19(7):1–22.

[167] Zasadzka E, Borowicz AM, Roszak M, Pawlaczyk M. Assessment of the risk of falling with the use of timed up and go test in the elderly with lower extremity osteoarthritis. Clin Interv Aging 2015;10:1289–98.

[168] Persson CU, Danielsson A, Sunnerhagen KS, Grimby-Ekman A, Hansson PO. Timed Up & Go as a measure for longitudinal change in mobility after stroke—Postural Stroke Study in Gothenburg (POSTGOT). J Neuroeng Rehabil 2014;11:83.

[169] Nguyen H, Lebel K, Boissy P, Bogard S, Goubault E, Duval C. Auto detection and segmentation of daily living activities during a Timed Up and Go task in people with Parkinson's disease using multiple inertial sensors. J Neuroeng Rehabil 2017;14(1):26.

[170] Podsiadlo D, Richardson S. The timed "Up & Go": a test of basic functional mobility for frail elderly persons. J Am Geriatr Soc 1991;39(2):142–8.

Chapter 12

Diagnosis of osteosarcopenia—Imaging

Ebrahim Bani Hassan[a], Mahdi Imani[a,b], and Ali Ghasem-Zadeh[c]

[a]*Department of Medicine, Western Health and Australian Institute for Musculoskeletal Science (AIMSS), The University of Melbourne, Melbourne, VIC, Australia,* [b]*Faculty of Medicine, Dentistry and Health Sciences, The University of Melbourne, Melbourne, VIC, Australia,* [c]*Endocrinology and Medicine, Austin Health, The University of Melbourne, Heidelberg, VIC, Australia*

Diagnosis of osteosarcopenia—Quantitative imaging

Introduction

The prevalence, importance, and impact of osteosarcopenia and its constituent syndromes (osteoporosis and sarcopenia) have been covered in previous chapters. Here, we briefly focus on the role of imaging in osteosarcopenia diagnosis. The science of quantitative imaging of all tissues, including the musculoskeletal system, is still an evolving field. However, due to the bone architecture complexity, including heterogeneity pattern of materials, in addition to imaging challenges such as beam hardening and edge effects, imaging and image analyses of musculoskeletal tissues becomes a complex task. In addition, gradual deposition of fat into muscle fibers creates an intermediate tissue between fat and muscle, that to our knowledge, no in vivo imaging technique is still capable of differentiating.

Regarding the above limitations and several others, we briefly review the current in vivo imaging-based techniques of osteosarcopenia diagnosis.

Learning outcomes

After reading the chapter, you may

- know the imaging-based current methods for diagnosis of osteosarcopenia
- understand the usefulness and potential of the common imaging tools in diagnosing osteosarcopenia
- know the major limitations of the existing imaging tools in diagnosing osteosarcopenia
- understand the possible roles of fat infiltration into bone and muscle in driving their decline by age

Osteosarcopenia. https://doi.org/10.1016/B978-0-12-820088-9.00001-9

Nonimaging techniques

Bioelectrical impedance analysis (BIA) and bioelectrical impedance spectroscopy (BIS), although not imaging techniques, deserve a brief discussion in this chapter. The indirect quantification of bone, muscle, and fat masses by BIA is based on the electric conductivity of the tissues, which is dependent on their water and electrolyte content [1]. Therefore, the hydration status of the subjects significantly impacts the estimation of tissue masses [2]. Also, the presence of metals that are very common in older adults (e.g., large orthopedic prostheses, surgical staples, etc.) can significantly impact the estimation of tissue masses. As BIA scales require the person to stand for a few seconds, the technique can prove to be a challenge in older adults with severe weakness and balance problems.

Nevertheless, where imaging modalities are not available, after considering the limitations, BIA can prove helpful in the primary care setting, especially in remote areas where direct imaging is not available. Both BIA and BIS show a reasonable correlation with muscle function in uncomplicated cases [3,4]. However, BIA has not been standardized on a large scale for the diagnosis of sarcopenia [5].

Two-dimensional imaging techniques

Quantitative ultrasonography (QUS): Ultrasound imaging is a well-established modality to assess soft tissue [6,7]. Also, ultrasound wave velocity in bone (usually the calcaneal bone) has been used to evaluate bone mineral density (BMD) and fracture risk prediction [8–10].

The issue with all quantitative ultrasound techniques is low sensitivity and specificity. For example, flexor and extensor muscles of the knee have a very low association with muscle volume determined by magnetic resonance imaging (MRI) [11]. In the authors' hands, the repeatability of the ultrasound measurements has been proven low. This might be the reason for the contradiction in the validity for muscle mass quantification by the technique [7], as the operator seems to be a critical factor in the measurements. There is also a lack of agreement on the regions of interest for the assessment of sarcopenia using QUS. Currently, two major protocols that include 9-site and 5-site are not considered practical in the clinical setting due to their complexity [12,13]. At best, the bone mineral density (BMD) measured by OUS shows a modest association [14] with dual-energy X-ray absorptiometry (DXA) (as a gold standard) [15] and very low sensitivity for the assessment of bone density; therefore, QUS is not recommended for the evaluation of bone fragility [16]. Considering the lack of sensitivity and specificity for both osteoporosis and sarcopenia, QUS is consequently also not recommended as a standard tool to diagnose osteosarcopenia.

Dual-energy X-ray absorptiometry (DXA): DXA (two-dimensional quantitative imaging that has been partly standardized) uses two X-ray beams with different energies to differentiate soft tissue (including fat and lean mass) from the bone [17]. As per definition, any subject with a T-score of −1 and below (osteopenic or osteoporotic) and sarcopenic (irrespective of the definition used) is osteosarcopenic. Currently, the most common tool used to measure bone and muscle mass is DXA. Below, we discuss the drawbacks and advantages of the technique and the current status of the research and clinical use of DXA in diagnosing osteosarcopenia.

DXA technology is half a century old, and assessing BMD has poor sensitivity and moderate specificity for predicting fragility fractures [18,19]. As a consequence, the majority (up to 82%) of people with fractures do not have osteoporosis according to their BMD [20,21] and, therefore, are not classified at risk of fractures, nor treated for osteoporosis. In addition, BMD improvement due to osteoporosis treatment only explains 16%–25% of reductions in fracture risk [22–24]; thus, BMD does not explain the remaining 75%–84% reduction in fractures secondary to treatment. Consequently, DXA is not recommended as an osteoporosis screening tool [19]. In other words, additional factors such as family history, clinical conditions such as specific diseases, fall history, personal habits (smoking and alcohol intake), and medications can all impact prediction of adverse outcomes [25,26]. Therefore, sensitive, specific, and noninvasive alternative methods for the diagnosis of osteoporosis, sarcopenia, and osteosarcopenia are imperative.

In the absence of better tools, DXA has been nominated as the gold standard for the diagnosis of osteoporosis by estimating BMD [15]. Due to its wider availability compared to other techniques, high repeatability, and being relatively less costly, it is still very popular—as there is effectively no competitive technology. As per the World Health Organization guidelines, BMD T-scores below −1 and −2.5 at the hip and/or lumbar spine, or forearm in the absence, or marginality of the previous two are considered osteopenic and osteoporotic. T-scores are the number of standard variations from the mean BMD of young adults at peak bone mass (30- to 35-year-old people) [15].

DXA technology also does an acceptable job in estimating the lean mass (the tissue mass excluding bone and fat). However, blood, vasculature, tendons and ligaments, gut, and most of its contents have similar X-ray absorption coefficients to muscle. Also, since other connective tissues, as well as most of the intramuscular fat, are included in the calculation of lean mass, the DXA-derived lean mass does not essentially always reflect the muscle properties, including mass and strength, performance, and clinical outcomes. Hence, appendicular lean muscle mass corrected for height or body mass index (BMI) is commonly used to partially remove other tissues' masses as much as possible. Separate studies show that adjusting appendicular lean mass for BMI is superior to adjusting for height squared in predicting main outcomes like strength and muscle performance and balance in older adults [27,28].

Nevertheless, appendicular lean mass shows high correlations with MRI-derived muscle mass [29]. Currently, the American (FNIH) [30], European (EWGSOP2) [31,32], and Asian consensuses use DXA-derived appendicular mass corrected for BMI and height, respectively, to determine sarcopenia. For the diagnostic algorithms and thresholds, please see Table 1.

Recently, research has shown that measurements of BMD, lean mass, and fat mass in the mid-thigh region using DXA technology [27,28] or other techniques - such as CT and MR scanning [33,34] are moderate to very highly correlated with the hip, spine, and forearm BMD, appendicular lean mass and total/android/gynoid fat mass. In addition, the tissue masses in the mid-thigh region are generally a potential predictor of muscle function, strength, balance, falls, and fractures [27,28]. Mid-thigh contains most of the major muscles responsible for weight-bearing with relatively less connective tissue (tendons and ligaments). Also, mid-thigh is at or close to the femur's center of bending (bone is preserved maximally due to Wolff's law), and largely overlaps with gynoid fat (Fig. 1). The above makes the mid-thigh almost ideal for lean and fat mass assessment by DXA.

Three-dimensional imaging techniques

X-ray based imaging

X-ray-based imaging modalities, like computed tomography (CT), rely on X-ray beam attenuation while crossing various tissues—the same principle that drives the DXA technology. Despite the good sensitivity and specificity for BMD and acceptable precision in assessing muscle mass, several major factors have limited the general application of the technique as a clinical diagnostic tool for osteoporosis and sarcopenia: high radiation dose per scan, low resolution, and the price and consequently the availability of the technique [35]. Nevertheless, it has commonly been used to measure bone and muscle volumes

TABLE 1 The summary of the recommended thresholds for sarcopenia according to the appendicular lean mass (ALM) adjusted for height-squared (h^2) or body mass index (BMI).

	Cut-points for men	Cut-points for women
American consensus (FNIH; ALM/BMI)	<0.789	<0.512
European consensus (ALM/height^2)	<7 kg/m^2	<6 kg/m^2
Asian consensus (AWGS; ALM/height^2)	<7.0 kg/m^2	<5.4 kg/m^2

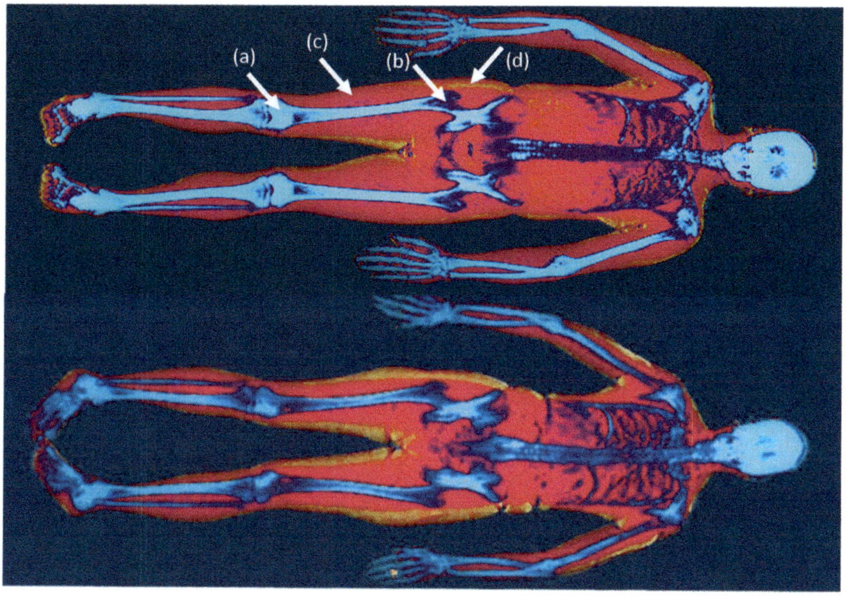

FIG. 1 A whole-body DXA scan of an older healthy man (age ~ 80) and his hip, spine, and forearm scans (top) vs an older woman (age ~ 80) suffering from low bone mass, low muscle mass (bottom). Dense bone is highlighted in whole-body scans as *turquoise green/blue* (a), and low density is *navy/royal blue* (b). Muscle and fat have been highlighted as *red* (c) and *yellow* (d), respectively.

for research purposes [36]. Single slice cross-sectional CT at the lumbar spine level to estimate whole-body lean tissue and skeletal muscle and sarcopenia has been suggested [37]. Fig. 2 displays a CT image of healthy and osteosarcopenic subjects that have been scanned by clinical CT-Scanner and axial images segmented to display muscle, bone, intramuscular fat, marrow adipose tissue, and hematopoietic marrow. Differentiating tissues with similar X-ray attenuation coefficients is a major limitation of X-ray based techniques. Considering the roles of ectopic fat infiltration into the muscle and bone that possibly drives the decline of bone and muscle with aging [35,38–40], one expects a reliable quantification of the infiltrating ectopic fat in tissues. However, differentiating marrow adipose tissue from hematopoietic tissue is still a challenge. Albeit, with sensitive image analysis technique, this issue can be addressed to a great extent (Fig. 2) [35,38–41].

Due to low resolution, bone microstructure (trabecular properties of bone) cannot be studied by conventional CT scans. However, the improvements in CT technology have led to the development of peripheral quantitative CT (pQCT) and high-resolution pQCT (HR-pQCT). The commercially available machines have an apparent maximum resolution of ~41–200 μm, and allow human distal limbs to be scanned with radiation doses under 5 μSv per scan [35], which enable the assessment of human bone trabeculae (around 100–250 μm thickness at distal

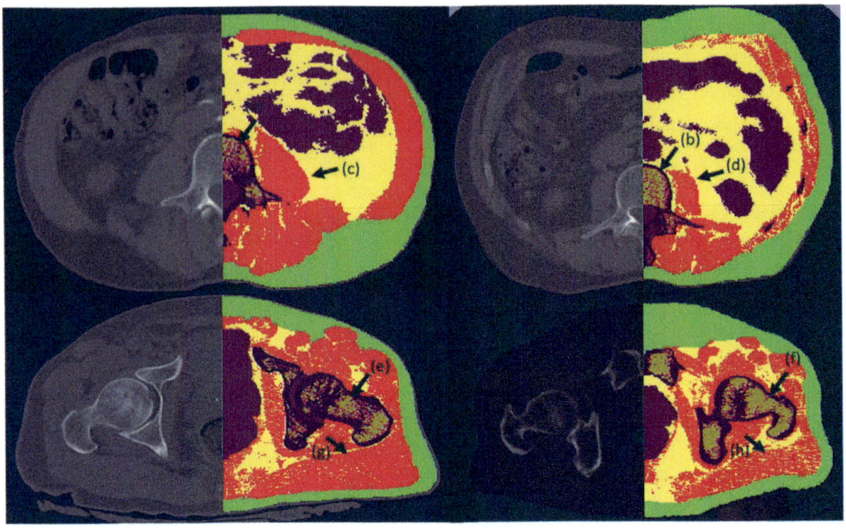

FIG. 2 CT scans of a healthy older man (age ~ 80) (right panels) compared to a man of the same age with osteosarcopenia (left panels). The top row displays abdominal CTs at the level of the L4 vertebra, and the lower panels have been taken at the level of the hip/femoral neck. The healthy subject displays higher bone *(blue)*, muscle *(red)*, and hematopoietic marrow *(pink/magenta)* volume compared to the osteosarcopenic person. Infiltration of intramuscular fat *(yellow)* and marrow adipose tissue *(khaki)* as well as accumulation of subcutaneous fat *(green)* is associated with a severe decline in musculoskeletal tissue. As an example, (a) and (e) contains much less marrow adipose tissue compared to (b) and (f), respectively. Also, muscle volume in (c) and (g) is much higher than (d) and (h), respectively. Joint spaces, rectum, prostate, major vessels, and viscera have been labeled *purple*.

tibia and radius) and the cortical bone compartment [42]; which has slightly improved the ability of the technique in predicting the fracture risk [43] (Fig. 3).

Dual-energy CT may prove helpful in osteosarcopenia diagnosis, as it better differentiates fat from other soft tissues. However, due to the limitations listed for CT-based images, there are still no widely used clinical protocols to diagnose osteosarcopenia or its components using dual-energy CT.

Further limitations of CT-based methods include sensitivity to patient motion and lack of reference values and standards. In addition, the ability of CT in quantifying marrow fat and particularly in contrast to red marrow and, especially in humans, has not been validated yet.

Magnetic resonance-based imaging

Magnetic resonance imaging (MRI) generally uses a strong magnetic field and high-frequency electromagnetic pulse sequence to excite hydrogen atoms in tissues and measures the relaxing time for different tissues [44]. MRI appears to be the best (gold-standard) imaging technique to assess muscle volumes and their volumetric and geographical associations with intramuscular fat due to

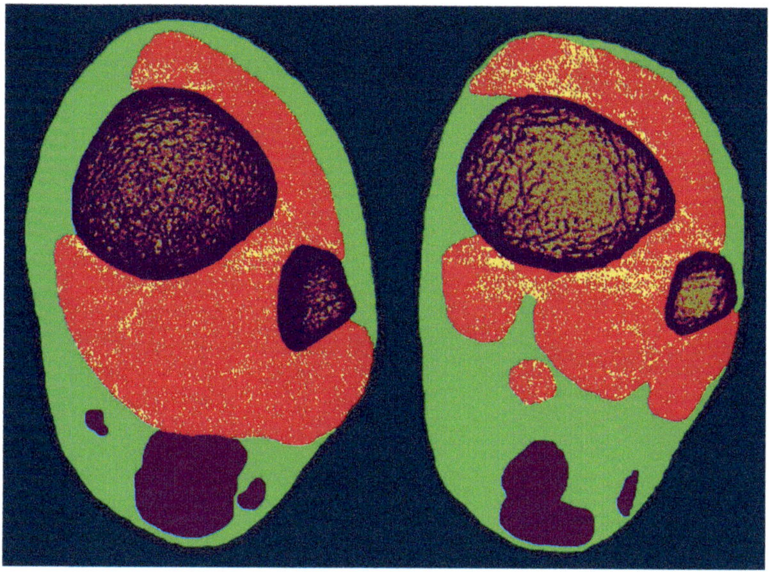

FIG. 3 HR-pQCT images of a young, healthy athletic person (age ~40) (left) at distal tibia shows much higher bone *(blue)*, muscle *(red)*, and hematopoietic marrow *(pink/magenta)* volume compared to an older person (age ~80) with osteosarcopenia (right), where the infiltration of intramuscular fat *(yellow)* and marrow adipose tissue *(khaki)* as well as accumulation of subcutaneous fat *(green)* seemingly induces a severe decline in musculoskeletal tissue. Tendons and major vessels have been labeled *purple*.

their stark differences in the proton content, making it a suitable method for the assessment of body composition [45]. However, bone-specific MRI sequences (ultrashort or zero echo time sequences) are still primitive and have not been validated broadly [46]. Regarding the importance of marrow fat in the pathogenesis of osteoporosis, along with good proton contrast between marrow fat versus bone and hematopoietic marrow, appropriate sequences of MRI may provide a potential diagnostic method for predicting future bone loss or fracture risk based on marrow fat volume quantification [35,38–40]. In addition to volume, marrow fat saturation increases as we age and lose bone [47,48]. Magnetic resonance spectroscopy, which quantifies the chemical composition of tissue, can prove useful in determining tissue composition content. Chemical shifts encoding-based water-fat imaging (based on spectroscopy) has the advantage of overcoming spatial resolution problems and may have a future in predicting falls and fractures associated with osteosarcopenia (Fig. 4).

MR-based techniques are still a research modality rather than actual clinical tools to determine adipose tissue composition or even bone structure. However, MRI images can be opportunistically used to assess muscle composition in patients imaged for other comorbidities, whereas standardization of the regions of interest in the musculoskeletal system is still required.

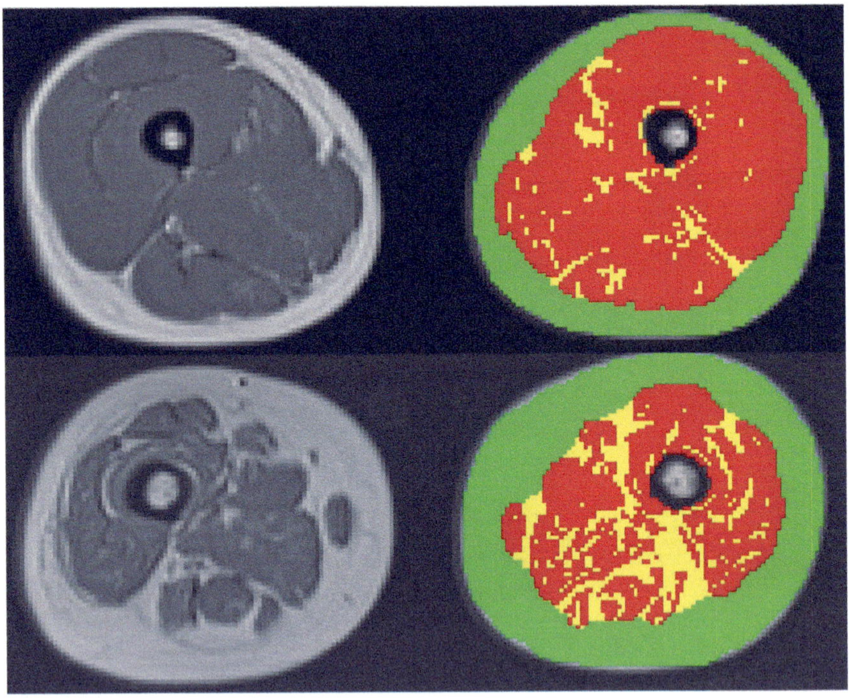

FIG. 4 T1 MRI images of the mid-thigh of an active and healthy adult (age ~40) (top) vs an osteosarcopenic subject (age ~80) (bottom). Note the fat infiltration into the muscle and increased subcutaneous fat mask the decline of muscle. Dilation of the femoral medulla in the osteosarcopenic subject is a prominent feature in this subject. However, as bone and hematopoietic marrow cannot be differentiated in T1 sequences, bone marrow and bone have not been analyzed.

Fracture risk prediction tools (FRAX)

Out of the two primary fracture risk tools, i.e., FRAX (https://www.sheffield.ac.uk/FRAX/) by the Sheffield University and Garvan institute (https://www.garvan.org.au/promotions/bone-fracture-risk/calculator/) tools, only the latter gives weight to the number of falls, and neither include lean/muscle mass or performance/strength in the calculation of the fracture risk. Considering that osteosarcopenic subjects are at greater risk of falls and fractures, it is expected that in the near future fracture risk algorithms will include muscle as a predictor of adverse outcomes.

Image analysis

Image analysis is as critical as image acquisition—if not more. Here, we very briefly touch on a couple of image analysis tools that we have found helpful in determining the volume of bone, muscle, and their components:

ImageJ is a freely available software (by the National Institute of Health, United States) [49] that can quantify images (mainly by thresholding); those with coding backgrounds may find the software helpful in quantifying certain voxels/pixels within medical images. However, most biologists of the current generation lack advanced programming skills. In addition, assigning the voxels to particular ranges (e.g., Hounsfield units) has no to minimal flexibility in ImageJ, and the visual presentation of the image segmentation, as well as the options of automatic segmentation techniques for osteosarcopenia regions of interest, are lacking in ImageJ.

Slice-O-Matic (by Tomovision, Montreal, CA) is an approved image analysis software that allows "tagging" particular voxel values to a certain color, as well as multiple ranges of voxel values, different segmentation techniques (e.g., thresholding versus watershed), and a 3D display of the segmented volumes. However, as image analysis of 3D medical images usually involves multiple stacks of images, the mostly manual protocols of Slice-O-Matic are very time-consuming.

Considering the limitations of the above image analysis software, we have developed a Tissue Compass that significantly increases the image analysis speed by semiautomation to automation of the segmentation steps. It also provides the most commonly used segmentation techniques, as well as simultaneous segmentation of multiple tissues together [50]. This tool is being improved for automatic diagnosis of osteosarcopenia using 3D medical images.

Conclusion

Imaging and image analysis techniques for quantifying bone, muscle, and their components is a young field. It requires significant investment to develop new imaging modalities with higher resolution, higher specificity/sensitivity, and better precision in the acquisition and analysis of the imaged tissues. Until then, we "have to" rely on the available modalities, particularly DXA, that at least partially provide a picture of musculoskeletal health, including for osteosarcopenia.

References

[1] Kushner RF. Bioelectrical impedance analysis: a review of principles and applications. J Am Coll Nutr 1992;11(2):199–209.

[2] Kuchnia A, Earthman C, Teigen L, et al. Evaluation of bioelectrical impedance analysis in critically ill patients: results of a multicenter prospective study. J Parenter Enter Nutr 2017;41(7):1131–8.

[3] Nescolarde L, Yanguas J, Lukaski H, Alomar X, Rosell-Ferrer J, Rodas G. Effects of muscle injury severity on localized bioimpedance measurements. Physiol Meas 2014;36(1):27.

[4] Siglinsky E, Buehring B, Krueger D, Binkley N, Yamada Y. Could bioelectric impedance spectroscopy (BIS) measured appendicular intracellular water serve as a lean mass measurement in sarcopenia definitions? A pilot study. Osteoporos Int 2018;29(7):1653–7.

[5] Gonzalez MC, Heymsfield SB. Bioelectrical impedance analysis for diagnosing sarcopenia and cachexia: what are we really estimating? J Cachexia Sarcopenia Muscle 2017;8(2):187–9.

[6] Anon, https://pubmed.ncbi.nlm.nih.gov/?term=muscle+cross-section++ultrasound.
[7] Sanada K, Kearns CF, Midorikawa T, Abe T. Prediction and validation of total and regional skeletal muscle mass by ultrasound in Japanese adults. Eur J Appl Physiol 2006;96(1):24–31.
[8] Anon, https://pubmed.ncbi.nlm.nih.gov/?term=bone+density+ultrasound.
[9] Oo WM, Vasikaran Naganathan MTB, Hunter DJ. Clinical utilities of quantitative ultrasound in osteoporosis associated with inflammatory rheumatic diseases. Quant Imaging Med Surg 2018;8(1):100.
[10] Amaral Filho JC, Pinheiro MM, de Moura Castro CH, Szejnfeld VL. Prevalence and risk factors associated with low-impact fractures in men with rheumatoid arthritis. Clin Rheumatol 2014;33(10):1389–95.
[11] Miyatani M, Kanehisa H, Ito M, Kawakami Y, Fukunaga T. The accuracy of volume estimates using ultrasound muscle thickness measurements in different muscle groups. Eur J Appl Physiol 2004;91(2):264–72.
[12] Abe T, Kondo M, Kawakami Y, Fukunaga T. Prediction equations for body composition of Japanese adults by B-mode ultrasound. Am J Hum Biol 1994;6(2):161–70.
[13] Paris MT, Lafleur B, Dubin JA, Mourtzakis M. Development of a bedside viable ultrasound protocol to quantify appendicular lean tissue mass. J Cachexia Sarcopenia Muscle 2017;8(5):713–26.
[14] Beerhorst K, Tan J, Tan IY, Verschuure P, Aldenkamp AP. Dual-energy X-ray absorptiometry versus quantitative ultrasonography in diagnosing osteoporosis in patients with refractory epilepsy and chronic antiepileptic drug use. Ther Adv Musculoskelet Dis 2013;5(2):59–66.
[15] World Health Organisation, editor. WHO scientific group on the assessment of osteoporosis at primary health care level meeting report; 2004.
[16] Panichkul S, Sripramote M, Sriussawaamorn N. Diagnostic performance of quantitative ultrasound calcaneus measurement in case finding for osteoporosis in Thai postmenopausal women. J Obstet Gynaecol Res 2004;30(6):418–26.
[17] Bazzocchi A, Ponti F, Albisinni U, Battista G, Guglielmi G. DXA: technical aspects and application. Eur J Radiol 2016;85(8):1481–92.
[18] Kanis JA. Diagnosis of osteoporosis and assessment of fracture risk. Lancet 2002; 359(9321):1929–36.
[19] Marshall D, Johnell O, Wedel H. Meta-analysis of how well measures of bone mineral density predict occurrence of osteoporotic fractures. BMJ 1996;312(7041):1254–9.
[20] Siris ES, Chen Y, Abbott TA, et al. Bone mineral density thresholds for pharmacological intervention to prevent fractures. Arch Intern Med 2004;164(10):1108–12.
[21] Schuit SCE, van der Klift M, Weel AEAM, et al. Fracture incidence and association with bone mineral density in elderly men and women: the Rotterdam study. Bone 2004;34(1):195–202.
[22] Small RE. Uses and limitations of bone mineral density measurements in the management of osteoporosis. Medscape Gen Med 2005;7(2):3.
[23] Cummings SR, Karpf DB, Harris F, et al. Improvement in spine bone density and reduction in risk of vertebral fractures during treatment with antiresorptive drugs. Am J Med 2002;112(4):281–9.
[24] Watts NB, Cooper C, Lindsay R, et al. Relationship between changes in bone mineral density and vertebral fracture risk associated with risedronate: greater increases in bone mineral density do not relate to greater decreases in fracture risk. J Clin Densitom 2004;7(3):255–61.
[25] Kanis JA, Melton III LJ, Christiansen C, Johnston CC, Khaltaev N. The diagnosis of osteoporosis. J Bone Miner Res 1994;9(8):1137–41.
[26] Kanis JA, Borgstrom F, De Laet C, et al. Assessment of fracture risk. Osteoporos Int 2005;16(6):581–9.

[27] Bani Hassan E, Phu S, Vogrin S, et al. Diagnostic value of mid-thigh and mid-calf bone, muscle, and fat mass in Osteosarcopenia: a pilot study. Calcif Tissue Int 2019;105(4):392–402.

[28] Bani Hassan E, Suriyaarachchi P, Boersma D, Duque G. Mid-thigh muscle and bone mass: new indices of bone and muscle loss in older fallers. In: Australia and New Zealand Bone and Mineral Society (ANZBMS) conference, Brisbane; 2017.

[29] Chen Z, Wang Z, Lohman T, et al. Dual-energy X-ray absorptiometry is a valid tool for assessing skeletal muscle mass in older women. J Nutr 2007;137(12):2775–80.

[30] Studenski SA, Peters KW, Alley DE, et al. The FNIH sarcopenia project: rationale, study description, conference recommendations, and final estimates. J Gerontol A Biol Sci Med Sci 2014;69(5):547–58.

[31] Cruz-Jentoft AJ, Bahat G, Bauer J, et al. Sarcopenia: revised European consensus on definition and diagnosis. Age Ageing 2018;afy169.

[32] Phu S, Vogrin S, Zanker J, Bani Hassan E, Al Saedi A, Duque G. Agreement between initial and revised European working group on sarcopenia in older people definitions. J Am Med Dir Assoc 2019;20(3):382–383.e1.

[33] Hansen RD, Williamson DA, Finnegan TP, et al. Estimation of thigh muscle cross-sectional area by dual-energy X-ray absorptiometry in frail elderly patients. Am J Clin Nutr 2007;86(4):952–8.

[34] Lee SJ, Janssen I, Heymsfield SB, Ross R. Relation between whole-body and regional measures of human skeletal muscle. Am J Clin Nutr 2004;80(5):1215–21.

[35] Bani Hassan E, Ghasem-Zadeh A, Imani M, et al. Bone marrow adipose tissue quantification by imaging. Curr Osteoporos Rep 2019;17(6):416–28.

[36] Chalhoub D, Boudreau R, Greenspan S, et al. Associations between lean mass, muscle strength and power, and skeletal size, density and strength in older men. J Bone Miner Res Off J Am Soc Bone Miner Res 2018;33(9):1612–21.

[37] Shen W, Punyanitya M, Wang Z, et al. Total body skeletal muscle and adipose tissue volumes: estimation from a single abdominal cross-sectional image. J Appl Physiol 2004;97(6):2333–8.

[38] Al Saedi A, Bani Hassan E, Duque G. The diagnostic role of fat in osteosarcopenia. J Lab Precis Med 2019;4:7.

[39] Bani Hassan E, Alderghaffar M, Wauquier F, et al. The effects of dietary fatty acids on bone, hematopoietic marrow and marrow adipose tissue in a murine model of senile osteoporosis. Aging (Albany NY) 2019;11(18):7938–47.

[40] Bani Hassan E, Demontiero O, Vogrin S, Ng A, Duque G. Marrow adipose tissue in older men: association with visceral and subcutaneous fat, bone volume, metabolism, and inflammation. Calcif Tissue Int 2018;103(2):164–74.

[41] Demontiero O, Li W, Thembani E, Duque G. Validation of non-invasive quantification of bone marrow fat volume with microCT in aging rats. Exp Gerontol 2011;46(6):435–40.

[42] Zebaze RMD, Ghasem-Zadeh A, Bohte A, et al. Intracortical remodelling and porosity in the distal radius and post-mortem femurs of women: a cross-sectional study. Lancet 2010;375(9727):1729–36.

[43] Bala Y, Zebaze R, Ghasem-Zadeh A, et al. Cortical porosity identifies women with osteopenia at increased risk for forearm fractures. J Bone Miner Res 2014;29(6):1356–62.

[44] McRobbie DW, Moore EA, Graves MJ, Prince MR. MRI from picture to proton. Cambridge University Press; 2017.

[45] Messina C, Maffi G, Vitale JA, Ulivieri FM, Guglielmi G, Sconfienza LM. Diagnostic imaging of osteoporosis and sarcopenia: a narrative review. Quant Imaging Med Surg 2018;8(1):86.

[46] Chang G, Boone S, Martel D, et al. MRI assessment of bone structure and microarchitecture. J Magn Reson Imaging 2017;46(2):323–37.

[47] Yeung DK, Griffith JF, Antonio GE, Lee FK, Woo J, Leung PC. Osteoporosis is associated with increased marrow fat content and decreased marrow fat unsaturation: a proton MR spectroscopy study. J Magn Reson Imaging 2005;22(2):279–85.
[48] Patsch JM, Li X, Baum T, et al. Bone marrow fat composition as a novel imaging biomarker in postmenopausal women with prevalent fragility fractures. J Bone Miner Res 2013;28(8):1721–8.
[49] Schneider CA, Rasband WS, Eliceiri KW. NIH image to ImageJ: 25 years of image analysis. Nat Methods 2012;9(7):671–5.
[50] Anon, https://www.researchsquare.com/article/rs-650019/v1.

Chapter 13

Genetics of osteosarcopenia

Iryna Khrystoforova[a], **Ching-Ti Liu**[b], **and David Karasik**[a,c]
[a]*The Azrieli Faculty of Medicine, Bar-Ilan University, Safed, Israel,* [b]*Department of Biostatistics, Boston University School of Public Health, Boston, MA, United States,* [c]*Marcus Institute for Aging Research, Hebrew SeniorLife, Boston, MA, United States*

Introduction

Osteosarcopenia (OSP) is a geriatric syndrome characterized by systemic loss of bone (osteopenia/osteoporosis), muscle strength, and muscle mass (sarcopenia) [1]. The age-related loss of bone and muscle tissues is known to be interconnected and usually occurs comorbidly. Low parameters of both lean mass and grip strength affect the bone stability and may cause the propensity to fall with a high fracture risk [2–4]. Taking into account these two comorbid events, the diagnostics of osteosarcopenia is dichotomous and comprises the assessment of bone and muscle parameters, such as strength and quality [5]. Bone mineral density (BMD) is one of the main markers of bone strength and can be easily measured by dual X-ray absorptiometry (DXA). By World Health Organization (WHO) definition, the "low bone mass" is considered as osteopenia when the T-score of BMD is between -1 and -2.5 SD from a young adult reference population, therefore for more severe condition—osteoporosis—BMD lower than -2.5 SD is a diagnostic criterion [6]. The assessment of muscle health is more complex and requires multistep-based diagnostic strategies [7]. According to the European Working Group of Sarcopenia in Older People (EWGSOP), the sarcopenia (low muscle mass) diagnostic procedure has to be built on muscle strength assessment and characterization of muscle quality. Later on, in 2019 EWGSOP2 working group provided an algorithm to diagnose and quantify the severity of sarcopenia [8]. Muscle quantity can be measured by DXA, bioelectric impedance analysis (BIA), computed tomography, and magnetic resonance imaging (MRI); muscle strength by grip strength and chair stand test. If the sarcopenia is confirmed, its severity can be estimated by physical performance tests, such as gait, speed, short physical performance battery (SPPB), etc. Taken together if the patient is diagnosed with both osteoporosis and sarcopenia, it is considered an osteosarcopenic condition. Currently, therapeutic options for preventing osteosarcopenia are limited and mostly based on nonpharmacological therapies with lifestyle modifications including regular exercising and

Osteosarcopenia. https://doi.org/10.1016/B978-0-12-820088-9.00010-X

nutritional strategies. A further search of pharmacological agents preserving both the strength and the quality of bone and muscles is required [9].

Heritability of musculoskeletal traits

In investigating the genetic associations with osteosarcopenia the understanding of the musculoskeletal phenotypic heritability (h^2) is necessary. Heritability is a proportion of measured variance in the trait of interest determined by genetic factors; it ranges in value from 0 to 1. Heritability can be defined, as "broad-sense" or "narrow-sense": broad-sense heritability comprises all genetic influences on variation, such as epistasis, dominance, gene-environmental interaction; the "narrow-sense" heritability includes just additive genetic variance. Traditionally the heritability of traits can be estimated by genetic similarity within the family and twin data; however, it is also possible to be extracted from genome-wide SNP data of unrelated individuals [10].

Since in 1973 Smith et al. demonstrated the significant contribution of genetic factors on bone mass of forearm, numerous heritability studies revealed the genetic contribution for different quantitative bone parameters, such as BMD of spine and hip, bone size, which confirmed them as high heritable traits (h^2=0.5 to 0.8) [11]. Similar to bone traits, it has been shown that muscle traits such as hand-grip strength are also highly heritable (h^2=30%–52%). Twin studies showed the additive genetic correlation (ρ_g) between lean mass and BMD within the range from 30% to 45% and in pediatric cohorts, a shared genetic component was shown around 43% [12]. Altogether, this shared significant correlation between bone and muscle traits triggered further studies of pleiotropy [11].

Genome-wide association studies

The pursuit of the genetic determinants of common phenotypes is essentially a quest for better prevention and treatment of heritable diseases. Genome-wide association studies (GWAS) are a relatively new way but have been instrumental in identifying genomic regions that harbor genetic determinants of human diseases or traits including bone and muscle. This approach equals a hypothesis-free evaluation to scan DNA sequence variation, specifically the single nucleotide polymorphisms (SNPs), across the human genome, evaluating their association with the traits of interest. For over a decade, GWAS have reported an impressive number of reproducible genomic regions associated with various common traits. To date, the NHGRI-EBI GWAS Catalog [13] has documented more than 71,673 variant-trait associations. The clinical utility from this success in GWAS may lie in many aspects, such as improving the disease prediction, better understanding response to treatment, and developing more personalized approaches to disease management.

Univariate GWAS

Over a decade since the first GWAS emerged, GWAS have provided numerous compelling genetic associations for human complex traits including musculoskeletal disorders. Specifically, by 2018 GWAS have identified more than 100 loci which are associated with DXA-derived BMD at the femoral neck, lumbar spine, or total body BMD [14]. In addition, more than 300 novel loci which are associated with estimated BMD based on heel ultrasound were added in 2019, by leveraging the large collection of the sample from UK Biobank [15]. On the other hand, relatively fewer GWAS efforts have been devoted to muscle-related traits, such as total body lean mass, appendicular lean mass, and handgrip strength. Specifically, more than 200 loci have been associated with these muscle-related traits [16–20].

Common genetic loci are observed to be associated with both bone and muscle, indicating the potential pleiotropy, which occurs when one locus affects multiple traits. Pleiotropy, either horizontal, vertical, or spurious (defined below), may result in *genetic correlations* [21]. Traditionally, the calculation of genetic correlation (ρ_g) requires the collection of family samples, and researchers can estimate ρ_g based on resemblance among family members. Recent development in cross-trait linkage disequilibrium (LD) score regression provides an alternative way to estimate genetic correlation by leveraging GWAS association summary statistics [22]. Although genetic correlation may mainly result from pleiotropy, vanished genetic correlation between two traits does not exclude the possibility of pleiotropy [23,24]. Intuitively, the overall genetic correlation can be considered as the averaged effect of genetic factors across the genome, which may include positive pleiotropy or negative pleiotropy at different loci [25]. Studying genetically correlated traits may offer insight into complex disease-related traits and lead to tremendous clinical implications because they may reveal genetic variation that contributes to both diseases.

GWAS uncover genetic determinants across the genome in an unbiased way, which implies that GWAS may uncover previously unsuspected, yet important loci that could be useful for further analysis. With this property, GWAS offer the opportunity for researchers to evaluate the commonly shared genetic determinants between bone and muscle. Several genomic loci identified in GWAS of bone-related traits have been also found to be associated with muscle-related traits [26]. Cross-trait association, which searches for the significant association with another trait for the loci associated with the trait of interest, may be the simplest and most intuitive approach to investigate cross-trait effect. However, such an ad hoc cross-trait association approach can be underpowered [27]. Besides, such screening will severely depend on the LD structure and may more likely identify spurious pleiotropy.

Bivariate GWAS and co-localization

Multivariate statistical approaches have direct applications in the analysis of multiple phenotypes. Many approaches have been proposed beyond the classic multivariate methods. For example, based on generalized estimating equations, Lange et al. [28] proposed a multivariate extension of the family-based association test to model multiple phenotypes. Zhang et al. [29] presented a nonparametric approach to testing the association for multiple traits together based on the generalized Kendall's Tau. Ray et al. [30] and Deng et al. [31] constructed a unified score-based association test for detecting pleiotropy that combines multivariate analysis of variance (MANOVA) and the sum of squared score (SSU) test, while Hartley et al. [32] modeled the pleiotropic association with Bayesian networks. These multivariate approaches can jointly model multiple traits under a certain statistical framework to increase the power compared to each single trait analyzed separately. However, through using the individual-level data, these approaches require the phenotypic and genotypic information from all or majority of the participants, ignoring the existing resources generated by large-scale trait-specific GWAS.

GWAS conventionally scans the DNA genome for the association with one trait at a time; however, recently, researchers have advanced the approach to leverage the single-trait derived association *summary statistics* and jointly examine the association with multiple traits. Besides, compared to directly modeling multiple phenotypes simultaneously, utilizing GWAS summary statistics involves less assumption about the relationship among the individual phenotypes. Therefore, such a combined summary statistic approach is instrumental to identify pleiotropic loci associated with multiple traits. For example, motivated by stratified false discovery rate (FDR) methods, a genetic pleiotropy-informed conditional FDR (cFDR) [33] method was proposed to identify the SNPs associated with multiple traits by applying this method to GWAS summary statistics data in order to minimize the association driven by a single phenotype. Intuitively, it is more likely to observe smaller *P*-values for the association with one trait of interest for the subsets of SNPs determined by the nominal *P*-values of their associations with another trait of interest being as small or smaller than a given threshold if there is a pleiotropic effect for the traits of interest. Therefore, the authors calculated conjunction FDR for the identification of pleiotropy, which is defined as the posterior probability to obtain the *P*-values for all the traits simultaneously as small or smaller than the observed *P*-values under the assumption of null association. This approach does not take the association effect into consideration.

Yang et al. [34] proposed the extension of O'Brien's statistics [35] by sample splitting or cross-validation method to gain the power in the scenario with the potentially heterogeneous effect of association with some computing expense for cross-validation method. However, there is one downside for Yang's approach requiring individual-level data to estimate the optimal weight of association, limiting its application. Therefore, the data-driven empirical linear combining approach (eLC) was proposed to overcome this limitation by combining correlated test statistics [12]. The eLC approach applied permutation techniques to construct the empirical null distribution of test statistics, and empirically optimize the overall association signals while accounting for the association between phenotypes. Similar to Yang et al.'s [34] approach, the eLC also allows for mixed directions of effects. There are many other methods to identify multivariate phenotypes simultaneously by leveraging the GWAS summary statistics, such as meta-SCOPA, metaUSAT, and so on [36–38].

The aforementioned bivariate analysis intends to identify genetic variants that are associated with multiple phenotypes. However, the underlying mechanism of interrelationship among the traits of interest and identified genetic variants remains unknown. The pleiotropy relationship between two traits can be classified into different categories: (1) biological pleiotropy or horizontal pleiotropy where the SNP affects both traits through different paths; (2) mediated or vertical pleiotropy where the SNP affects one of the traits, which lies on the causal path to another trait; and (3) spurious pleiotropy where the identified SNP is in LD with two different—not colocalized—causal variants (even different genes) that affect different traits, respectively. Spurious pleiotropy is usually less of interest. However, the other two pleiotropy phenomena have attracted much attention. For example, Phenome-wide association (PheWAS) studies have been conducted to explore the biological pleiotropy, and the Mendelian randomization [39,40] approach has been widely used to delineate the causal relationship of traits in the vertical pleiotropy. Along the same line, some researchers have also explored pleiotropy with polygenic risk scores (PRS [41,42]). These approaches have been proven to be a useful tool to shed the light to usher the new discoveries which require experimental validation eventually. It is obvious that with the extension of current bivariate applications to really multivariate ones (e.g., combining BMD, lean mass, and grip strength), the scenarios—increasing the number of hypotheses regarding interrelationship among identified genetic variants and our traits of interest—will become even more convoluted, possibly affecting the interpretability [43].

Current status of OSP-related genetics in humans

During the last decade, multiple tools were developed to analyze the pleiotropic regulation of complex traits and to shed light on genetic interaction between comorbid diseases. However, only a few studies were done for musculoskeletal traits. For example, a bivariate GWAS study for bone size phenotypes (hip bone size and appendicular lean mass identified variants mapped near *GLYAT* gene [44]. Bivariate GWAS metaanalysis of pediatric musculoskeletal traits revealed variants with pleiotropic effect in eight loci. Seven loci: *WNT4, GALNT3, MEPE, CPED1/WNT16, TNFSF11, RIN3*, and *PPP6R3/LRP5* are established BMD loci [12]. The variants in the eighth—novel—locus (*TOM1L2/SREBF1*) demonstrated the opposing effect on total-body lean mass and total-body BMD. In addition to that, *SREBF1* was pointed out as a strong candidate driving the correlation between two traits. It was shown that *SREBF1* is highly expressed during osteoblasts mineralization in human MSCs. Also, SREBP1 protein regulates myogenesis via indirect inhibition of MYOD1, MYOG, and MEF2C [45,46].

OSP genetics might reflect shared mechanisms underlying MSK-related comorbidity and the relationship between anthropometry and metabolic traits, and even neurodegenerative diseases (especially if a neuromuscular junction is involved [47,48]. Identification of a candidate gene requires additional experimental validation to establish causality, for example, by validating candidate genes with gene-editing technologies in the cell cultures or model organisms. Therefore, we focus here only on several genes, which have been validated in animal models or human cells [26].

Candidate genes

In an early study, by combining the data from the inbred strains of mice with the human GWAS data from the GEFOS consortium, we were able to narrow a quantitative trait locus (QTL) on the mouse Chr 15—which contained 131 annotated genes—to one gene, *Trps1* [49] (then called "trichorhinophalangeal syndrome I" gene). In humans, *TRPS1* SNPs were significantly associated with femoral neck BMD. Therefore, combining association studies in humans with murine models [49] may bear fruits. At the same time, it was demonstrated that *TRPS1* is a target for miR-133a/b during chondrogenesis [50] and underlies a QTL for carcass weight and muscle area in Korean Cattle [51]. More recently, *TRPS1* was identified among potentially pleiotropic loci for bone and obesity metabolism [52], lean mass [16], and handgrip strength [20], again supporting its possible involvement with body weight and muscle properties.

The METTL21 protein family has been implicated in the pathogenesis of some muscle (e.g., inclusion Body Myositis) and bone (Paget's) diseases [53]. In a bivariate (muscle-bone) GWAS study of the Framingham Study, we identified an intronic SNP in *METTL21C* [54]. Functional validation was performed in both C2C12 myoblasts and MLO-Y4 osteocyte cells, and the consequences in both were remarkable. It was further shown that ablation of the *Mettl21c* reduces endurance capacity and leads to age-dependent accumulation of autophagic vacuoles in skeletal muscles [55]. METTL21C mediates the trimethylation and stabilizes the heat shock protein Hspa8/Hsp70, a chaperone required for protein import into mitochondria [56]. A recent study identifies that Mettl21c is a type I myofiber specific protein, and functions to tri-methylate valosin-containing protein (Vcp/p97), a protein required for autophagy. VCP in turn affects both muscle and bone [57], as its defect is associated with Inclusion Body Myopathy and Paget Disease of Bone.

In Table 1, we provide the existing mouse KO models from the Mouse Genome Informatics database for GWAS-derived candidate genes associated with musculoskeletal phenotypes in humans. The annotated bone and or muscle phenotypes for these mutants are highlighted. For some candidates, as *GALNT3* the mutant murine model is annotated with alteration in both bone and muscle parameters. However, for the majority of candidates, the mutants display either bone or muscle phenotype. Similarly, to date, Srebf1^{tm2Jdh}/Srebf1^{tm2Jdh} mouse mutant line is annotated just with decreased levels of triglyceride and cholesterol while MSK phenotypes are not reported.

Rare conditions/monogenic diseases

Rare monogenic conditions also known as Mendelian diseases provide a good source of gene candidates and pathways they are involved in Refs. [58,59]. There is no conceptual dichotomy between common and rare diseases if a causal variant is known (usually common for the former and less common for the latter). Muscular dystrophies are known to affect the skeletal system as well [60]. The most prominent is Duchenne Muscular Dystrophy (DMD) and Becker Muscular Dystrophy, where muscle impairment is accompanied by low BMD or increased fracture propensity (reviewed in Ref. [61]). Both are associated with the dystrophin (DMD) locus on the X chromosome.

Fibrodysplasia ossificans progressiva (FOP) is a rare autosomal dominant disease, which is caused by a mutation in ACVR1 (activin a receptor, Type I) gene. It is characterized by extraosseous ossification which does not only affect muscles, but also ligaments, tendons, and connective tissue leading to severe restriction of movements. Also, skeletal muscle myopathies, characterized by various patterns of weakness and dysfunction, sometimes also affect bones. For example, a mutation in methylthioadenosine phosphorylase (MTAP) gene causes an autosomal dominant bone dysplasia, along with a limb-girdle myopathy; there might be both muscle weakness and atrophy and pathologic fractures due to abnormal cortical growth. Congenital generalized lipodystrophy type 4 has prominent muscular dystrophy, probably due to mutated Caveolae Associated Protein 1 (CAVIN1, a.k.a. Polymerase I and Transcript Release Factor). This recessive disorder also is characterized by impaired bone formation, lordosis, or scoliosis. Also, inclusion body myopathy associated with Paget's disease, which seems to be caused by a defect in valosin-containing protein, VCP [57], affects both muscle and bone.

By perusing the OMIM database with a search keyword: "sarcopenia," one finds several additional diseases and genes, such as ERCC1 (excision repair, complementing defective); this gene is also associated with "estimated BMD" (eBMD [15,62]). Of note, this gene is located on 19q13.32 near the *APOE* gene, raising the likely possibility that these associations reflect the influence of variants in that well-established longevity-associated locus [63]. Also, POLG (polymerase, DNA, gamma) was associated with eBMD [15]. The $PolgA^{(D257A/D257A)}$ mice were described above. A gene responsible for spinal muscular atrophy with congenital bone fractures 1, TRIP4 (thyroid hormone receptor interactor 4), was similarly associated with heel BMD [15].

These disease-related genes provide new insights into biological pathways that can become the target of intervention for more complex musculoskeletal conditions like osteosarcopenia [61]. Some of the persons with the rare musculoskeletal conditions if their symptoms are mild might be misclassified as "normal" (so-called "phenocopies") and therefore to be included in the population-based GWAS. However, it is difficult to imagine anyone who survives for a long time without a correct diagnosis to make it to the older-age GWAS effort.

TABLE 1 Murine mutant models for human GWAS-derived candidate genes associated with musculoskeletal parameters.

Gene	Animal model	Bone phenotype	Muscle phenotype	Mouse Genome Informatics database
WNT16 (wingless-type MMTV integration site family, member 16)	$Wnt16^{tm1Lex}/Wnt16^{tm1Lex}$	Decreased cortical bone volume	No data	http://www.informatics.jax.org/marker/phenotypes/MGI:2136018
LRP5 (low density lipoprotein receptor-related protein 5)	$Lrp5^{Gt(OST164883)Lex}/Lrp5^{Gt(OST164883)Lex}$	Abnormal bone morphology, decreased BMD	No data	http://www.informatics.jax.org/marker/phenotypes/MGI:1278315
MC4R (melanocortin 4 receptor)	$Mc4r^{tm1.1Fbz}/Mc4r^{tm1.1Fbz}$	No data	Altered lean body mass	http://www.informatics.jax.org/marker/phenotypes/MGI:99457
	$Mc4r^{tm1Dhu}/Mc4r^{tm1Dhu}$	Decreased osteoclast cell number, increased BMD	No data	
TRPS1 (transcriptional repressor GATA binding 1)	$Trps1^{tm1.1Shiv}/Trps1^{tm1.1Shiv}$	Abnormal rib formation, thorax cage, scoliosis	No data	http://www.informatics.jax.org/marker/phenotypes/MGI:1927616
WNT4 (wingless-type MMTV integration site family, member 4)	$Gt(ROSA)26Sor^{tm1(Wnt4)Bhr}$	Shortened limbs; abnormal axial skeleton	No data	http://www.informatics.jax.org/marker/phenotypes/MGI:98957
GALNT3 (polypeptide N-acetylgalactosaminyltransferase 3)	$Galnt3^{tcal}/Galnt3^{tcal}$	Increased BMD	Calcification of muscles	http://www.informatics.jax.org/marker/phenotypes/MGI:894695
MEPE (matrix extracellular phosphoglycoprotein with ASARM motif (bone))	$Mepe^{tm1Tbrw}/Mepe^{tm1Tbrw}$	Abnormal skeleton morphology; increased BMD	No data	http://www.informatics.jax.org/marker/phenotypes/MGI:2137384

METTL21C (methyltransferase like 21C)	$Mettl21c^{tm1.1Krug}$/$Mettl21c^{tm1.1Krug}$	No data	Abnormal muscle physiology; impaired exercise endurance; muscle weakness	http://www.informatics.jax.org/marker/phenotypes/MGI:3611450
TNFSF11 (tumor necrosis factor (ligand) superfamily, member 11)	Tg(APCS-Tnfsf11*)#aKhs/0 C57BL/6J-Tg(APCS-Tnfsf11*)#aKhs	Decreased BMD; osteoporotic phenotype	No data	http://www.informatics.jax.org/marker/phenotypes/MGI:1100089
	$Tnfsf11^{gum}$/$Tnfsf11^{gum}$	Osteopetrosis; small cranium; mandible hypoplasia	Dystrophic muscle; decreased lean body mass	
SREBF1 (sterol regulatory element binding transcription factor 1)	$Srebf1^{tm2Jdh}$/$Srebf1^{tm2Jdh}$	No data	No data	http://www.informatics.jax.org/marker/phenotypes/MGI:107606
TOM1L2 (target of myb1-like 2)	$Tom1l2^{Gt(XG909)Byg}$/$Tom1l2^{+}$	Malocclusion; kyphosis	No data	http://www.informatics.jax.org/marker/phenotypes/MGI:2443306

Effect of environment on musculoskeletal quality and tissue-specific aging

Different tissues of the human body undergo DNA methylation during the lifespan and musculoskeletal tissues are not an exception [64]. The effect of tissue-environment interactions on tissue quality and its decline with age is measurable. For example, an epigenetic clock—a mathematical algorithm—was established to predict the biological age of tissue, based on DNA methylation level [65]. Specifically for the musculoskeletal application, the epigenetic clock may help to evaluate the effect of environmental factors, such as exercise and diet on the biological aging of muscles and bones. Multiple studies in humans and animals (even in the small fish models) have explored that exercise promotes the gain in muscle as well as bone mass, thus preventing musculoskeletal degradation [66]. Within the human population, the regularly exercising cohort of people are usually athletes, dancers, and soldiers [67]. Moreover, it was shown that retired athletes and dancers after cessation of high physical exercising still have higher BMD than people with a sedentary lifestyle [68,69]. Therefore, people with a physically active lifestyle are more protected against impaired musculoskeletal conditions. The mechanical loading on the skeletal system induces the process of bone remodeling, by increasing the number of bone-forming cells, BMD and bone volume; however, the continuous loading can lead to impaired energy availability and increase the (stress) fracture risk [70]. Further GWAS studies of elite athletes, who endure much higher mechanical stress than most of the people, can elucidate the genetic peculiarities underlying the musculoskeletal abilities of such an extreme population [68]. As an example, a candidate gene *ACTN3* came out from such studies and further was confirmed as a regulator of muscle and bone phenotype in the mouse model [71,72]. In addition, the SNP polymorphism in *ACTN3* appears to influence muscle phenotype in elite athletes [73], BMD, muscle impairment, and metabolic disorder risk in older people [7]. Also, the polymorphism in *VDR* was shown to be associated with higher BMD in weight-bearing athletes compared to the control group [68]. However, at the present, both these genes have not been replicated in extant GWAS for musculoskeletal traits. This might mean that either they are not as relevant for the majority of the population or that GWAS should be attempted in a case-control fashion, e.g., comparing athletes with nonexercising adults.

Besides physical activity, there are still many other factors affecting musculoskeletal homeostasis. For example, insufficient protein intake, low vitamin D level, and calcium deficiency may substantially affect the quality of bone and muscle tissues [74]. The loss of each or both tissues may appear subsequently as a result of behavioral influences, including a balance of activity and resting (including sleeping [75]). It is known that physiology and behavior are rhythmically orchestrated by circadian rhythms. The disruption of circadian rhythms in humans may change the DNA methylation of clock genes in key metabolic tissues, such as skeletal muscles, thereby altering their epigenetic age [75]. A recent study had shown that muscle-specific disruption of core molecular clock protein BMAL1 significantly affects muscle/bone metabolism in a paracrine manner [76]. The microarray analysis of BmaL1 muscle-specific KO in mice revealed the significant expression change of myokines involved in bone formation/resorption processes, such as myostatin, TGFB1, IGFB5, irisin, and GDF11 [77]. These findings hint at a possible direction for further discovery of new pathways controlling these relationships which may lead to intervention strategies directed to alter clock genes in muscles.

Pleiotropy for bone-and-muscle-related phenotypes in animals

Animals have been used to identify genes underlying bone-and-muscle traits; the most prominent animal models are rodent, ovine, porcine, and piscine [78–80]. The International Knockout Mouse Consortium [81] and the International Mouse Phenotyping Consortium [82] generated a wealth of genetic information on MSK phenotypes [83]. The advantages of these animal models are numerous, including controlled genetic background and testing of advanced phenotypes (e.g., biomechanical properties) that cannot be assessed in humans in vivo. Models of co-occurring sarcopenia and osteoporosis exist, usually in senescence-accelerated mice [84]. Strategies for mapping of genes in mice traditionally relied largely on intercross or backcross approaches or the use of recombinant inbred lines, to facilitate the forward genetic discovery. For example, in advanced intercross lines (AIL) of mice, Gonzales et al. [85] identified 126 significant associations for 50 traits, including bone length and muscle mass. Also, in mice, the investigators explored the QTL intervals to identify genes that potentially affect muscle mass and bone length; they revealed human-mouse genetic convergence specifically for the myogenesis loci [16] (see also Ref. [86] for human muscle regulation).

GWAS is widely used in farmed animals, e.g., cattle and other livestock, for MSK traits [87]. Many putatively pleiotropic QTLs affecting traits of biomedical importance have been discovered in farmed animals [88], although the aims of the discovery were obviously of agricultural interest. The animal genetic terminology differs somehow, but in the essence, traits such as "bony carcass" or "body frame size" refer to bone-and-muscle-related phenotypes. For example, a recent GWAS identified an SNP within the diacylglycerol *O*-acyltransferase 1 (*DGAT1*) gene that was significantly associated with the "quality" of long bones [89]. Besides being pleiotropic for multiple bovine traits, *DGAT1* was shown to function in rodent skeletal muscle cells [90]. In humans, SNP rs7838717 in the *DGAT1* locus was associated with Dupuytren's disease [91].

Dogs and horses continue to serve as best helpers for humans also for genome-mapping purposes. Musculoskeletal phenotypes were studied in the domestic dog [92], given this species amenability for morphological genetic study [93]. Similarly, although muscle performance is the most studied trait in the thoroughbred racing horse, it was realized that susceptibility to fracture risk is also genetically-determined [94]. In thoroughbreds, among regions selected for inbreeding using the pan-genomic SNP-based genotypes, genes relating to musculoskeletal form and function were identified [95]. These include the deleted lymphocytic leukemia 7 gene (*DLEU7*) associated with growth traits and eBMD in humans [15]. The other was the von Willebrand factor C domain containing 2 gene (*VWC2*), a bone morphogenic protein, which promotes bone formation, regeneration, and healing [95,96].

Forward genetics is also feasible in a small teleost, the zebrafish (*Danio rerio*) [78,79]. Screens for MSK phenotypes were performed by Harris' group [97] to identify genes of interest for skeletogenesis. *D. rerio* is also helpful to validate human-first GWAS discovery (reverse genetics) [78]. However, a lion's share of such studies is still done in mice. Relevant to the GWAS of MSK phenotype, Tanaka et al. [98] recently noted that human polymorphisms in *FAM210a* were strongly associated with fracture risk and BMD, as well as also nominally associated with lean mass. The authors created genetically modified mice; they showed that *Fam210a* was expressed in muscle mitochondria and cytoplasm but not in bone. Notably, grip strength and limb lean mass were reduced in both tamoxifen-inducible *Fam210a* homozygous global knockout mice (*TFam210a−/−*) and skeletal muscle cell-specific knockout mice (*Fam210aMus−/−*). In parallel, decreased BMD, bone biomechanical strength and bone formation, and elevated osteoclast activity were observed in *TFam210a−/−* mice [98]. Therefore, *Fam210a* seems to play an important role in bone quality and quantity, as well as in muscle bulk and power.

More recently, Scheuren et al. [99] aimed to evaluate the PolgA$^{(D257A/D257A)}$ mouse, which due to elevated mitochondrial DNA point mutations and systemic mitochondrial dysfunction, exhibits an accelerated aging phenotype, as a model of frailty and osteosarcopenia. Longitudinal assessment of the PolgA$^{(D257A/D257A)}$ mice displayed progressive MSK deterioration such as reduced bone and muscle mass as well as impaired MSK function. Specifically, PolgA$^{(D257A/D257A)}$ had lower grip strength and concentric muscle forces as well as reduced bone turnover. In addition, PolgA$^{(D257A/D257A)}$ mutation altered the sensitivity to anabolic stimuli in skeletal muscle, muscle progenitors, and bone. While compared to WT, PolgA$^{(D257A/D257A)}$ caudal vertebrae were not responsive to a cyclic loading regime. Overall, PolgA$^{(D257A/D257A)}$ mutation leads to hallmarks of age-related frailty and osteosarcopenia and, thus, provides a powerful model to better understand the relationship between frailty and the OSP for human study.

Animal models of bone-muscle interaction are frequently using mechanobiology approaches, with the loading of both muscles/bones [99] or artificial immobilization and disuse. Relevant for the MSK regeneration in older age would be a study of hibernating mammals [100]. There is a diverse array of species that may conserve muscle mass despite prolonged inactivity. It is interesting to compare them to the artificial immobilization/prolonged disuse in nonhibernating mammals, as a source of genetic factors responsible for musculoskeletal regeneration and maintenance [100].

In summary, this is an exciting time for the construction of an extensive catalog of a range of model species, of a variety of genomes and conserved genetic loci, focused on the osteosarcopenia-relevant mechanisms.

Sex-specificity of disease: Is there any genetic predisposition?

Osteosarcopenia's definition (thresholds) might seem arbitrary; however, the difference between the sexes exists in OSP occurrence. It means that sex-specific genetics has to be tested. Recently, the role of sex in the genomics of human complex traits was well described [101]. Such body-composition-related phenotypes as BMD, lean mass, and body shape demonstrate an evident sexual dimorphism [102]. Therefore, the Genetic Investigation of Anthropometric Traits (GIANT) Consortium performed a metaanalysis in order to study the BMI and waist-to-hip ratio (WHR), with sex-specific genetic effects (G x sex) modeled [102]. No sex-dependent effects were identified for BMI. However, for WHR they identified 44 sex-specific loci, 11 of which showed opposite effects between sexes [102]. This study's findings of sexual dimorphism in body shape are important for the OSP, since it might partly explain the male-to-female differences in the OSP prevalence.

There is mounting evidence that all adult tissues exhibit sex-specific expression patterns, some of which are independent of hormonal influence [103]. Sexually dimorphic differences in gene expression across adult tissues may be modulated by sex-specific cis-regulatory elements, alternative splicing, and differentially methylated sites. This calls for a transcriptome-wide study with sex interaction terms.

One might assume that for sex dimorphic traits, sex differences may be simply explained by differences in the sex chromosome. However, Traglia and colleagues [104] did not find a consistent disproportionate role for the X-chromosome in disease risk, despite sex-heterogeneity on the X for several anthropometric traits. Here to remind that *DMD* and *AR* genes are mapped on the X chromosome, as well as *FAM9B*—the latter associated with testosterone concentrations [105] and BMD [106]. Unfortunately, X-chromosome was not systematically studied during the first GWAS decade, thus even metaanalysis of age at menopause [107] included only autosomal SNPs.

Sex chromosomes start to program autosomal gene expression and establish sex-specific epigenetic patterns very soon after fertilization [103]. Differences in the male and female epigenomes include distinct methylated patterns such as imprinting and result in differential gene expression [108]. As such, the presence or absence of the Y-linked SRY locus is noted in the early fetus. Then, the life-long sex-specific environment seems to play a role in changing genotype expression across a range of human complex traits. The role of sex steroids and sex steroid receptors (e.g., ESRs and AR) is well known both for BMD and muscle mass regulation. Testosterone is an androgen, which is produced in the fetus and controls the sexual fate of the early gonads. Of note, myostatin is an androgen target gene in skeletal muscle [109].

For those traits where sexual dimorphism is obvious, sex-specific statistical approaches may aid in future gene-finding efforts [104]. However, some predictions show that for most of the traits the number of sex-specific genetic variants will be small [110]. Furthermore, this may be a challenging endeavor due to the likely small effects of the interactions at individual loci. In an earlier study, we suggested that gene-by-sex interactions probably have weak effects on BMD, accounting for less than 0.08% of the BMD variation per implicated SNP [111].

The presence of sex-specific effects would require sex-stratified analysis, as well as the study of enrichment in sex-hormone-related functional categories. If successful, sex-specific approaches may aid in future gene-finding efforts. Then, in clinical practice, sex-specific diagnostic markers or targeted treatments would be warranted.

Translational perspectives

Genetic discoveries are important for drug target identification and repurposing; pharmacogenetics is also helpful in assigning a drug to a disease. This is especially true for the loci with the opposite effect in bone vs. muscle that become a target for a drug: a lack of pleiotropic effects from such analysis supports their safety and efficacy.

Clinical applications might be possible for a genetic risk score (GRS, a.k.a. polygenic risk score, PRS). Whether GRS based on pleiotropic signals have more effective prediction is still unclear. However, it was shown that PRS might serve as a genetic instrument for MR analyses. Results of a preliminary simulation study [112] indicated that, although using a PRS provides higher statistical power, it also suffers from substantive false positive rates due to horizontal pleiotropy (defined above). A single SNP which is known to be pleiotropic with large effects on different and diverse traits had been found to distort findings from PRS analyses [112,113].

Challenges and solutions

The complex and pleiotropic genetic architecture of MSK disorders poses some challenges for work in model systems as we discussed above. The absence of a clear-cut definition or diagnosis of OSP instructs us to use multivariate and bivariate statistics. It is important to take into consideration that osteosarcopenia, as a dichotomous phenotype, is useful for clinical use; however, for the study of genetics this is not optimal, commanding the investigators to keep looking for additional (endo)phenotypes. The presence of pleiotropy implies the need for a search of a particular endophenotype that mediates the effect of risk on the clinical phenotype of OSP. There is also a need in the phenotypes of "change," to capture a trajectory of bone and muscle loss. Ideally, a longitudinal study should be a good answer, paralleled by (multi)omics data, to reflect an individual rate of bone and muscle loss and to test whether a combination of omics data correlates with this trajectory rather than a one-time measure of OSP. This corresponds to the logistical challenge to generate gene expression data for muscle and bone of the same individual (although material left over from the surgical procedures can be a good source, for example, from the hip replacement operations).

A substrate of metabolic communications between bone and muscle can be pointed out by the cross-phenotype study. The ensuing issue would then be a cell(s) with regulatory potential—whose origin can be either in bone or in muscle; the answer for this question is important to correctly allocate the resources for a functional study following the genomic approaches [43]. Again, Big Data/omics should help identify cell(s) of origin for these molecules. They might be neither bone nor muscle, but some other organs/tissues (e.g., liver, adipose).

Furthermore, the effects of relevant variants are often found to be environment-specific and to have different temporal patterns [114]. This necessitates a conduct of age-dependent time-to-event analyses to investigate temporal patterns of the genetic effects, where age can be considered an environment and used to stratify the population accordingly. A related problem is the lack of GWAS specifically focused on the aged population—or trying to analyze mid- to older persons transition or to model age × gene interaction. To date, animal genetic models as well as orchid- or ovariectomy models exist; however, they are insufficient to model the organism's aging in its entirety.

It was proposed that a pleiotropic analysis combined with annotation with various expression and regulatory database resources can serve as a substantive tool to elucidate a causality behind the association between SNPs and diseases [114].

Detecting pleiotropic effects is just the 1st step. After the initial discovery, *replication is a must*: the ability to reproduce results is a cornerstone of science, especially due to the exponential growth of the amount of scientific data [115]. Frequently the inability to reproduce findings is seriously dampening chances of correct applications. A "triangulation" approach is a gold standard in the field—where human discovery is followed by functional analysis with various means—e.g., cells and animal models. This is where the wealth of (multi)-omics and biology/laboratory follow-up is required.

Summary and future directions

With prolonged lifespan, the importance of quality of life in older persons is growing exponentially. Even though there is still an uncertainty in the definition of OSP, it is clear that this aging-related condition comprises the impairment of bones and muscles that coincide. Genome-wide association studies substantially contributed to our understanding of the genetic architecture of osteoporosis;

however, there are still gaps in genetic insight into the sarcopenia phenotypes, either muscle mass or strength. Univariate GWAS is therefore still of value. The bi- and multivariate analyses are expected to contribute to additional discoveries of metabolic communications between bone and muscle, beyond biomechanical links between these tissues.

Recent GWAS findings produced large numbers of candidates with possible functions in musculoskeletal homeostasis, demonstrating the benefit of synthesizing data on related traits to uncover potential new disease-associated loci. This search of candidate genes with possible pleiotropic effects on bones and muscles successfully reveals numerous candidates that have to be further validated. Some of these candidates have been examined in human cells and animal models, exemplified by FAM210A, SREBF1, METTL21C, and other genes. However, to evaluate the genetic landscape of OSP, further GWAS for osteoporosis and sarcopenia in the older population are necessary in order to decipher the genetic contribution of senescence-related factors. In addition, the implementation of sex-specific approaches could shed the light on the pathogenesis of OSP, which seems to have different etiology in men and women. Furthermore, retired athletes, dancers, and people with active physical backgrounds with non-traumatic experience in the past display a better quality of MSK parameters compared to people with a sedentary lifestyle. Together with experimental studies of exercising impact on MSK system in animal models, this may provide a strong statement about the necessity of physical activity in order to prevent the OSP symptoms—or to contribute the understanding of their peculiar genetics. Thus, to find out whether there is a genetic predisposition for "preserved" MSK health, the GWAS of retired athletes is required. Together with multiomics, the study of human disease's genetics may pave the way for precision medicine in the prevention or the treatment of osteoporosis and sarcopenia. Beyond knowledge of etiology, it is destined to provide new drug target(s) for pharmacy and improve the strategies of nonpharmacological intervention.

References

[1] Kirk B, Al Saedi A, Duque G. Osteosarcopenia: a case of geroscience. Aging Med 2019;2(3):147–56.

[2] Tagliaferri C, Wittrant Y, Davicco MJ, Walrand S, Coxam V. Muscle and bone, two interconnected tissues. Ageing Res Rev 2015;21:55–70.

[3] Bhasin S, Apovian CM, Travison TG, Pencina K, Moore LL, Huang G, et al. Effect of protein intake on lean body mass in functionally limited older men: a randomized clinical trial. JAMA Intern Med 2018;178(4):530–41.

[4] Norman K, Stobäus N, Gonzalez MC, Schulzke J-D, Pirlich M. Hand grip strength: outcome predictor and marker of nutritional status. Clin Nutr 2011;30(2):135–42.

[5] Hirschfeld HP, Kinsella R, Duque G. Osteosarcopenia: where bone, muscle, and fat collide. Osteoporos Int 2017;28(10):2781–90.

[6] WHO. WHO_TRS_843_eng.pdf; 1994.

[7] Yoo J-I, Ha Y-C. Review of epidemiology, diagnosis, and treatment of osteosarcopenia in Korea. J Bone Metab 2018;25(1):1–7.

[8] Cruz-Jentoft AJ, Bahat G, Bauer J, Boirie Y, Bruyère O, Cederholm T, et al. Sarcopenia: revised European consensus on definition and diagnosis. Age Ageing 2019;48(1):16–31.
[9] Fatima M, Brennan-Olsen SL, Duque G. Therapeutic approaches to osteosarcopenia: insights for the clinician. Ther Adv Musculoskelet Dis 2019;11, 1759720X19867009.
[10] Evans LM, Tahmasbi R, Jones M, Vrieze SI, Abecasis GR, Das S, et al. Narrow-sense heritability estimation of complex traits using identity-by-descent information. Heredity 2018;121(6):616–30.
[11] Karasik D, Demissie S, Zhou Y, Lu D, Broe KE, Bouxsein ML, et al. Heritability and genetic correlations for bone microarchitecture: the Framingham study families. J Bone Miner Res 2017;32(1):106–14.
[12] Medina-Gomez C, Kemp JP, Dimou NL, Kreiner E, Chesi A, Zemel BS, et al. Bivariate genome-wide association meta-analysis of pediatric musculoskeletal traits reveals pleiotropic effects at the SREBF1/TOM1L2 locus. Nat Commun 2017;8(1):121.
[13] Buniello A, MacArthur JAL, Cerezo M, Harris LW, Hayhurst J, Malangone C, et al. The NHGRI-EBI GWAS catalog of published genome-wide association studies, targeted arrays and summary statistics 2019. Nucleic Acids Res 2019;47(D1):D1005–d12.
[14] Yang T-L, Shen H, Liu A, Dong S-S, Zhang L, Deng F-Y, et al. A road map for understanding molecular and genetic determinants of osteoporosis. Nat Rev Endocrinol 2020;16(2):91–103.
[15] Morris JA, Kemp JP, Youlten SE, Laurent L, Logan JG, Chai RC, et al. An atlas of genetic influences on osteoporosis in humans and mice. Nat Genet 2019;51(2):258–66.
[16] Hernandez Cordero AI, Gonzales NM, Parker CC, Sokoloff G, Vandenbergh DJ, Cheng R, et al. Genome-wide associations reveal human-mouse genetic convergence and novel modifiers of myogenesis, CPNE1 and STC2. bioRxiv 2019;370312.
[17] Zillikens MC, Demissie S, Hsu YH, Yerges-Armstrong LM, Chou WC, Stolk L, et al. Large meta-analysis of genome-wide association studies identifies five loci for lean body mass. Nat Commun 2017;8(1):80.
[18] Matteini AM, Tanaka T, Karasik D, Atzmon G, Chou W-C, Eicher JD, et al. GWAS analysis of handgrip and lower body strength in older adults in the CHARGE consortium. Aging Cell 2016;15(5):792–800.
[19] Willems SM, Wright DJ, Day FR, Trajanoska K, Joshi PK, Morris JA, et al. Large-scale GWAS identifies multiple loci for hand grip strength providing biological insights into muscular fitness. Nat Commun 2017;8:16015.
[20] Tikkanen E, Gustafsson S, Amar D, Shcherbina A, Waggott D, Ashley EA, et al. Biological insights into muscular strength: genetic findings in the UK biobank. Sci Rep 2018;8(1):6451.
[21] van Rheenen W, Peyrot WJ, Schork AJ, Lee SH, Wray NR. Genetic correlations of polygenic disease traits: from theory to practice. Nat Rev Genet 2019;20(10):567–81.
[22] Bulik-Sullivan B, Finucane HK, Anttila V, Gusev A, Day FR, Loh PR, et al. An atlas of genetic correlations across human diseases and traits. Nat Genet 2015;47(11):1236–41.
[23] Gratten J, Visscher PM. Genetic pleiotropy in complex traits and diseases: implications for genomic medicine. Genome Med 2016;8(1):78.
[24] Cheverud JM. Developmental integration and the evolution of pleiotropy. Am Zool 1996;36(1):44–50.
[25] Hughes KA, Leips J. Pleiotropy, constraint, and modularity in the evolution of life histories: insights from genomic analyses. Ann NY Acad Sci 2017;1389(1):76–91.
[26] Trajanoska K, Rivadeneira F, Kiel DP, Karasik D. Genetics of bone and muscle interactions in humans. Curr Osteoporos Rep 2019;17(2):86–95.

[27] Salinas YD, Wang Z, DeWan AT. Statistical analysis of multiple phenotypes in genetic epidemiologic studies: from cross-phenotype associations to pleiotropy. Am J Epidemiol 2018;187(4):855–63.
[28] Lange C, Silverman EK, Xu X, Weiss ST, Laird NM. A multivariate family-based association test using generalized estimating equations: FBAT-GEE. Biostatistics 2003;4(2):195–206.
[29] Zhang H, Liu CT, Wang X. An association test for multiple traits based on the generalized Kendall's Tau. J Am Stat Assoc 2010;105(490):473–81.
[30] Ray D, Pankow JS, Basu S. USAT: a unified score-based association test for multiple phenotype-genotype analysis. Genet Epidemiol 2016;40(1):20–34.
[31] Deng X, Wang B, Fisher V, Peloso G, Cupples A, Liu CT. Genome-wide association study for multiple phenotype analysis. BMC Proc 2018;12(Suppl 9):55.
[32] Hartley SW, Monti S, Liu CT, Steinberg MH, Sebastiani P. Bayesian methods for multivariate modeling of pleiotropic SNP associations and genetic risk prediction. Front Genet 2012;3:176.
[33] Andreassen OA, Thompson WK, Schork AJ, Ripke S, Mattingsdal M, Kelsoe JR, et al. Improved detection of common variants associated with schizophrenia and bipolar disorder using pleiotropy-informed conditional false discovery rate. PLoS Genet 2013;9(4):e1003455.
[34] Yang Q, Wu H, Guo CY, Fox CS. Analyze multivariate phenotypes in genetic association studies by combining univariate association tests. Genet Epidemiol 2010;34(5):444–54.
[35] O'Brien PC. Procedures for comparing samples with multiple endpoints. Biometrics 1984;40(4):1079–87.
[36] Li X, Zhu X. Cross-phenotype association analysis using summary statistics from GWAS. Methods Mol Biol 2017;1666:455–67.
[37] Ray D, Boehnke M. Methods for meta-analysis of multiple traits using GWAS summary statistics. Genet Epidemiol 2018;42(2):134–45.
[38] Liu Z, Lin X. Multiple phenotype association tests using summary statistics in genome-wide association studies. Biometrics 2018;74(1):165–75.
[39] Smith GD, Ebrahim S. 'Mendelian randomization': can genetic epidemiology contribute to understanding environmental determinants of disease? Int J Epidemiol 2003;32(1):1–22.
[40] Lawlor DA, Harbord RM, Sterne JA, Timpson N, Davey Smith G. Mendelian randomization: using genes as instruments for making causal inferences in epidemiology. Stat Med 2008;27(8):1133–63.
[41] Zheutlin AB, Dennis J, Karlsson Linner R, Moscati A, Restrepo N, Straub P, et al. Penetrance and pleiotropy of polygenic risk scores for schizophrenia in 106,160 patients across four health care systems. Am J Psychiatry 2019;176(10):846–55.
[42] Purcell SM, Wray NR, Stone JL, Visscher PM, O'Donovan MC, Sullivan PF, et al. Common polygenic variation contributes to risk of schizophrenia and bipolar disorder. Nature 2009;460(7256):748–52.
[43] Cano-Gamez E, Trynka G. From GWAS to function: using functional genomics to identify the mechanisms underlying complex diseases. Front Genet 2020;11:424.
[44] Guo YF, Zhang LS, Liu YJ, Hu HG, Li J, Tian Q, et al. Suggestion of GLYAT gene underlying variation of bone size and body lean mass as revealed by a bivariate genome-wide association study. Hum Genet 2013;132(2):189–99.
[45] Dessalle K, Euthine V, Chanon S, Delarichaudy J, Fujii I, Rome S, et al. SREBP-1 transcription factors regulate skeletal muscle cell size by controlling protein synthesis through myogenic regulatory factors. PLoS One 2012;7(11):e50878.
[46] Lecomte V, Meugnier E, Euthine V, Durand C, Freyssenet D, Nemoz G, et al. A new role for sterol regulatory element binding protein 1 transcription factors in the regulation of muscle mass and muscle cell differentiation. Mol Cell Biol 2010;30(5):1182–98.

[47] Larsson L, Degens H, Li M, Salviati L, Lee YI, Thompson W, et al. Sarcopenia: aging-related loss of muscle mass and function. Physiol Rev 2019;99(1):427–511.

[48] Drey M, Hasmann SE, Krenovsky J-P, Hobert MA, Straub S, Elshehabi M, et al. Associations between early markers of Parkinson's disease and sarcopenia. Front Aging Neurosci 2017;9:53.

[49] Ackert-Bicknell CL, Demissie S, Tsaih SW, Beamer WG, Cupples LA, Paigen BJ, et al. Genetic variation in TRPS1 may regulate hip geometry as well as bone mineral density. Bone 2012;50(5):1188–95.

[50] Zhang Y, Xie RL, Gordon J, LeBlanc K, Stein JL, Lian JB, et al. Control of mesenchymal lineage progression by microRNAs targeting skeletal gene regulators Trps1 and Runx2. J Biol Chem 2012;287(26):21926–35.

[51] Lee SH, van der Werf JH, Kim NK, Lee SH, Gondro C, Park EW, et al. QTL and gene expression analyses identify genes affecting carcass weight and marbling on BTA14 in Hanwoo (Korean cattle). Mamm Genome 2011;22(9–10):589–601.

[52] Hu Y, Tan L-J, Chen X-D, Liu Z, Min S-S, Zeng Q, et al. Identification of novel potentially pleiotropic variants associated with osteoporosis and obesity using the cFDR method. J Clin Endocrinol Metab 2018;103(1):125–38.

[53] Cloutier P, Lavallée-Adam M, Faubert D, Blanchette M, Coulombe B. A newly uncovered group of distantly related lysine methyltransferases preferentially interact with molecular chaperones to regulate their activity. PLoS Genet 2013;9(1), e1003210.

[54] Huang J, Hsu YH, Mo C, Abreu E, Kiel DP, Bonewald LF, et al. METTL21C is a potential pleiotropic gene for osteoporosis and sarcopenia acting through the modulation of the NF-kappaB signaling pathway. J Bone Miner Res 2014;29(7):1531–40.

[55] Wiederstein JL, Nolte H, Gunther S, Piller T, Baraldo M, Kostin S, et al. Skeletal muscle-specific methyltransferase METTL21C trimethylates p97 and regulates autophagy-associated protein breakdown. Cell Rep 2018;23(5):1342–56.

[56] Wang C, Arrington J, Ratliff AC, Chen J, Horton HE, Nie Y, et al. Methyltransferase-like 21c methylates and stabilizes the heat shock protein Hspa8 in type I myofibers in mice. J Biol Chem 2019;294(37):13718–28.

[57] Badadani M, Nalbandian A, Watts GD, Vesa J, Kitazawa M, Su H, et al. VCP associated inclusion body myopathy and Paget disease of bone knock-in mouse model exhibits tissue pathology typical of human disease. PLoS One 2010;5(10):e13183.

[58] Rivadeneira F, Makitie O. Osteoporosis and bone mass disorders: from gene pathways to treatments. Trends Endocrinol Metab 2016;27(5):262–81.

[59] De Ridder R, Boudin E, Mortier G, Van Hul W. Human genetics of sclerosing bone disorders. Curr Osteoporos Rep 2018;16(3):256–68.

[60] Buckner JL, Bowden SA, Mahan JD. Optimizing bone health in duchenne muscular dystrophy. Int J Endocrinol 2015;2015:928385.

[61] Trajanoska K, Rivadeneira F. Genetics of osteosarcopenia. In: Duque G, editor. Osteosarcopenia: bone, muscle and fat interactions. Cham: Springer; 2019.

[62] Kemp JP, Morris JA, Medina-Gómez M, Gregson CL, Forgetta V, Trajanoska K, et al. Genome-wide association study of bone mineral density in the UK Biobank Study identifies over 376 loci associated with osteoporosis. Vancouver, CA: American Society for Human Genetics; 2016, October 20.

[63] Deelen J, Evans DS, Arking DE, Tesi N, Nygaard M, Liu X, et al. A meta-analysis of genome-wide association studies identifies multiple longevity genes. Nat Commun 2019;10(1):3669.

[64] Horvath S, Raj K. DNA methylation-based biomarkers and the epigenetic clock theory of ageing. Nat Rev Genet 2018;19(6):371–84.

[65] Voisin S, Harvey NR, Haupt LM, Griffiths LR, Ashton KJ, Coffey VG, et al. An epigenetic clock for human skeletal muscle. J Cachexia Sarcopenia Muscle 2020;11(4):887–98.
[66] Tagliaferri C, Wittrant Y, Davicco MJ, Walrand S, Coxam V. Muscle and bone, two interconnected tissues. Elsevier Ireland Ltd; 2015. p. 55–70.
[67] Hadid A, Epstein Y, Shabshin N, Gefen A. Biomechanical model for stress fracture-related factors in athletes and soldiers. Med Sci Sports Exerc 2018;50(9):1827–36.
[68] Herbert AJ, Williams AG, Hennis PJ, Erskine RM, Sale C, Day SH, et al. The interactions of physical activity, exercise and genetics and their associations with bone mineral density: implications for injury risk in elite athletes. Springer Verlag; 2019. p. 29–47.
[69] Keay N. Bone mineral density in professional female dancers. Br J Sports Med 1997;31(2):143–7.
[70] Hart NH, Nimphius S, Rantalainen T, Ireland A, Siafarikas A, Newton RU. Mechanical basis of bone strength: influence of bone material, bone structure and muscle action. J Musculoskelet Neuronal Interact 2017;17(3):114–39.
[71] Yang N, MacArthur DG, Gulbin JP, Hahn AG, Beggs AH, Easteal S, et al. ACTN3 genotype is associated with human elite athletic performance. Am J Hum Genet 2003;73(3):627–31.
[72] Yang N, Schindeler A, McDonald MM, Seto JT, Houweling PJ, Lek M, et al. α-Actinin-3 deficiency is associated with reduced bone mass in human and mouse. Bone 2011;49(4):790–8.
[73] Pickering C, Kiely J. ACTN3, morbidity, and healthy aging. Frontiers Media SA; 2018.
[74] Verlaan S, Maier AB, Bauer JM, Bautmans I, Brandt K, Donini LM, et al. Sufficient levels of 25-hydroxyvitamin D and protein intake required to increase muscle mass in sarcopenic older adults—the PROVIDE study. Clin Nutr 2018;37(2):551–7.
[75] Cedernaes J, Osler ME, Voisin S, Broman J-E, Vogel H, Dickson SL, et al. Acute sleep loss induces tissue-specific epigenetic and transcriptional alterations to circadian clock genes in men. J Clin Endocrinol Metab 2015;100(9):E1255–61.
[76] Riley LA, Esser KA. The role of the molecular clock in skeletal muscle and what it is teaching us about muscle-bone crosstalk. Curr Osteoporos Rep 2017;15(3):222–30.
[77] McDearmon EL, Patel KN, Ko CH, Walisser JA, Schook AC, Chong JL, et al. Dissecting the functions of the mammalian clock protein BMAL1 by tissue-specific rescue in mice. Science 2006;314(5803):1304–8.
[78] Kwon RY, Watson CJ, Karasik D. Using zebrafish to study skeletal genomics. Bone 2019;126:37–50.
[79] Daya A, Donaka R, Karasik D. Zebrafish models of sarcopenia. Dis Model Mech 2020;13(3):DMM/042689.
[80] Bergen DJM, Kague E, Hammond CL. Zebrafish as an emerging model for osteoporosis: a primary testing platform for screening new osteo-active compounds. Front Endocrinol 2019;10:6.
[81] Ringwald M, Iyer V, Mason JC, Stone KR, Tadepally HD, Kadin JA, et al. The IKMC web portal: a central point of entry to data and resources from the international knockout mouse consortium. Nucleic Acids Res 2011;39(Database issue):D849–55.
[82] Consortium IMP, https://www.mousephenotype.org/understand/the-data.
[83] Freudenthal B, Logan J, Sanger Institute Mouse P, Croucher PI, Williams GR, Bassett JHD. Rapid phenotyping of knockout mice to identify genetic determinants of bone strength. J Endocrinol 2016;231(1):R31–46.
[84] Zhang N, Chow SKH, Leung KS, Lee HH, Cheung WH. An animal model of co-existing sarcopenia and osteoporotic fracture in senescence accelerated mouse prone 8 (SAMP8). Exp Gerontol 2017;97:1–8.

[85] Gonzales NM, Seo J, Hernandez Cordero AI, St. Pierre CL, Gregory JS, Distler MG, et al. Genome wide association analysis in a mouse advanced intercross line. Nat Commun 2018;9(1):5162.
[86] Williams K, Ingerslev LR, Bork-Jensen J, Wohlwend M, Hansen AN, Small L, et al. Skeletal muscle enhancer interactions identify genes controlling whole-body metabolism. Nat Commun 2020;11(1):2695.
[87] Leal-Gutiérrez JD, Elzo MA, Johnson DD, Hamblen H, Mateescu RG. Genome wide association and gene enrichment analysis reveal membrane anchoring and structural proteins associated with meat quality in beef. BMC Genomics 2019;20(1):151.
[88] Erickson PA, Baek J, Hart JC, Cleves PA, Miller CT. Genetic dissection of a supergene implicates Tfap2a in craniofacial evolution of threespine sticklebacks. Genetics 2018;209(2):591–605.
[89] Abo-Ismail MK, Brito LF, Miller SP, Sargolzaei M, Grossi DA, Moore SS, et al. Genome-wide association studies and genomic prediction of breeding values for calving performance and body conformation traits in Holstein cattle. Genet Sel Evol 2017;49(1):82.
[90] Yu J, Li Y, Zou F, Xu S, Liu P. Phosphorylation and function of DGAT1 in skeletal muscle cells. Biophys Rep 2015;1:41–50.
[91] Divers J, Palmer ND, Langefeld CD, Brown WM, Lu L, Hicks PJ, et al. Genome-wide association study of coronary artery calcified atherosclerotic plaque in African Americans with type 2 diabetes. BMC Genet 2017;18(1):105.
[92] Hayward JJ, Castelhano MG, Oliveira KC, Corey E, Balkman C, Baxter TL, et al. Complex disease and phenotype mapping in the domestic dog. Nat Commun 2016;7(1):10460.
[93] Plassais J, Kim J, Davis BW, Karyadi DM, Hogan AN, Harris AC, et al. Whole genome sequencing of canids reveals genomic regions under selection and variants influencing morphology. Nat Commun 2019;10:1489.
[94] Blott SC, Swinburne JE, Sibbons C, Fox-Clipsham LY, Helwegen M, Hillyer L, et al. A genome-wide association study demonstrates significant genetic variation for fracture risk in thoroughbred racehorses. BMC Genomics 2014;15:147.
[95] McGivney BA, Han H, Corduff LR, Katz LM, Tozaki T, MacHugh DE, et al. Genomic inbreeding trends, influential sire lines and selection in the global thoroughbred horse population. Sci Rep 2020;10(1):466.
[96] Ohyama Y, Katafuchi M, Almehmadi A, Venkitapathi S, Jaha H, Ehrenman J, et al. Modulation of matrix mineralization by Vwc2-like protein and its novel splicing isoforms. Biochem Biophys Res Commun 2011;418:12–6.
[97] Harris M, Henke K, Hawkins M, Witten P. Fish is fish: the use of experimental model species to reveal causes of skeletal diversity in evolution and disease. J Appl Ichthyol 2014;30(4):616–29.
[98] Tanaka KI, Xue Y, Nguyen-Yamamoto L, Morris JA, Kanazawa I, Sugimoto T, et al. FAM210A is a novel determinant of bone and muscle structure and strength. Proc Natl Acad Sci USA 2018;115(16):E3759–68.
[99] Scheuren AC, D'Hulst G, Kuhn GA, Masschelein E, Wehrle E, De Bock K, et al. Hallmarks of frailty and osteosarcopenia in prematurely aged PolgA((D257A/D257A)) mice. J Cachexia Sarcopenia Muscle 2020;11(4):1121–40.
[100] Reilly BD, Franklin CE. Prevention of muscle wasting and osteoporosis: the value of examining novel animal models. J Exp Biol 2016;219(17):2582–95.
[101] Khramtsova EA, Davis LK, Stranger BE. The role of sex in the genomics of human complex traits. Nat Rev Genet 2019;20(3):173–90.

[102] Winkler TW, Justice AE, Graff M, Barata L, Feitosa MF, Chu S, et al. The influence of age and sex on genetic associations with adult body size and shape: a large-scale genome-wide interaction study. PLoS Genet 2015;11(10):e1005378.

[103] Deegan DF, Engel N. Sexual dimorphism in the age of genomics: how, when, where. Front Cell Dev Biol 2019;7:186.

[104] Traglia M, Bseiso D, Gusev A, Adviento B, Park DS, Mefford JA, et al. Genetic mechanisms leading to sex differences across common diseases and anthropometric traits. Genetics 2017;205(2):979–92.

[105] Ohlsson C, Wallaschofski H, Lunetta KL, Stolk L, Perry JR, Koster A, et al. Genetic determinants of serum testosterone concentrations in men. PLoS Genet 2011;7(10):e1002313.

[106] Estrada K, Styrkarsdottir U, Evangelou E, Hsu YH, Duncan EL, Ntzani EE, et al. Genome-wide meta-analysis identifies 56 bone mineral density loci and reveals 14 loci associated with risk of fracture. Nat Genet 2012;44(5):491–501.

[107] Stolk L, Perry JRB, Chasman DI, He C, Mangino M, Sulem P, et al. Meta-analyses identify 13 loci associated with age at menopause and highlight DNA repair and immune pathways. Nat Genet 2012;44(3):260–8.

[108] Zheng HF, Forgetta V, Hsu YH, Estrada K, Rosello-Diez A, Leo PJ, et al. Whole-genome sequencing identifies EN1 as a determinant of bone density and fracture. Nature 2015;526:112.

[109] Dubois V, Laurent MR, Sinnesael M, Cielen N, Helsen C, Clinckemalie L, et al. A satellite cell-specific knockout of the androgen receptor reveals myostatin as a direct androgen target in skeletal muscle. FASEB J 2014;28(7):2979–94.

[110] Stringer S, Polderman TJC, Posthuma D. Majority of human traits do not show evidence for sex-specific genetic and environmental effects. Sci Rep 2017;7(1):8688.

[111] Liu CT, Estrada K, Yerges-Armstrong LM, Amin N, Evangelou E, Li G, et al. Assessment of gene-by-sex interaction effect on bone mineral density. J Bone Miner Res 2012;27(10):2051–64.

[112] Richardson TG, Harrison S, Hemani G, Davey SG. An atlas of polygenic risk score associations to highlight putative causal relationships across the human phenome. elife 2019;8:e43657.

[113] Felsky D, Patrick E, Schneider JA, Mostafavi S, Gaiteri C, Patsopoulos N, et al. Polygenic analysis of inflammatory disease variants and effects on microglia in the aging brain. Mol Neurodegener 2018;13(1):38.

[114] He L, Kernogitski Y, Kulminskaya I, Loika Y, Arbeev KG, Loiko E, et al. Pleiotropic meta-analyses of longitudinal studies discover novel genetic variants associated with age-related diseases. Front Genet 2016;7:179.

[115] Altbach PG, Wit HD. Too much academic research is being published. Internet High Educ 2018;(96):2–3.

Chapter 14

Frailty: The end of the osteosarcopenia continuum?

Kenneth Ladd Seldeen, Brian Alexander MacDonald, and Bruce Robert Troen
Division of Geriatrics and Palliative Medicine, Jacobs School of Medicine and Biomedical Sciences, University at Buffalo and Research Service, Veterans Affairs Western New York Healthcare System, Buffalo, NY, United States

Introduction

Individuals 65 years of age and older represent the fastest-growing demographic worldwide—accounting for 703 million individuals in 2019 and expected to reach 1.5 billion by 2050 [1]. This rectangularization of the population age pyramid presents significant societal challenges, including the daunting task of addressing age-associated health declines. Of particular concern for older adults is the condition of frailty, defined as a "biologic syndrome of decreased reserve and resistance to stressors, resulting from cumulative declines across multiple physiologic systems, and causing vulnerability to adverse outcomes" [2]. Frailty incidence increases with age, and in the absence of intervention, can be marked by significant functional impairments (Fig. 1) [3]. Frail individuals also have higher rates of disability, institutionalization, and mortality [4]. Therefore, characterizing frailty can provide critical insights that allow for targeted and individually tailored treatment strategies to maintain healthspan, improve quality of life, and reduce healthcare system costs [5]. In this chapter, we examine whether frailty represents the end of an osteosarcopenia continuum resulting in markedly diminished muscle mass and strength, fractures, and impaired functional capacity and quality of life. We further discuss common mechanisms that may lay the foundation for therapeutic strategies.

History of frailty detection and assessment

Frailty has often been considered easy to identify, yet difficult to define. Early characterization of frailty recognized core elements, including a continuum of functional decline, failure to thrive, and vulnerability to challenges [6,7]. Efforts to explore the underlying science of frailty took an important step forward in 2001 with the introduction of the physical frailty phenotype by Fried et al. [2].

Osteosarcopenia. https://doi.org/10.1016/B978-0-12-820088-9.00002-0

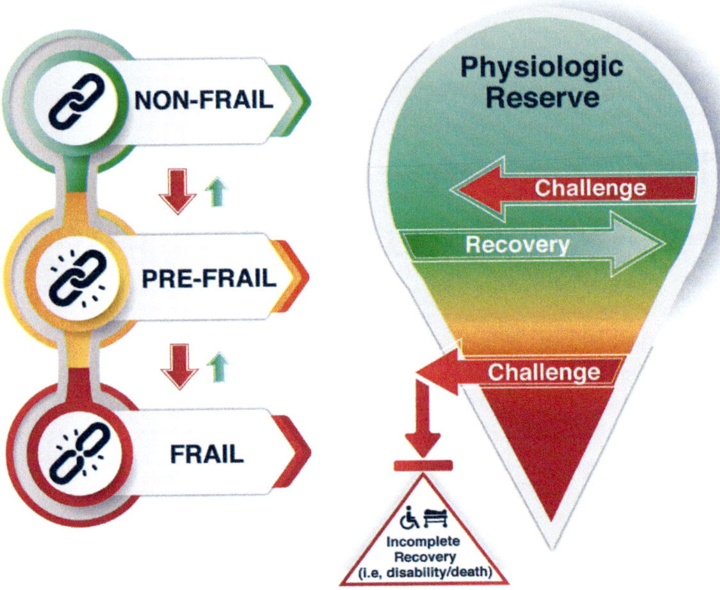

FIG. 1 The progression of frailty represents a decline of physiologic reserve leading to greater susceptibility to health challenges (i.e., illness, falls, stress) and an increased risk for adverse events. *(Based on concepts and findings from Fried LP, et al. Frailty in older adults: evidence for a phenotype. J Gerontol A Biol Sci Med Sci 2001;56(3):M146–56; Fernandez-Garrido J, et al. Clinical features of prefrail older individuals and emerging peripheral biomarkers: a systematic review. Arch Gerontol Geriatr 2014;59(1):7–17; Pujos-Guillot E, et al. Identification of pre-frailty sub-phenotypes in elderly using metabolomics. Front Physiol 2018;9:1903.)*

For the first time, measurable components were established, which included five factors: unintentional weight loss—10 pounds in the past year, self-reported exhaustion, weakness—lowest quintile of grip strength, slow walking speed, and low physical activity [2]. The presence of 3 of 5 of the factors indicated frailty, and 1 or 2 factors represented prefrailty. In this landmark study involving over 5000 community-dwelling older adults from the Cardiovascular Health Study, frailty was more prevalent with increasing age, in women, and in minority populations [2]. Further, the authors linked frailty status with an increased risk of mortality (Fig. 2). The Fried physical frailty scale has since been used in multiple other studies, and others have linked frailty to a variety of outcomes such as loss of independence, increased disability, and greater morbidity and mortality [2,8,9].

Around this same time, an alternative strategy for the determination of frailty was introduced based upon a deficit accumulation model, whereby a wide range of parameters are taken into account that range from the ability to perform daily activities, coordination and gait, mental components, physiological problems and history, and the presence of medical morbidities [9]. In total, the instrument termed the clinical frailty index, applied 70 parameters in

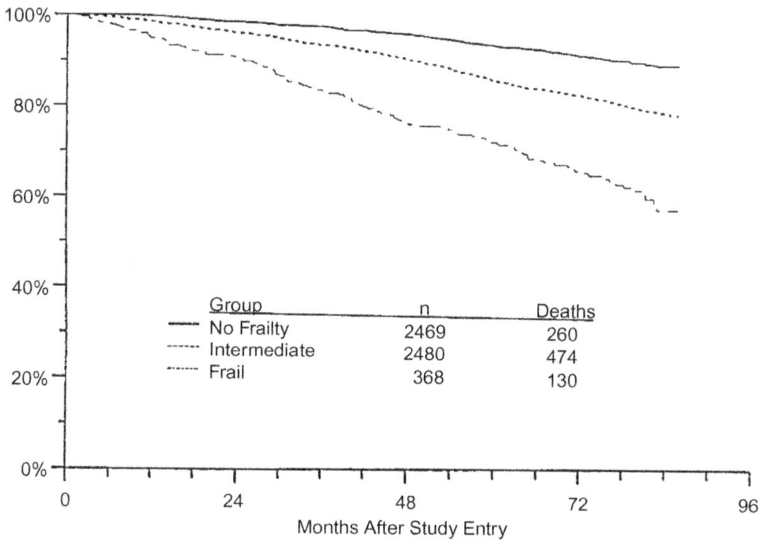

FIG. 2 Physical frailty status predicted survival across a cohort of 5317 men and women aged 65–101. *(Reproduced with permission from Fried LP, et al. Frailty in older adults: evidence for a phenotype. J Gerontol A Biol Sci Med Sci 2001;56(3):M146–56.)*

the initial use [9] and identified that frailty index scores increased with age, the severity of impairment when comparing well and unwell groups and that survival probability could be estimated [9]. Subsequently, the 70 parameters were pared down to 36 parameters in an effort to improve clinical utility [10]. Similar to the Fried physical frailty scale, the frailty index has laid a foundation for future research, and together these frailty tools characterize two major schools of thought for scientific frailty assessment that includes dozens of tools [11]. Furthermore, these concepts are echoed in preclinical mouse and rat models of frailty that can accelerate the translation of potential healthspan enhancing interventions [12,13].

Frailty detection in clinical situations

Despite the success of frailty assessment for elucidating the biological underpinnings of age-associated declines, the practical clinical utility was questionable due to both the time to administer the tests as well as needing patients to participate in physical performance challenges. In an effort to circumvent these difficulties, a new generation of frailty assessment tools has featured survey questions to replace physical tests. One such instrument is the FRAIL scale that transforms the Fried criteria (fatigue, resistance, ambulation, illnesses, and loss of weight) into 5 self-reported measures (Table 1) [14,15]. Other clinically useful frailty scales have been developed that feature a greater range of domains. Such scales include the Frailty Trait Scale that explores seven dimensions

TABLE 1 The FRAIL scale survey questionnaire.

1	**Fatigue**	How much of the time during the past four weeks did you feel tired?
2	**Resistance**	By yourself and not using any aids, do you have difficulty walking up one flight of stairs?
3	**Aerobic**	By yourself and not using any aids, do you have difficulty walking one block?
4	**Illnesses**	Did a doctor ever tell you that you have: (hypertention, diabetes, cancer...)
5	**Loss of weight**	Over the past years, would you say you have lost greater than 10 lbs without trying?

(energy balance-nutrition, physical activity, nervous system, vascular system, strength, endurance, and gait speed) [16], the Tilburg Frailty index that encompasses 15 questions within 3 domains (physical, psychological and social) [17], and the Groningen Frailty indicator that measures the loss of function through 15 questions in 4 domains (physical, cognitive, social and psychological) [18]. Additional tools include the 2-min Gill frailty instrument, the Gerontopole frailty screening tool, and the PRISMA questionnaire [11,19], as well as the frailty index for elders (FIFE) [20]. The proliferation of frailty instruments reflects the effort to implement clinically efficient screens in multiple settings. Furthermore, some individual measures such as gait speed or grip strength may inform future frailty susceptibility [11,19]. In particular, usual walking speed was found to be the most highly correlated across multiple fitness tests with frailty status [21].

Alternatively, some clinicians opt to conduct a comprehensive geriatric assessment (CGA), which often takes approximately 2 h per patient to complete [22]. The core domains of CGA are functional status, mobility, gait speed, cognition, mood, and emotional status, nutritional status, comorbidities and polypharmacy, geriatric syndromes (e.g., falls, dementia, delirium, urinary incontinence, dentition, visual, or hearing impairments), goals of care, and advanced care planning. A patient's social and environmental situation is also evaluated, focusing on the social interactions network, social support needs and resources, financial concerns, and environmental adequacy and safety. CGA produces a holistic inventory of health problems, which can then serve to develop an individualized geriatric intervention plan. In many settings, the CGA relies on a core team consisting of a physician (usually a geriatrician), a nurse, and a social worker. When appropriate, specialists in several other disciplines either take part in the basic assessment or act as consultants with an "extended" team of physical and occupational therapists, nutritionists, pharmacists, psychiatrists, psychologists, dentists, audiologists, podiatrists, and opticians. Program setting, goals of assessment, availability of resources, and caseload influence the size of the core and extended team. At present, CGA programs are moving toward a "virtual team" concept in which members are included as needed, assessments are conducted at different locations on different days, and team communication is completed via telephone or electronically. The strategy has emerged as the gold standard approach for ensuring optimal outcomes in older populations. Still, due to the clinician's time investment and the inability to provide CGA to all patients, uncertainty remains regarding who would benefit most [23]. Consequently, frailty instruments are increasingly being looked at as a possible screening tool in advance of a CGA [24,25]. In particular, the rapid geriatric assessment, which takes approximately 4 min and includes the FRAIL scale (Table 1), and screens for sarcopenia, nutrition, and cognition [26], can identify those who would benefit from a CGA and/or a geriatrician.

Frailty demographics and prognosis

Frailty is defined as a clinically recognizable state of increased vulnerability resulting from aging-associated declines in reserve and function across multiple physiologic systems that compromise the ability to cope with everyday or acute stressors [27]. The predominant risk factor for frailty is age (Fig. 3). Although the prevalence is lower at early old age (approximately 7%–10% of those around the age of 65 years [28,29]), this rapidly increases and can affect 25%–50% of those 85 years of age and older [2,10].

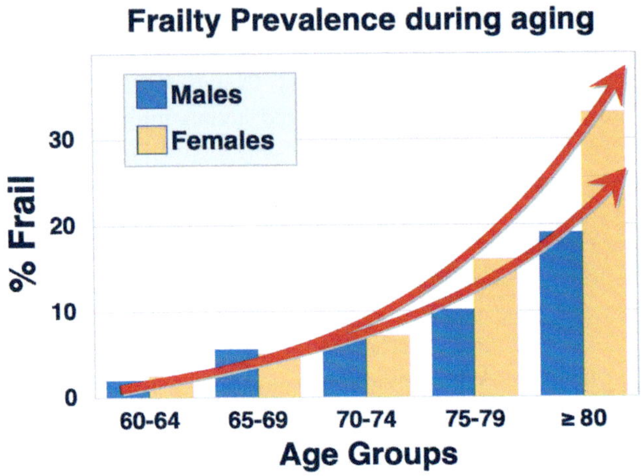

FIG. 3 Frailty prevalence increases progressively with age. *(Based on data from Ahmad NS, et al. Prevalence, transitions and factors predicting transition between frailty states among rural community-dwelling older adults in Malaysia. PLoS One 2018;13(11):e0206445.)*

Women are also at higher risk for frailty [29,30], but paradoxically can survive with frailty for more extended periods [31]. Frailty also is more pronounced in minority groups, including African Americans who can exhibit rates 4 times higher than Caucasians [32]. Other risk factors for frailty include smoking, obesity, loneliness [33], socio-economic status, malnourishment [34–36], and importantly, inactivity [37–39]. Inactivity, in particular, is a major risk factor for many factors that contribute to frailty, including obesity and osteosarcopenia [40,41], and may be a key trigger that initiates and accelerates the cycle of functional decline that culminates in frailty [42,43].

A frailty diagnosis carries a prognosis for adverse events and a higher risk of all-cause mortality. This relationship has been identified across multiple studies and frailty assessment tools [10,28,29,44–47]. Specifically, frailty increases mortality risk by over 150%, and even prefrailty increases the risk by 60%–80% [44,46,47]. Notably, frailty status was predictive of mortality in large patient cohorts, including nearly 500,000 UK Biobank participants [28] and 5000 participants in the National Health and Nutrition Examination Survey [44]. Very importantly, quality of life is diminished in frail older adults [48]. This may be due to approximately a twofold increase in physical limitations [49], as well as a twofold increased risk for impairment of activities of daily living [50]. As might be expected with the individual challenges of frailty, there is also a greater likelihood of hospitalization and need for institutional care [50,51]. Therefore, frailty in older adults places a significant burden on healthcare systems, as also exemplified by increases in expenditures of 50%–100% [52] and utilization of services [53,54]. The progression of frailty is best characterized as a collection

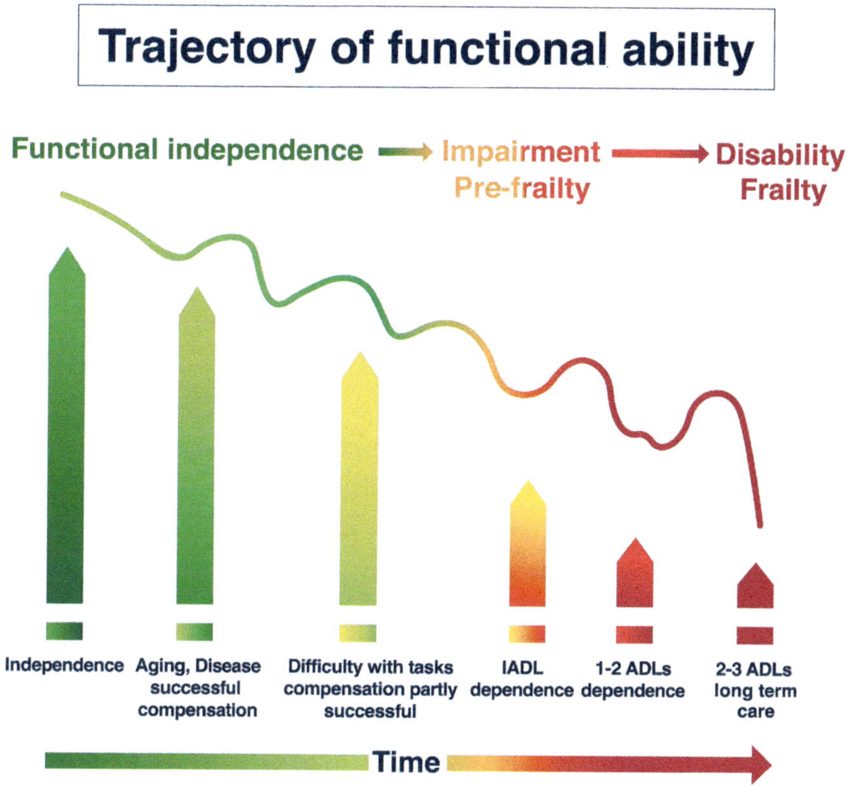

FIG. 4 The progression of frailty is often not linear, but rather features moments of loss of function due to challenges (i.e., illness, injury) followed by recovery—both complete and incomplete.

of health challenges, with failure to recover to previous baselines and resultant progressive declines, particularly concerning instrumental activities of daily living (IADLs: shopping, housework, finances, food preparation, medications, transportation) and subsequently to basic activities of daily living (ADLs: dressing, eating, ambulating, toileting, hygiene) (Fig. 4). This phenomenon has been reported in the literature by two studies that examined frailty status longitudinally and identified fluidity in the stages (transitioning bi-directionally between nonfrail, prefrail, and frail status), but with a trend toward increasing disability and frailty [3,55].

In addition, frailty status has been shown to be very important as a prognostic indicator for adverse events following surgery in multiple settings [56,57]. These studies demonstrate the potential of incorporating frailty determination to inform critical decision-making and risk assessment. In fact, the utility continues to expand and has also recently been used to identify at-risk patients exhibiting COVID-19 infection [58].

Underlying pathophysiology of frailty

Frailty is considered as one of the many syndromes of aging. Inherent in the aging process are systematic declines at both the cellular and tissue levels [59]. Hallmarks include genomic instability, telomere attrition, epigenetic alterations, loss of proteostasis, deregulated nutrient sensing, mitochondrial dysfunction, and cellular senescence [59]. These factors play a role in the onset of frailty, but of particular interest are chronic inflammation, a dysregulated gut microbiome, and underlying miRNA signaling in mediating age-related declines. Chronic inflammation, often labeled "inflammaging," refers to the lingering and frequently subclinical elevation of serum and tissue cytokines including interleukin-6 (IL-6), IL-8, IL-1, tumor necrosis factor (TNF) alpha, and C-reactive protein (CRP) [60]. The combination of obesity and sarcopenia can be a dual path to frailty [61]. Notably, adipose tissue produces more inflammatory cytokines that exert a catabolic effect, reducing muscle mass and quality, thereby leading to greater functional decline and frailty [61]. One potential driver of chronic inflammation stems from deleterious alterations in the gut microbiome during aging [62,63], which increase vulnerability to malnutrition, inactivity, disease, or response to drug treatments [64,65]. This in turn diminishes anabolic responses [63] and can reduce muscle mass, and again lead to both sarcopenia and frailty [62,63,65].

Frailty is often thought of as a decline of resilience or the physiological "bounce back" from an acute stressor. Although the microbiome contributes to resilience [66], epigenetic changes are another key factor that can amplify the deleterious impacts of stressors [67]. Serum microRNA profiles are salient indicators and drivers of epigenetic changes. MicroRNAs are 18–22 base pair fragments of noncoding RNA that can silence messenger RNA expression as well as block gene expression via heterochromatin formation [68]. Specific microRNAs have been implicated in both sarcopenia and other muscle wasting diseases [69,70]. MicroRNAs are also being investigated as potential biomarkers for frailty [71], and may well underlie many of the pathologic mechanisms of frailty [72]. Together, the encompassing hallmarks of aging that include chronic inflammation, microbiome dysbiosis, and altered microRNA signaling appear to represent long-term factors leading to the presentation of geriatric syndromes in late life such as frailty (Fig. 5).

Frailty lies at the end of the osteosarcopenia continuum

As alluded to above, the underlying pathophysiology of frailty is shared in large part with osteosarcopenia—suggesting a close relationship between the two age-related conditions. Binkley and Buehring first coined the term "sarco-osteopenia" to characterize a combination of factors that predisposed to falls and fractures [73]. They recognized that age-related losses in both muscle and bone contributed to morbidity, reduced quality of life, and ultimately mortality [73]. Underlying mechanistic elements of osteosarcopenia are similar to those

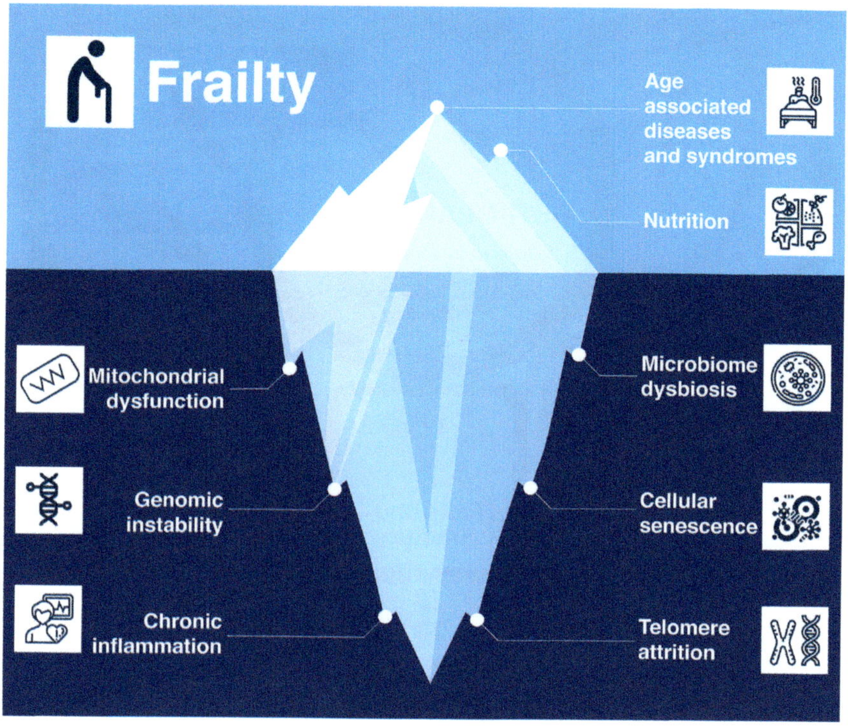

FIG. 5 Geriatric syndromes such as frailty sit atop long periods of underlying dysregulation. *(Based upon concepts from Franceschi C, et al. The continuum of aging and age-related diseases: common mechanisms but different rates. Front Med (Lausanne) 2018;5:61.)*

of frailty and include impaired mitochondrial metabolism, diminished stem cell response, reduced adaptation to stress, as well as increased subclinical inflammation, and alterations in the epigenetic landscape [74]. In addition, microbiome dysbiosis [65,75,76] and microRNA signaling [77] also contribute to the onset of sarcopenia. Furthermore, the role of bone health in mediating frailty status is increasingly being recognized, as well as the use of frailty assessment to evaluate strategies in treating osteoporosis [78]. In addition, as with frailty and sarcopenia, damage responses with repair and maintenance at the tissue and cellular levels underlie the osteoporosis and frailty phenotypes [79].

Thus, the closely aligned pathophysiology between osteosarcopenia and frailty has led to reconceptualizing the intricate relationships between these age-related syndromes [80]. In particular, sarcopenia is a critical contributor to the downward cycle of frailty progression, whereby inactivity decreases caloric intake, which in turn increases sarcopenia leading to reduced muscle function and subsequently even more inactivity [81]. Likewise, osteoporosis is also being recognized for contributing to frailty via increased risk for fracture from falls and subsequent disability and inactivity [82,83]. Frailty thus lies at the end of

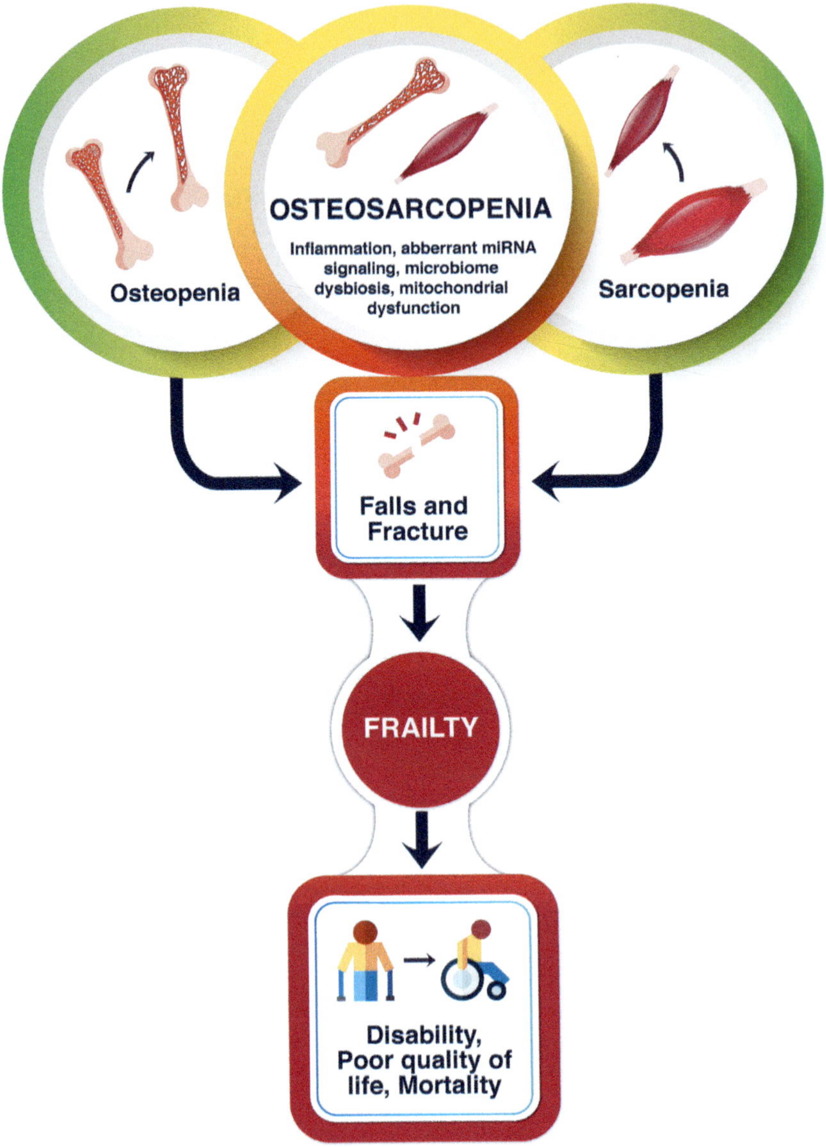

FIG. 6 Frailty lies at the end of the osteosarcopenia continuum—the culmination of musculoskeletal declines that lead to adverse outcomes, including mortality.

this osteosarcopenia continuum, where the accumulation of functional deficits increases susceptibility to adverse outcomes (Fig. 6).

Although frailty and osteosarcopenia have many similarities, it is important to recognize the inherent differences. In the review of these relationships, geriatrician investigator Matteo Cesari writes, "I believe the frailty phenotype finds in sarcopenia a substantial, but not exhaustive pathogenetic explanation [84]." This distinction lies in frailty being a whole-body multifactorial syndrome, that not only includes musculoskeletal decline, but also cardiovascular, and even cognitive decline. In particular, the manifestation of cognitive frailty is considered by some as a focal point for subsequent disability, poor quality of health, and ultimately mortality [85].

Therapeutic strategies—Overlap with those of osteosarcopenia

Similar to osteosarcopenia, there are few proven therapeutic interventions for frailty. Exercise represents the most effective strategy to delay the onset of and even potentially reverse frailty [86]. However, as with the application of geroscience to understand osteosarcopenia [74], therapeutic strategies, including senolytics [87] or NAD+ restoration [88], may also yield promising avenues of therapy for frailty in the future. The importance of other nonpharmacologic strategies, including protein supplementation and vitamin D repletion, may also play a role in slowing the progression of frailty [89]. Perhaps even more importantly, the combination of such strategies with exercise, particularly high-intensity interval training [90,91], may yield complementary and even synergistic benefits. Therapeutic strategies for osteosarcopenia will be discussed in detail in the following two chapters.

Acknowledgments

The authors report no relevant disclosures or conflicts of interest. Dr. Troen is supported by grants from the National Institutes of Health (K07 AG060266), Veterans Affairs (BX004369), and the Indian Trail Foundation. Dr. Seldeen is supported by grants from Veteran Affairs (RX003396). Illustrations by Sidra Aslam.

References

[1] Anon. World population aging 2019: highlights. United Nations, Department of Economic and Social Affairs, Population Division; 2019.
[2] Fried LP, et al. Frailty in older adults: evidence for a phenotype. J Gerontol A Biol Sci Med Sci 2001;56(3):M146–56.
[3] Fernandez-Garrido J, et al. Clinical features of prefrail older individuals and emerging peripheral biomarkers: a systematic review. Arch Gerontol Geriatr 2014;59(1):7–17.
[4] Lee DH, et al. Frail patients are at increased risk for mortality and prolonged institutional care after cardiac surgery. Circulation 2010;121(8):973–8.
[5] Hoogendijk EO, et al. Frailty: implications for clinical practice and public health. Lancet 2019;394(10206):1365–75.
[6] Buchner DM, Wagner EH. Preventing frail health. Clin Geriatr Med 1992;8(1):1–17.
[7] Hamerman D. Toward an understanding of frailty. Ann Intern Med 1999;130(11):945–50.
[8] Lin CC, et al. Reduced health-related quality of life in elders with frailty: a cross-sectional study of community-dwelling elders in Taiwan. PLoS One 2011;6(7):e21841.

[9] Rockwood K, et al. A global clinical measure of fitness and frailty in elderly people. CMAJ 2005;173(5):489–95.
[10] Song X, Mitnitski A, Rockwood K. Prevalence and 10-year outcomes of frailty in older adults in relation to deficit accumulation. J Am Geriatr Soc 2010;58(4):681–7.
[11] Walston J, Buta B, Xue QL. Frailty screening and interventions: considerations for clinical practice. Clin Geriatr Med 2018;34(1):25–38.
[12] Banga S, Heinze-Milne SD, Howlett SE. Rodent models of frailty and their application in preclinical research. Mech Ageing Dev 2019;179:1–10.
[13] Baumann CW, Kwak D, Thompson LV. Phenotypic frailty assessment in mice: development, discoveries, and experimental considerations. Physiology (Bethesda) 2020;35(6):405–14.
[14] Abellan van Kan G, et al. Frailty: toward a clinical definition. J Am Med Dir Assoc 2008;9(2):71–2.
[15] Morley JE, Malmstrom TK, Miller DK. A simple frailty questionnaire (FRAIL) predicts outcomes in middle aged African Americans. J Nutr Health Aging 2012;16(7):601–8.
[16] Garcia-Garcia FJ, et al. A new operational definition of frailty: the Frailty Trait Scale. J Am Med Dir Assoc 2014;15(5):371 e7–371 e13.
[17] Gobbens RJ, et al. The Tilburg Frailty Indicator: psychometric properties. J Am Med Dir Assoc 2010;11(5):344–55.
[18] Peters LL, et al. Measurement properties of the Groningen Frailty Indicator in home-dwelling and institutionalized elderly people. J Am Med Dir Assoc 2012;13(6):546–51.
[19] Kim H, et al. Frailty assessment in the geriatric outpatient clinic. Geriatr Gerontol Int 2014;14(1):78–83.
[20] Tocchi C, et al. Development of a frailty measure for older adults: the frailty index for elders. J Nurs Meas 2014;22(2):223–40.
[21] Navarrete-Villanueva D, et al. Frailty and physical fitness in elderly people: a systematic review and meta-analysis. Sports Med 2021;51(1):143–60.
[22] Pilotto A, et al. Three decades of comprehensive geriatric assessment: evidence coming from different healthcare settings and specific clinical conditions. J Am Med Dir Assoc 2017;18(2):192 e1–192 e11.
[23] Parker SG, et al. What is comprehensive geriatric assessment (CGA)? An umbrella review. Age Ageing 2018;47(1):149–55.
[24] Lee H, Lee E, Jang IY. Frailty and comprehensive geriatric assessment. J Korean Med Sci 2020;35(3):e16.
[25] Vettoretti S, et al. Frailty phenotype and multi-domain impairments in older patients with chronic kidney disease. BMC Geriatr 2020;20(1):371.
[26] Morley JE, Adams EV. Rapid geriatric assessment. J Am Med Dir Assoc 2015;16(10):808–12.
[27] Xue QL. The frailty syndrome: definition and natural history. Clin Geriatr Med 2011;27(1):1–15.
[28] Hanlon P, et al. Frailty and pre-frailty in middle-aged and older adults and its association with multimorbidity and mortality: a prospective analysis of 493 737 UK Biobank participants. Lancet Public Health 2018;3(7):e323–32.
[29] Saum KU, et al. Frailty prevalence and 10-year survival in community-dwelling older adults: results from the ESTHER cohort study. Eur J Epidemiol 2014;29(3):171–9.
[30] Ahmad NS, et al. Prevalence, transitions and factors predicting transition between frailty states among rural community-dwelling older adults in Malaysia. PLoS One 2018;13(11):e0206445.
[31] Gordon EH, Peel NM, Hubbard RE. The male-female health-survival paradox in hospitalized older adults. Maturitas 2018;107:13–8.
[32] Hirsch C, et al. The association of race with frailty: the cardiovascular health study. Ann Epidemiol 2006;16(7):545–53.

[33] Gale CR, Westbury L, Cooper C. Social isolation and loneliness as risk factors for the progression of frailty: the English Longitudinal Study of Ageing. Age Ageing 2018;47(3):392–7.
[34] Chang SF. Frailty is a major related factor for at risk of malnutrition in community-dwelling older adults. J Nurs Scholarsh 2017;49(1):63–72.
[35] Verlaan S, et al. High prevalence of physical frailty among community-dwelling malnourished older adults-a systematic review and meta-analysis. J Am Med Dir Assoc 2017;18(5):374–82.
[36] Wei K, et al. Frailty and malnutrition: related and distinct syndrome prevalence and association among community-dwelling older adults: Singapore longitudinal ageing studies. J Am Med Dir Assoc 2017;18(12):1019–28.
[37] da Silva Coqueiro R, et al. Cross-sectional relationships between sedentary behavior and frailty in older adults. J Sports Med Phys Fitness 2017;57(6):825–30.
[38] da Silva VD, et al. Association between frailty and the combination of physical activity level and sedentary behavior in older adults. BMC Public Health 2019;19(1):709.
[39] da Silva VD, et al. Time spent in sedentary behaviour as discriminant criterion for frailty in older adults. Int J Environ Res Public Health 2018;15(7):1336.
[40] Kirk B, Zanker J, Duque G. Osteosarcopenia: epidemiology, diagnosis, and treatment-facts and numbers. J Cachexia Sarcopenia Muscle 2020;11(3):609–18.
[41] Sultana S, et al. Associations of lifestyle risk factors with overweight or obesity among adolescents: a multicountry analysis. Am J Clin Nutr 2021;113(3):742–50.
[42] Heppenstall CP, et al. Frailty: dominos or deliberation? N Z Med J 2009;122(1299):42–53.
[43] Rezus E, et al. Inactivity and skeletal muscle metabolism: a vicious cycle in old age. Int J Mol Sci 2020;21(2):592.
[44] Crow RS, et al. Mortality risk along the frailty spectrum: data from the national health and nutrition examination survey 1999 to 2004. J Am Geriatr Soc 2018;66(3):496–502.
[45] Kelly SG, et al. Frailty is an independent risk factor for mortality, cardiovascular disease, bone disease, and diabetes among aging adults with human immunodeficiency virus. Clin Infect Dis 2019;69(8):1370–6.
[46] Kojima G. Frailty defined by FRAIL scale as a predictor of mortality: a systematic review and meta-analysis. J Am Med Dir Assoc 2018;19(6):480–3.
[47] Yuki A, et al. Physical frailty and mortality risk in Japanese older adults. Geriatr Gerontol Int 2018;18(7):1085–92.
[48] Kojima G, et al. Association between frailty and quality of life among community-dwelling older people: a systematic review and meta-analysis. J Epidemiol Community Health 2016;70(7):716–21.
[49] Nascimento CM, et al. Sarcopenia, frailty and their prevention by exercise. Free Radic Biol Med 2019;132:42–9.
[50] Vermeiren S, et al. Frailty and the prediction of negative health outcomes: a meta-analysis. J Am Med Dir Assoc 2016;17(12):1163 e1–1163 e17.
[51] Owodunni OP, et al. Preoperative frailty assessment, operative severity score, and early postoperative loss of independence in surgical patients age 65 years or older. J Am Coll Surg 2021;232(4):387–95.
[52] Hajek A, et al. Frailty and healthcare costs-longitudinal results of a prospective cohort study. Age Ageing 2018;47(2):233–41.
[53] Bock JO, et al. Associations of frailty with health care costs—results of the ESTHER cohort study. BMC Health Serv Res 2016;16:128.
[54] Ensrud KE, et al. Frailty phenotype and healthcare costs and utilization in older women. J Am Geriatr Soc 2018;66(7):1276–83.

[55] Pujos-Guillot E, et al. Identification of pre-frailty sub-phenotypes in elderly using metabolomics. Front Physiol 2018;9:1903.
[56] Harris DG, et al. A frailty-based risk score predicts morbidity and mortality after elective endovascular repair of descending thoracic aortic aneurysms. Ann Vasc Surg 2020;67:90–9.
[57] Mogal H, et al. Modified frailty index predicts morbidity and mortality after pancreaticoduodenectomy. Ann Surg Oncol 2017;24(6):1714–21.
[58] Bellelli G, et al. Frailty index predicts poor outcome in COVID-19 patients. Intensive Care Med 2020;46(8):1634–6.
[59] Lopez-Otin C, et al. The hallmarks of aging. Cell 2013;153(6):1194–217.
[60] Vatic M, von Haehling S, Ebner N. Inflammatory biomarkers of frailty. Exp Gerontol 2020;133, 110858.
[61] Florez H, Troen BR. Fat and inflammaging: a dual path to unfitness in elderly people? J Am Geriatr Soc 2008;56(3):558–60.
[62] Casati M, et al. Gut microbiota and physical frailty through the mediation of sarcopenia. Exp Gerontol 2019;124:110639.
[63] Ni Lochlainn M, Bowyer RCE, Steves CJ. Dietary protein and muscle in aging people: the potential role of the gut microbiome. Nutrients 2018;10(7):929.
[64] Bana B, Cabreiro F. The microbiome and aging. Annu Rev Genet 2019;53:239–61.
[65] Ticinesi A, et al. Aging gut microbiota at the cross-road between nutrition, physical frailty, and sarcopenia: is there a gut-muscle axis? Nutrients 2017;9(12):1303.
[66] Fassarella M, et al. Gut microbiome stability and resilience: elucidating the response to perturbations in order to modulate gut health. Gut 2021;70(3):595–605.
[67] Brivio P, et al. From healthy aging to frailty: in search of the underlying mechanisms. Curr Med Chem 2019;26(20):3685–701.
[68] Matsuyama H, Suzuki HI. Systems and synthetic microRNA biology: from biogenesis to disease pathogenesis. Int J Mol Sci 2020;21(1):132.
[69] Fan J, et al. MicroRNA-regulated proinflammatory cytokines in sarcopenia. Mediat Inflamm 2016;2016:1438686.
[70] Sannicandro AJ, Soriano-Arroquia A, Goljanek-Whysall K. Micro(RNA)-managing muscle wasting. J Appl Physiol (1985) 2019;127(2):619–32.
[71] Cardoso AL, et al. Towards frailty biomarkers: candidates from genes and pathways regulated in aging and age-related diseases. Ageing Res Rev 2018;47:214–77.
[72] Rusanova I, et al. Involvement of plasma miRNAs, muscle miRNAs and mitochondrial miRNAs in the pathophysiology of frailty. Exp Gerontol 2019;124:110637.
[73] Binkley N, Buehring B. Beyond FRAX: it's time to consider "sarco-osteopenia". J Clin Densitom 2009;12(4):413–6.
[74] Kirk B, Al Saedi A, Duque G. Osteosarcopenia: a case of geroscience. Aging Med (Milton) 2019;2(3):147–56.
[75] Steves CJ, et al. The microbiome and musculoskeletal conditions of aging: a review of evidence for impact and potential therapeutics. J Bone Miner Res 2016;31(2):261–9.
[76] Ticinesi A, Microbiota G, et al. Muscle mass and function in aging: a focus on physical frailty and sarcopenia. Nutrients 2019;11(7):1633.
[77] Yin J, et al. MicroRNA regulatory networks in the pathogenesis of sarcopenia. J Cell Mol Med 2020;24(9):4900–12.
[78] Li G, et al. An overview of osteoporosis and frailty in the elderly. BMC Musculoskelet Disord 2017;18(1):46.

[79] van der Spoel E, van Vliet NA, van Heemst D. Viewpoint on the role of tissue maintenance in ageing: focus on biomarkers of bone, cartilage, muscle, and brain tissue maintenance. Ageing Res Rev 2019;56:100964.

[80] Cesari M, et al. Sarcopenia and physical frailty: two sides of the same coin. Front Aging Neurosci 2014;6:192.

[81] Xue QL, et al. Initial manifestations of frailty criteria and the development of frailty phenotype in the Women's Health and Aging Study II. J Gerontol A Biol Sci Med Sci 2008;63(9):984–90.

[82] Bartosch P, et al. In community-dwelling women frailty is associated with imminent risk of osteoporotic fractures. Osteoporos Int 2021;32(9):1735–44.

[83] Greco EA, Pietschmann P, Migliaccio S. Osteoporosis and sarcopenia increase frailty syndrome in the elderly. Front Endocrinol (Lausanne) 2019;10:255.

[84] Cesari M. The frailty phenotype and sarcopenia: similar but not the same. Aging Med (Milton) 2019;2(2):97–8.

[85] Arai H, Satake S, Kozaki K. Cognitive frailty in geriatrics. Clin Geriatr Med 2018;34(4):667–75.

[86] Angulo J, et al. Physical activity and exercise: strategies to manage frailty. Redox Biol 2020;35:101513.

[87] Xu M, et al. Senolytics improve physical function and increase lifespan in old age. Nat Med 2018;24(8):1246–56.

[88] Zhang H, et al. NAD(+) repletion improves mitochondrial and stem cell function and enhances life span in mice. Science 2016;352(6292):1436–43.

[89] Morley JE. Frailty and sarcopenia: the new geriatric giants. Rev Investig Clin 2016;68(2):59–67.

[90] Losa-Reyna J, et al. Effect of a short multicomponent exercise intervention focused on muscle power in frail and pre frail elderly: a pilot trial. Exp Gerontol 2019;115:114–21.

[91] Seldeen KL, et al. High intensity interval training improves physical performance in aged female mice: a comparison of mouse frailty assessment tools. Mech Ageing Dev 2019;180:49–62.

Chapter 15

Nonpharmacologic intervention for osteosarcopenia

Debra L. Waters
Department of Medicine and School of Physiotherapy, University of Otago, Dunedin, New Zealand

Introduction

This chapter reviews the nonpharmaceutical interventions for the treatment of osteosarcopenia in older adults. Modifiable risk factors such as exercise, nutrition, nutritional supplements, supplements plus nutrition, and complex interventions will be covered. Other factors such as intentional weight loss/regain, and circadian rhythms will also be discussed. Both skeletal muscle and bone have a mesodermal origin making these tissues respond to stimulus such as resistance and aerobic exercise and nutritional interventions, in some similar, but also unique manners. Although genetic factors significantly contribute to the attainment of peak bone mineral density and muscle mass, the impact of modifiable factors such as exercise and nutrition, also play a role in the loss of these tissues with aging [1,2]. Other lesser studied factors such as rest periods in resistance training, weight loss and regain, and circadian rhythms may also play a role.

The relationship between muscle and bone has been described as a mechanostat model where deformations of the bone in response to muscle contractions are monitored by osteocytes, which in turn signal osteoblasts and osteoclasts to begin modifying bone architecture and mass to maintain bone homeostasis [3]. Thus, it is biologically plausible that the loss of muscle could result in the reduction of bone mass leading to osteosarcopenia [4]. In order to understand the context of designing effective and appropriate nonpharmaceutical interventions, a brief review of the physiological changes in skeletal muscle and bone and their response to external forces (e.g., resistance exercise) and nutrition are addressed followed by more specific recommendations for exercise prescription and nutritional recommendations.

Osteosarcopenia. https://doi.org/10.1016/B978-0-12-820088-9.00007-X

Age-related changes in skeletal muscle and bone

Changes in skeletal muscle

The loss of skeletal muscle involves both the atrophy of fast-twitch muscle fibers (type IIa and IIx) [4] and the total number of myofibers [5]. Resistance training (also called weight or strength training) can be an effective stimulus for hypertrophy of myofibers. The physiological response to resistance training in older adults' results in a myofiber type redistribution (IIx to IIa) and myofiber hypertrophy across fiber types, which is preferential to type II fiber types [6–8]. However, the loss of myofiber number does not appear to be reversed by resistance training [9]. Thus, the main adaptation to resistance training in older adults is type II myofiber hypertrophy [6,10]. Concurrent with the loss of muscle mass, there is a change in neuromuscular function, which occurs faster than changes in muscle mass [11]. There may be ~30%–40% fewer motor units in older adults compared with young adults [12–16], and the surviving motor units are both larger [14–16] and undergo remodeling in type I myofibers [17–19]. It has been suggested that neural activation of the larger type I motor units may also play a role in reduced muscular power in older adults [20]. It is beyond the scope of this chapter to discuss the accumulation of adipocytes in skeletal muscle and bone marrow, which is now recognized as a common feature of aging in these tissues and could impact on response to interventions discussed in this chapter [21,22].

Changes in bone mass

Cortical and trabecular bone microarchitecture is essential to the strength of bone. In normal/nonosteoporotic bone the trabeculae are plate-like structures, but these become thinner and more rod shaped with osteoporotic changes [23]. Osteoporotic changes include microarchitecture defects of the trabeculae, defective intrinsic material properties of bone tissue, and defective repair of microdamage to bone [24]. In adults, bone remodeling is the primary mechanism for bone renewal. The remodeling is triggered by signaling from osteoblasts or their matured form osteocytes, which in turn activate osteoclasts. The osteocyte is replaced by bone remodeling and can result in increased hypermineralized calcium phosphate blockages that decrease canalicular fluid flow and negatively impact the osteocyte's sensing of mechanical loading, which can subsequently lead to microdamage [25,26].

Skeletal muscle and bone: Cross talk

Although the "mechanostat" hypothesis in the interaction between skeletal muscle and bone is important, there are also paracrine and/or endocrine factors involved [27]. Muscle secretes myokines and bone secretes osteokines that play a role in the cross-communication between muscle and bone [28]. For example,

Myostatin inhibits skeletal muscle growth but also affects tendons and bone [29]. In skeletal muscle, the age-related bone changes of the lacuno-canalicular system, that was described above, result in fewer factors produced to support muscle myogenesis and function [30]. Skeletal muscle contractions also result in the production of factors that maintain osteocytes, but this is decreased or lost with aging [30,31]. Other signaling pathways include the Wnt-β-catenin pathway that controls osteoblast activity and is also involved with muscle regeneration [32]. The receptor activator of nuclear factor kappa-B ligand (RANKL), is produced by osteocytes to activate osteoclasts, and the receptor for RANKL, (RANK) is expressed by both osteoclasts and skeletal muscle [33,34]. In skeletal muscle, RANKL appears to regulate Ca^{2+} storage and sarcoendoplasmic reticulum Ca^{2+}-ATPase, activity, which has implications for exercise [35]. The Growth Hormone/Insulin-like Growth Factor axis is also involved with the regulation of both muscle and bone [28]. So it is clear that skeletal muscle and bone do not respond and adapt in isolation, but rather cross-talk between these tissues underlies their ability to respond to stimulus.

Research has clearly shown that loading of both skeletal muscle and bone is critical for not only achieving peak muscle and bone mass but also for maintaining these tissues during aging and that there are complex biochemical and signaling pathways involved in the cross-talk between muscle and bone. Unfortunately, in more developed countries low physical activity/exercise is pervasive not only in older adults, but across the life course, leading to an increased risk of not achieving peak skeletal muscle and bone mass and then not maintaining it during aging. There is evidence in community-dwelling older adults that BMI and physical activity are inversely associated with osteosarcopenia and that higher fat mass increases the risk in both men and women with a greater than twofold increased risk in women [36]. Thus, both age and sex may be risk factors for developing osteosarcopenia, but the modifiable risk factors are physical activity/exercise and nutrition. The next section will focus on physiological responses to exercise and nutrition in skeletal muscle and bone.

Exercise

Physiological responses to exercise in skeletal muscle and bone

Acute exercise stimulates the secretion of exosomes with cargo molecules that can mediate the endocrine effects between muscle and bone. Conversely, long-term exercise induces adaptations of the tissue secretome in order to maintain a homeostatic environment [37]. Thus, acute, and long-term adaptations to exercise may not be the same [38,39]. Both muscle and bone need exercise that is dynamic (rather than static), and that exceeds a threshold of intensity, with adequate nutrition to support adaptation [40].

As discussed earlier in this chapter, the strain placed on the musculoskeletal system is sensed through cells and translated into biochemical and/or physiochemical responses, which result in bone formation, myofiber hypertrophy, and increased production of the components of the extracellular matrix, adhesion molecules, and elements of the cytoskeletal. Both bone and skeletal muscle secret growth and differentiation factors in response to this stimulus [37]. A stimulus such as resistance exercise changes the tension and compression of skeletal muscle, which stimulates the rapamycin complex 1 (mTORC1) that in turn integrates mechanical strains, nutrients, and growth factors, leading to the activation of signaling pathway that initiates muscle protein translation [41,42]. Insulin-like growth factor 1 also increases in response to resistance training and activates a PI3K-Akt-mTORC1 signaling pathway to stimulate muscle protein synthesis [43,44]. The Wnt-catenin signaling pathway is also stimulated by exercise which initiates osteogenesis, either by direct stimulation of bone transcription factor RUNX2 or by cross-talk with Parathyroid hormone or protein signaling pathways [45]. The release of Parathyroid hormone stimulated by exercise also downregulates sclerostin in osteocytes at the same time it upregulates fibroblast growth factor-23 expression, which in turn influences phosphatase homeostasis and vitamin D metabolism [45]. Exercise also increases the OPG/RANKL ratio and downstream inhibition of osteoclast differentiation, promotion of osteoblast differentiation, and bone formation [46].

As noted in the previous section, acute and chronic exercise training responses are not the same and one does not predict the other. Moreover, the magnitude of the response in skeletal muscle to resistance training is different in younger and older adults [47–49]. Acute bouts of resistance training may increase muscle protein synthesis lasting up to 48h [38,50–52] whereas repeated bouts of resistance training stimulate the rapamycin complex 1 (mTORC1), which directly promotes protein synthesis via phosphorylation of specific downstream effectors (S6K1, rpS6, eEF2, and 4EBP1). A single bout of resistance training can increase the muscle protein anabolic response to nutritional stimuli [53,54] and specific myofiber hypertrophy is reported to be partially mediated by differential induction of ribosome biogenesis [55]. Long-term resistance training may increase basal muscle protein synthesis, but in older adults does not further improve the muscle protein anabolic response to amino acids [56].

As described earlier, bone has an extensive network of cell processes located in the canaliculi, and loading of the skeletal system causes shifts in fluid flow in the lacunae and canaliculi [57]. However, microcracks can transect canaliculi disrupting communication and triggering osteocyte apoptosis. This has a flow-on effect on RANKL and other cytokines to be transmitted to bone surfaces which in turn signals osteoclast precursors to differentiate into osteoclasts for removal and repair by osteoblasts [58]. Liu and colleagues nicely summarized a large number of genes and polymorphisms that are possible candidates for regulating bone mass. This included transforming growth factor B1 (TGF-B1), bone morphogenic proteins (BMPs), sclerostin (SOST), transcription factors such as Runx2, cathepsin K, type 1 collagen (TCIRG1), chloride channel 7 (CLCN7), vitamin D receptor (VDR), and estrogen receptor (ER-a) [59].

This section has described some of the known cellular responses and adaptations for exercise. Now we will turn to more practical implications of exercise prescription for skeletal muscle and bone.

Exercise modalities

At present, there is no scientific consensus regarding the optimal mode and dose (type, frequency, duration, and intensity) of exercise that can simultaneously enhance bone and muscle health and improve functional ability in older adults with osteosarcopenia. As such this section will address training programs for muscle and bone separately and identify potential overlaps in the training that could be applied to osteosarcopenia.

Skeletal muscle training programs

Resistance training has been shown to be safe and effective for older adults, with rates of injuries extremely low and similar across all ages and intensities as long as exercise sessions progressively increase intensity and the movements are performed with the correct form [9]. Training dose is made up of the frequency (number of days per week), intensity (% of a 1 repetition maximum (RM)), and volume (number of sets and repetitions within a set). The American College of Sports Medicine (ACSM) recommends a minimum of two resistance training sessions per week [60], although a minimal effective dose of once-weekly has also been shown to elicit adaptations [61,62]. Other investigations have reported no difference in training response across different training frequencies [61,63] although the lack of consensus could be the often-overlooked aspect of exercise training which is rest periods both within and between exercise sessions. Stec and colleagues conducted a four-arm, randomized dose-response trial and reported substantially greater gains in total lean body mass, thigh muscle mass, and strength using 3 day/week training, with the second training day at a lower intensity, compared to 3 days that were all high-intensity training [8].

Most resistance exercise programs use isotonic contractions, which is a concentric contraction where the contracting muscle shortens to overcome an external force [64]. Power training is characterized by rapid concentric movement followed by a slower eccentric (lowering) phase. A review and metaanalyses on power training in older adults reported that it is feasible and safe and has similar gains in muscle strength but better functional outcomes (e.g., chair rising time, stair climbing, walking speed) [65]. Despite this, the majority of resistance training programs utilize slow velocity concentric contractions (2–4 s concentric phase) at a moderate to high intensity [66]. There are even fewer studies that have used isometric (static contractions) or isokinetic (controlled contractions at constant angular velocity using dynamometers).

Looking at the influence of duration of the resistance training program on skeletal muscle mass and strength, a metaanalysis of 49 studies averaging

20 weeks in duration reported the number of sets and repetitions was positively associated with increases in lean body mass [67]. Others reported that using constant intensity for 6–10 weeks showed gains in muscle mass and strength that were similar between higher (3 sets) and lower (1 set) [68,69], but by the 20th week there was more benefit from sessions that used a higher number of sets and repetitions [70]. Villareal and colleagues have used high-intensity resistance exercise training (85% 1RM 3× week) in older obese frail adults and have demonstrated this feasible and effective for mitigating the loss of lean body mass while dieting [71,72].

Bone exercise training programs

The current national and international consensus guidelines for osteoporosis recommend a combination of weight-bearing and resistance training with challenging balance exercises to improve falls risk [73,74]. As discussed in the physiological adaptations to exercise, the stimulation of bone remodeling requires some unique training aspects. A metaanalysis of randomized controlled trials in older adults reported a combination of impact producing weight-bearing impact exercise such as jogging, stair-climbing, and jumping, along with resistance training were most effective for maintaining bone mineral density or preventing bone loss at clinically relevant sites such as the hip and spine [75]. Sufficient loading is needed to stimulate osteogenic bone remodeling and it must be dynamic (i.e., not isometric), with fast high-frequency strains that are progressed over time [40,45,76,77]. As well as the speed of the movement, higher loading intensity requires fewer repetitions to stimulate an osteogenic response [77]. The recommendation is high mechanical load with high velocity (around 80%–85% of 1 RM with fast movements) [40,78], performed at least twice a week, and using large muscles targeting the hip and spine [40,66,77,79]. A recently published RCT using Osteo-cise: Strong Bones for Life multicomponent exercise program that consisted of progressive resistance, weight-bearing impact, and balance training (3 days/week) demonstrated significant improvement in the lumbar spine and femoral neck BMD, muscle strength, and physical measures. However, there was no difference in falls incidence or trabecular bone microarchitecture of the distal femur or proximal tibia [80].

Aerobic training such as swimming, cycling, and walking provide inadequate stimulus to increase bone mass [66,81,82]. The message that weight-bearing exercise, such as walking, can preserve bone mass is confusing given walking alone in not an adequate stimulus for bone remodeling. Only if the aerobic exercise includes high-impact or multidirectional weight-bearing is there evidence for maintaining or increasing hip and spine bone mineral density- in older adults [83–85].

Current exercise guidelines for people with or at high risk for osteoporosis is moderate-intensity exercises (70%–80% 1 RM, 8–15 repetitions) for individual muscle groups, which are likely insufficient to generate mechanical strain to stimulate an osteogenic response in the hip [86]. Initiating the types of exercise that will increase BMD or slow the loss in people with diagnosed osteoporosis, particularly severe osteoporosis needs to be undertaken with extreme caution due to the risk of low trauma fracture. Similar to the physiological response to resistance exercise in skeletal muscle, recovery or rest periods are also needed for the bone to physiologically respond. Repetitive skeletal loading can desensitize the osteocytes and it has been reported that shorter bouts with rest intervals are more beneficial than the same number of loads performed all at once [87].

Although skeletal muscle and bone require different interventions to stimulate muscle hypertrophy and osteogenesis, respectively, it has been recommended that a combination of resistance exercise with weight-bearing aerobic exercise (e.g., running, skipping, jumping, or high-impact aerobics) can provide muscular loading while weight-bearing aerobic exercise provides additional mechanical loading to the bone above gravity alone. This approach has been demonstrated in individual studies, systematic reviews, and metaanalyses to increase lumbar spine and femoral neck BMD, and to increase muscle mass, and strength, in older women as well as men [40,75,79,85,88,89]. Thus this may be the type of exercise that would be appropriate for people with osteosarcopenia.

In summary resistance exercise either alone or in combination with other exercise interventions increases muscle mass and strength and appropriate high magnitude and intensity stimulus to the skeletal systems slows bone loss and/or increases BMD in both lumbar spine and femoral neck in older adults. Table 1 show summarizes the exercise recommendations for skeletal muscle and bone.

Now we will briefly discuss nutritional interventions for skeletal muscle and bone with a focus on calcium, vitamin D, and protein.

Calcium

Calcium plays a key role in muscle contraction through calcium-induced calcium release from the sarcoplasmic reticulum and contributes to the strength of bone, nerve impulses and transmission, regulation of heartbeat, and cellular fluid balance [90–92]. For most people, adequate calcium can be obtained through a balanced diet that includes dairy products (e.g., milk, yogurt, and cheese), nuts, dark-green leafy vegetables, dried peas, and beans [91,92]. Low dietary calcium intake, high sodium intake, and excessive alcohol and cola consumption are risk factors for low bone mass in older adults [93]. The absorption of calcium through the intestine is increased in people with obesity, but the physiological mechanisms are poorly understood [94] Conversely, caloric restriction resulting in weight loss is associated with decreased intestinal absorption of calcium independent from the effects of vitamin D and may be one mechanism underlying the loss of bone mass with weight loss [95]. In people with osteoporosis who have adequate vitamin D status and a normal calcium intake, routine calcium and vitamin D supplements are not required and

TABLE 1 Summary of resistance exercise training for skeletal muscle and bone.

	Exercise modality	Intensity	Speed of movement	Set and repetitions	Frequency	Rest periods
Skeletal muscle	Isotonic resistance training	High intensity 80%–85% 1RM	2–4 s contraction phase	3 sets 6–8 reps	2–3 times/weekly 1 × weekly minimum effective dose	Alternate high-intensity training days with low intensity
Bone	Resistance training or multidirectional high impact movements	High strain	Fast	3 sets 6–8 reps	2–3 times/week	Shorter intense bouts with rest intervals

supplementation does not appear to affect treatment efficacy for osteoporosis [92,96]. Calcium supplementation also can have side effects that include constipation, bloating and kidney stones, and a small increased risk of myocardial infarction [92]. Insufficient calcium intake during peak bone growth and mineralization periods may lead to suboptimal bone mass peak and low bone mineralization, possibly contributing to the risk of osteoporosis [97]. Current guidelines recommend an adequate intake of calcium (1000–1300 mg/day) from the diet for optimal bone health [91].

As noted above, calcium intake and supplementation are controversial. A review of randomized controlled trials and cohort studies concluded that increasing calcium intake from dietary sources cannot prevent fractures [92,98]. Reid and Bollard also concluded that "calcium supplements in healthy individuals are not needed, nor are they required in most people receiving treatment for osteoporosis" [92]. The European Society for Clinical and Economic Aspects of Osteoporosis, Osteoarthritis, and Musculoskeletal Diseases and the International Osteoporosis Foundation also concluded that current evidence on calcium supplementation alone does not reduce the risk of fracture [97].

Thus, for older adults, it appears that the main message is against taking calcium supplementation, but to try to achieve adequate calcium intake through the diet.

Vitamin D

Most of the circulating vitamin D is made in the skin when exposed to sunlight. Dietary sources include oily fish, liver, egg yolks, margarine, some yogurts, cheeses, cereals, and vitamin D-fortified milk and orange juice, but the major source of vitamin D3 comes from sunlight exposure [90,92,99]. Many studies have described the association of low vitamin D status with osteoporosis and increased risk of fracture [100] whereas for sarcopenia, Bruyère and colleagues reported that there was an association of low vitamin D levels with negative muscle-related outcomes [101]. Conversely, Reid and Bollard reviewed clinical trials and concluded that vitamin D supplementation had no benefits for nonskeletal endpoints. They also reviewed trials that showed vitamin D increases bone density only when winter 25-hydroxyvitamin D levels are below 25–30 nmol/L and that supplementation with 400–800 units per day was effective in restoring normal serum vitamin D levels [92]. These low daily doses appear to be safe; however, there is no evidence that loading, or bolus doses have a positive effect on falls or fracture outcomes [102], in fact, high doses have been shown to increase falls incidence and fractures [92,96]. Vitamin D toxicity can occur if > 10,000 IU of vitamin D are taken per day for more than 5 months [103,104].

One can conclude from these studies and reviews that vitamin D supplementation may only be warranted if 25-hydroxyvitamin D levels are below 25–30 nmol/L and that lower doses of vitamin D supplementation 400–800 IU/day is sufficient to restore levels to normal ranges.

Protein

There are reports that moderate or high consumption of protein (≥ 1.1 g/kg/day) in older adults (aged 70–79 years) attenuates age-related loss of skeletal muscle [105] and also preserves lower limb performance when compared with protein intake is lower than 0.8 g/kg/day [106]. Data from the Framingham Osteoporosis Study reported that low protein intake was also associated with bone loss at proximal femur and spine over 4 years [107] whereas protein supplements have been reported to increase BMD and decrease fracture risk [108,109]. An expert consensus for healthy adults have recommended a dietary intake of protein of 0.8 g per kg of body weight per day (g/kg/day), and somewhat surprisingly, this was irrespective of age or sex [110]. However, older postmenopausal women may need up to 1.2 g/kg/day [111] which is similar to the recommendation in older people with frailty living in residential aged care facilities with the additional recommendation to have the protein intake equally split across the meals [112].

It has been suggested that higher supplemental protein intake is more effective when vitamin D levels are in an optimal range [113]. The level of vitamin D supplementation that was recommended was at least 1000 IU/day, which is much higher than the recommendation by Reid and Bollard [92]. There are other sources of protein such as leucine, β-hydroxy-β-methylbutyrate, creatine, and whey, that are under investigation [36].

Weight loss and weight regain

Both intentional and unintentional weight loss, either with or without exercise, has been shown to decrease BMD at the hip [71,72,114,115]. Surprisingly, all weight loss/weight loss plus exercise RCTs with older obese people have reported no changes in lumbar spine BMD [71,114,116–120]. These results support an earlier metaanalysis of weight-loss trials that also concluded BMD at the lumbar spine is unaffected by weight loss [121]. The biological mechanisms behind the differential loss of bone at the hip versus the spine have yet to be elucidated. More concerning is that BMD lost with voluntary weight loss in older adults with obesity and in postmenopausal women is not regained with weight regain [122–125]. The biological mechanisms behind these changes are unknown, but it does suggest negative alterations in calcium balance during weight loss [126], which may be associated with increased calcium absorption in people with obesity.

Circadian rhythm

The circadian cycle is a molecular clock of approximately 24 h based on light/dark and works as a series of interconnected transcriptional-translational feedback loops [127,128]. Every cell in the body has a circadian rhythm including muscle and bone [35,128,129] and these rhythms are important for the maintenance of bone [130], regulation of skeletal muscle metabolic homeostasis [131–133] and possibly bone to muscle crosstalk [134,135]. Bone formation and resorption have circadian rhythmicity with C-terminal cross-linked telopeptide of type 1 collagen with a low point in the afternoon and a high point at night [136]. In mice, scheduled resistance exercise appears to entrain the circadian clocks [46], which is intriguing, but not considered in exercise or nutritional interventions in humans. The circadian clock becomes less synchronous with age, which may be associated with visual changes and reduced sensitivity to light, daytime sleeping, and low physical activity [137], which given the evidence in mice on exercise entraining circadian rhythms could be a new avenue to explore. It is intriguing to think that understanding these pathways might lead to specifically timed exercise and nutrition interventions aimed to alter clock genes in muscle to slow the loss or promote the growth of skeletal muscle mass and subsequently bone mass.

Conclusions

Age-related changes and loss of skeletal muscle and bone appear most responsive to exercise interventions and adequate nutrition is essential for a physiological response to exercise interventions. However, the role of calcium, vitamin D, and protein supplements either with or without exercise is still unclear. It is clear that physiological responses to acute and long-term exercise are not the same and that these mediate the endocrine effects between muscle and bone and adaptations of the tissue secretome. Both muscle and bone require relatively high-intensity resistance exercise (~85% 1 RM) for a physiological response. The differentiating factor is bone needing high intensity and speed movements to stimulate osteogenesis and bone remodeling, whereas for skeletal muscle high intensity seems more critical than the speed of the movement. For both bone and muscle walking alone, is not an adequate stimulus, but is an important component of an exercise training regime for older adults. Resistance exercise sessions require adequate recovery both within sessions and between sessions, which is an often-overlooked element of exercise training and requires more research. Another potentially overlooked area of resistance exercise training is the role of circadian rhythms and the impact of weight loss and weight gain, particularly on bone mass.

Based on the separate evidence for sarcopenia and osteopenia one could suggest that a nonpharmaceutical approach for people with, or at risk of, osteosarcopenia would be the approach used for maintaining or increasing bone mass. This should provide adequate stimulus for both muscle and bone and the limited available evidence reports that skeletal muscle/lean body mass does respond to exercise modalities targeting bone. More research is needed on including the other elements discussed in this chapter particularly the role of other proteins supplements and timing of the supplements, recovery during and after exercise sessions, and the timing of training sessions to optimize circadian rhythms.

References

[1] Chen L-R, Hou P-H, Chen K-H. Nutritional support and physical modalities for people with osteoporosis: current opinion. Nutrients 2019;11:2848. https://doi.org/10.3390/nu11122848.

[2] Chen LR, Ko NY, Chen KH. Medical treatment for osteoporosis: from molecular to clinical opinions. Int J Mol Sci 2019;20:2213.

[3] Frost HM. Bone's mechanostat: a 2003 update. Anat Rec A Discov Mol Cell Evol Biol 2003;275(2):1081–101. https://doi.org/10.1002/ar.a.10119.

[4] Go SW, Cha YH, Lee JA, Park HS. Association between sarcopenia, bone density, and health-related quality of life in Korean men. Korean J Fam Med 2013;34(4):281–8. https://doi.org/10.4082/kjfm.2013.34.4.281.

[5] Lexell J, Downham D, Sjöström M. Distribution of different fibre types in human skeletal muscles. Fibre type arrangement in m. vastus lateralis from three groups of healthy men between 15 and 83 years. J Neurol Sci 1986;72:211–22. https://doi.org/10.1016/0022-510X(86)90009-2.

[6] Bickel CS, Cross JM, Bamman MM. Exercise dosing to retain resistance training adaptations in young and older adults. Med Sci Sports Exerc 2011;43:1177–87. https://doi.org/10.1249/MSS.0b013e318207c15d.

[7] Stec MJ, Kelly NA, Many GM, Windham ST, Tuggle SC, Bamman MM. Ribosome biogenesis may augment resistance training-induced myofiber hypertrophy and is required for myotube growth in vitro. Am J Physiol Endocrinol Metab 2016;310:E652–61.

[8] Stec MJ, Thalacker-Mercer A, Mayhew DL, Kelly NA, Tuggle SC, Merritt EK, Brown CJ, Windham ST, Dell'Italia LJ, Bickel CS, Roberts BM, Vaughn KM, Isakova-Donahue I, Many GM, Bamman MM. Randomized, four-arm, dose-response clinical trial to optimize resistance exercise training for older adults with age-related muscle atrophy. Exp Gerontol 2017;99:98–109.

[9] Lavin KM, Roberts BM, Fry CS, Moro T, Rasmussen BB, Bamman MM. The importance of resistance exercise training to combat neuromuscular aging. Physiology (Bethesda) 2019;34(2):112–22. https://doi.org/10.1152/physiol.00044.2018 [published online 2019 Feb 6].

[10] Kosek DJ, Kim JS, Petrella JK, Cross JM, Bamman MM. Efficacy of 3 days/wk resistance training on myofiber hypertrophy and myogenic mechanisms in young vs. older adults. J Appl Physiol 2006;101:531–44. https://doi.org/10.1152/japplphysiol.01474.2005.

[11] McGregor RA, Cameron-Smith D, Poppitt SD. It is not just muscle mass: a review of muscle quality, composition and metabolism during ageing as determinants of muscle function and mobility in later life. Longev Healthspan 2014;3:9. https://doi.org/10.1186/2046-2395-3-9.

[12] Krantic S, Mechawar N, Reix S, Quirion R. Molecular basis of programmed cell death involved in neurodegeneration. Trends Neurosci 2005;28:670–6. https://doi.org/10.1016/j.tins.2005.09.011.

[13] Nilwik R, Snijders T, Leenders M, Groen BB, van Kranenburg J, Verdijk LB, van Loon LJ. The decline in skeletal muscle mass with aging is mainly attributed to a reduction in type II muscle fiber size. Exp Gerontol 2013;48:492–8. https://doi.org/10.1016/j.exger.2013.02.012.

[14] Piasecki M, Ireland A, Coulson J, Stashuk DW, Hamilton-Wright A, Swiecicka A, Rutter MK, McPhee JS, Jones DA. Motor unit number estimates and neuromuscular transmission in the tibialis anterior of master athletes: evidence that athletic older people are not spared from age-related motor unit remodeling. Physiol Rep 2016;4. https://doi.org/10.14814/phy2.12987, e12987.

[15] Piasecki M, Ireland A, Jones DA, McPhee JS. Age-dependent motor unit remodelling in human limb muscles. Biogerontology 2016;17:485–96. https://doi.org/10.1007/s10522-015-9627-3.

[16] Piasecki M, Ireland A, Stashuk D, Hamilton-Wright A, Jones DA, McPhee JS. Age-related neuromuscular changes affecting human vastus lateralis. J Physiol 2016;594:4525–36. https://doi.org/10.1113/JP271087.

[17] Hepple RT, Rice CL. Innervation and neuromuscular control in ageing skeletal muscle. J Physiol 2016;594:1965–78. https://doi.org/10.1113/JP270561.

[18] Kelly NA, Hammond KG, Stec MJ, Bickel CS, Windham ST, Tuggle SC, Bamman MM. Quantification and characterization of grouped type I myofibers in human aging. Muscle Nerve 2018;57:E52–9. https://doi.org/10.1002/mus.25711.

[19] Roberts BM, Lavin KM, Many GM, Thalacker-Mercer A, Merritt EK, Bickel CS, Mayhew DL, Tuggle SC, Cross JM, Kosek DJ, Petrella JK, Brown CJ, Hunter GR, Windham ST, Allman RM, Bamman MM. Human neuromuscular aging: sex differences revealed at the myocellular level. Exp Gerontol 2018;106:116–24. https://doi.org/10.1016/j.exger.2018.02.023.

[20] Ling SM, Conwit RA, Ferrucci L, Metter EJ. Age-associated changes in motor unit physiology: observations from the Baltimore longitudinal study of aging. Arch Phys Med Rehabil 2009;90:1237–40. https://doi.org/10.1016/j.apmr.2008.09.565.

[21] Hardouin P, Marie PJ, Rosen CJ. New insights into bone marrow adipocytes: report from the first European meeting on bone marrow adiposity (BMA 2015). Bone 2015;(15):414–7. https://doi.org/10.1016/j.bone.2015.11.013.

[22] Kirkland JL, Tchkonia T, Pirtskhalava T, Han J, Karagiannides I. Adipogenesis and aging: does aging make fat go MAD? Exp Gerontol 2002;37:757–67. https://doi.org/10.1016/S0531-5565(02)00014-1.

[23] Akhter MP, Lappe JM, Davies KM, et al. Transmenopausal changes in the trabecular bone structure. Bone 2007;41(1):111–6.

[24] Armas LAG, Recker RR. Pathophysiology of osteoporosis new mechanistic insights. Endocrinol Metab Clin North Am 2012;41:475–86. https://doi.org/10.1016/j.ecl.2012.04.006.

[25] Bell LS, Kayser M, Jones C. The mineralized osteocyte: a living fossil. Am J Phys Anthropol 2008;137(4):449–56. 18615594.

[26] Busse B, Djonic D, Milovanovic P, Hahn M, Puschel K, Ritchie RO, et al. Decrease in the osteocyte lacunar density accompanied by hypermineralized lacunar occlusion reveals failure and delay of remodeling in aged human bone. Aging Cell 2010;9(6):1065–75. 20874757.

[27] Paintin J, Cooper C, Dennison E. Osteosarcopenia. Br J Hosp Med (Lond) 2018;79(5):253–8. https://doi.org/10.12968/hmed.2018.79.5.253.

[28] Girgis CM, Mokbel N, Digirolamo DJ. Therapies for musculoskeletal disease: can we treat two birds with one stone? Curr Osteoporos Rep 2014;12:142–53. https://doi.org/10.1007/s11914-014-0204-5. 24633910.

[29] Kaji H. Interaction between muscle and bone. J Bone Metab 2014;21:29–40. https://doi.org/10.11005/jbm.2014.21.1.29. 24707465.

[30] Brotto M, Bonewald L. Bone and muscle: interactions beyond mechanical. Bone 2015;80:109–14. https://doi.org/10.1016/j.bone.2015.02.010.

[31] Pedersen BK. Muscle as a secretory organ. Compr Physiol 2013;3(3):1337–62. 23897689.

[32] Oliveira A, Vaz C. The role of sarcopenia in the risk of osteoporotic hip fracture. Clin Rheumatol 2015;34:1673–80. https://doi.org/10.1007/s10067-015-2943-9. 25912213.

[33] Bialek P, Parkington J, Li X, Gavin D, Wallace C, Zhang J, et al. A myostatin and activin decoy receptor enhances bone formation in mice. Bone 2014;60:162–71. 24333131.

[34] Karasik D, Zhou Y, Cupples LA, Hannan MT, Kiel DP, Demissie S. Bivariate genome-wide linkage analysis of femoral bone traits and leg lean mass: Framingham study. J Bone Miner Res 2009;24(4):710–8. 19063671.

[35] Bonewald L. Use it or lose it to age: a review of bone and muscle communication. Bone 2019;120:212–8. https://doi.org/10.1016/j.bone.2018.11.002.

[36] Kirk B, Zanker J, Duque G. Osteosarcopenia: epidemiology, diagnosis, and treatment—facts and numbers. J Cachexia Sarcopenia Muscle 2020. https://doi.org/10.1002/jcsm.12567. Published online in Wiley Online Library (wileyonlinelibrary.com).

[37] Herrmann M, Engelke K, Ebert R, Müller-Deubert A, Rudert M, Ziouti F, Jundt F, Felsenberg D, Jakob F. Interactions between muscle and bone—where physics meets biology. Biomolecules 2020;10:432. https://doi.org/10.3390/biom10030432.

[38] Damas F, Phillips SM, Libardi CA, Vechin FC, Lixandrão ME, Jannig PR, Costa LA, Bacurau AV, Snijders T, Parise G, Tricoli V, Roschel H, Ugrinowitsch C. Resistance training-induced changes in integrated myofibrillar protein synthesis are related to hypertrophy only after attenuation of muscle damage. J Physiol 2016;594:5209–22. https://doi.org/10.1113/JP272472.

[39] Mitchell CJ, Churchward-Venne TA, Parise G, Bellamy L, Baker SK, Smith K, Atherton PJ, Phillips SM. Acute post-exercise myofibrillar protein synthesis is not correlated with resistance training-induced muscle hypertrophy in young men. PLoS One 2014;9. https://doi.org/10.1371/journal.pone.0089431, e89431.

[40] Borer KT. Physical activity in the prevention and amelioration of osteoporosis in women: interaction of mechanical, hormonal and dietary factors. Sports Med 2005;35:779–830.

[41] Atherton PJ, Smith K. Muscle protein synthesis in response to nutrition and exercise. J Physiol 2012;590:1049–57.

[42] Laplante M, Sabatini DM. mTOR signaling in growth control and disease. Cell 2012;149:274–93.

[43] Musaro A, McCullagh K, Paul A, Houghton L, Dobrowolny G, Molinaro M, et al. Localized IGF-1 transgene expression sustains hypertrophy and regeneration in senescent skeletal muscle. Nat Genet 2001;27:195–200.

[44] Rommel C, Bodine SC, Clarke BA, Rossman R, Nunez L, Stitt TN, et al. Mediation of IGF-1-induced skeletal myotube hypertrophy by PI(3)K/Akt/mTOR and PI(3)K/Akt/GSK3 pathways. Nat Cell Biol 2001;3:1009–13.

[45] Santos L, Elliott-Sale KJ, Sale C. Exercise and bone health across the lifespan. Biogerontology 2017;18:931–46.

[46] Castrogiovanni P, Trovato FM, Szychlinska MA, Nsir H, Imbesi R, Musumeci G. The importance of physical activity in osteoporosis. From the molecular pathways to the clinical evidence. Histol Histopathol 2016;31(11):1183–94.

[47] Kumar V, Selby A, Rankin D, Patel R, Atherton P, Hildebrandt W, Williams J, Smith K, Seynnes O, Hiscock N, Rennie MJ. Age-related differences in the dose response relationship of muscle protein synthesis to resistance exercise in young and old men. J Physiol 2009;587:211–7. https://doi.org/10.1113/jphysiol.2008.164483.

[48] Moro T, Ebert SM, Adams CM, Rasmussen BB. Amino acid sensing in skeletal muscle. Trends Endocrinol Metab 2016;27:796–806. https://doi.org/10.1016/j.tem.2016.06.010.

[49] Shad BJ, Thompson JL, Breen L. Does the muscle protein synthetic response to exercise and amino acid-based nutrition diminish with advancing age? A systematic review. Am J Physiol Endocrinol Metab 2016;311:E803–17. https://doi.org/10.1152/ajpendo.00213.2016.

[50] Damas F, Phillips S, Vechin FC, Ugrinowitsch C. A review of resistance training-induced changes in skeletal muscle protein synthesis and their contribution to hypertrophy. Sports Med 2015;45:801–7. https://doi.org/10.1007/s40279-015-0320-0.

[51] Dreyer HC, Fujita S, Glynn EL, Drummond MJ, Volpi E, Rasmussen BB. Resistance exercise increases leg muscle protein synthesis and mTOR signalling independent of sex. Acta Physiol (Oxford) 2010;199:71–81. https://doi.org/10.1111/j.1748-1716.2010.02074.x.

[52] Fry CS, Drummond MJ, Glynn EL, Dickinson JM, Gundermann DM, Timmerman KL, Walker DK, Dhanani S, Volpi E, Rasmussen BB. Aging impairs contraction induced human skeletal muscle mTORC1 signaling and protein synthesis. Skelet Muscle 2011;1:11. https://doi.org/10.1186/2044-5040-1-11.

[53] Burd NA, Holwerda AM, Selby KC, West DW, Staples AW, Cain NE, Cashaback JG, Potvin JR, Baker SK, Phillips SM. Resistance exercise volume affects myofibrillar protein synthesis and anabolic signalling molecule phosphorylation in young men. J Physiol 2010;588:3119–30. https://doi.org/10.1113/jphysiol.2010.192856.

[54] Dickinson JM, Gundermann DM, Walker DK, Reidy PT, Borack MS, Drummond MJ, Arora M, Volpi E, Rasmussen BB. Leucine-enriched amino acid ingestion after resistance exercise prolongs myofibrillar protein synthesis and amino acid transporter expression in older men. J Nutr 2014;144:1694–702. https://doi.org/10.3945/jn.114.198671.

[55] Figueiredo VC, McCarthy JJ. Regulation of ribosome biogenesis in skeletal muscle hypertrophy. Physiology (Bethesda) 2019;34(1):30–42. https://doi.org/10.1152/physiol.00034.2018.

[56] Moro T, Brightwell CR, Deer RR, Graber TG, Galvan E, Fry CS, Volpi E, Rasmussen BB. Muscle protein anabolic resistance to essential amino acids does not occur in healthy older adults before or after resistance exercise training. J Nutr 2018;148:900–9. https://doi.org/10.1093/jn/nxy064.

[57] Bonewald LF. The amazing osteocyte. J Bone Miner Res 2011;26(2):229–38.

[58] Mulcahy LE, Taylor D, Lee TC, et al. RANKL and OPG activity is regulated by injury size in networks of osteocyte-like cells. Bone 2011;48(2):182–8.

[59] Liu Y, Liu Y, Recker R, et al. Molecular studies of identification of genes for osteoporosis: the 2002 update. J Endocrinol 2003;177(2):147–96.

[60] Chodzko-Zajko WJ, Proctor DN, Fiatarone Singh MA, Minson CT, Nigg CR, Salem GJ, Skinner JS. American College of Sports Medicine position stand. Exercise and physical activity for older adults. Med Sci Sports Exerc 2009;41:1510–30. https://doi.org/10.1249/MSS.0b013e3181a0c95c.

[61] DiFrancisco-Donoghue J, Werner W, Douris PC, McKenna RF. Comparison of once-weekly and twice-weekly strength training in older adults. Br J Sports Med 2007;41:19–22. https://doi.org/10.1136/bjsm.2006.029330.

[62] Taaffe DR, Duret C, Wheeler S, Marcus R. Once-weekly resistance exercise improves muscle strength and neuromuscular performance in older adults. J Am Geriatr Soc 1999;47:1208–14. https://doi.org/10.1111/j.1532-5415.1999.tb05201.x.

[63] Carneiro NH, Ribeiro AS, Nascimento MA, Gobbo LA, Schoenfeld BJ, Achour Júnior A, Gobbi S, Oliveira AR, Cyrino ES. Effects of different resistance training frequencies on flexibility in older women. Clin Interv Aging 2015;10:531–8. https://doi.org/10.2147/CIA.S77433.

[64] Hong RA, Kim SW. Effects of resistance exercise on bone health. Endocrinol Metab 2018;33:435–44. https://doi.org/10.3803/EnM.2018.33.4.435.

[65] Fielding RA, LeBrasseur NK, Cuoco A, Bean J, Mizer K, Fiatarone Singh MA. High-velocity resistance training increases skeletal muscle peak power in older women. J Am Geriatr Soc 2002;50(4):655–62.

[66] Daly RM, Duckham R, Tait JL, Rantalainen T, Nowson CA, Taaffe DR, Sanders K, Hill K, Kidgell DJ, Busija L. Effectiveness of dual-task functional power training for preventing falls in older people: study protocol for a cluster randomised controlled trial. Trials 2015;16:120. https://doi.org/10.1186/s13063-015-0652-y.

[67] Peterson MD, Sen A, Gordon PM. Influence of resistance exercise on lean body mass in aging adults: a meta-analysis. Med Sci Sports Exerc 2011;43:249–58. https://doi.org/10.1249/MSS.0b013e3181eb6265.

[68] Cannon J, Marino FE. Early-phase neuromuscular adaptations to high- and low-volume resistance training in untrained young and older women. J Sports Sci 2010;28:1505–14. https://doi.org/10.1080/02640414.2010.517544.

[69] Radaelli R, Wilhelm EN, Botton CE, Rech A, Bottaro M, Brown LE, Pinto RS. Effects of single vs. multiple-set short-term strength training in elderly women. Age (Dordr) 2014;36:9720. https://doi.org/10.1007/s11357-014-9720.

[70] Radaelli R, Botton CE, Wilhelm EN, Bottaro M, Brown LE, Lacerda F, Gaya A, Moraes K, Peruzzolo A, Pinto RS. Time course of low- and high-volume strength training on neuromuscular adaptations and muscle quality in older women. Age (Dordr) 2014;36:881–92. https://doi.org/10.1007/s11357-013-9611-2.

[71] Villareal DT, Aguirre L, Gurney AB, Waters DL, Sinacore DR, Colombo E, et al. Aerobic or resistance exercise, or both, in dieting obese older adults. N Engl J Med 2017;376(20):1943–55. https://doi.org/10.1056/NEJMoa1616338.

[72] Villareal DT, Chode S, Parimi N, Sinacore DR, Hilton T, Armamento-Villareal R, et al. Weight loss, exercise, or both and physical function in obese older adults. N Engl J Med 2011;364:1218–29.

[73] Gianoudis J, Bailey CA, Sanders KM, Nowson CA, Hill K, Ebeling PR, Daly RM. Osteocise: strong bones for life: protocol for a community-based randomised controlled trial of a multi-modal exercise and osteoporosis education program for older adults at risk of falls and fractures. BMC Musculoskelet Disord 2012;13:78. https://doi.org/10.1186/1471-2474-13-78.

[74] Kohrt WM, Bloomfield SA, Little KD, Nelson ME, Yingling VR, American College of Sports Medicine. Position stand: physical activity and bone health. Med Sci Sports Exerc 2004;36(11):1985–96.

[75] Martyn-St James M, Carroll S. A meta-analysis of impact exercise on postmenopausal bone loss: the case for mixed loading exercise programmes. Br J Sports Med 2009;43(12):898–908.

[76] Beck BR, Daly RM, Singh MA, Taaffe DR. Exercise and sports science Australia (ESSA) position statement on exercise prescription for the prevention and management of osteoporosis. J Sci Med Sport 2017;20:438–45.

[77] Robling AG, Bonewald LF. The osteocyte: new insights. Annu Rev Physiol 2020;(82):485–506. https://doi.org/10.1146/annurev-physiol-021119-034332.

[78] Steib S, Schoene D, Pfeifer K. Dose-response relationship of resistance training in older adults: a meta-analysis. Med Sci Sports Exerc 2010;42:902–14.

[79] Zhao R, Zhao M, Xu Z. The effects of differing resistance training modes on the preservation of bone mineral density in postmenopausal women: a meta-analysis. Osteoporos Int 2015;26:1605–18.

[80] Daly RM, Gianoudis J, Kersh ME, Bailey CA, Ebeling PR, Krug R, Nowson CA, Hill K, Sanders KM. Effects of a 12-month supervised, community-based, multimodal exercise program followed by a 6-month research-to-practice transition on bone mineral density, trabecular microarchitecture, and physical function in older adults: a randomized controlled trial. J Bone Miner Res 2020;35(3):419–29. https://doi.org/10.1002/jbmr.3865 [Epub 2019 Oct 24].

[81] Martyn-St James M, Carroll S. Meta-analysis of walking for preservation of bone mineral density in postmenopausal women. Bone 2008;43:521–31.

[82] Rector RS, Rogers R, Ruebel M, Hinton PS. Participation in road cycling vs running is associated with lower bone mineral density in men. Metabolism 2008;57:226–32.

[83] Allison SJ, Poole KE, Treece GM, Gee AH, Tonkin C, Rennie WJ, et al. The influence of high-impact exercise on cortical and trabecular bone mineral content and 3d distribution

across the proximal femur in older men: a randomized controlled unilateral intervention. J Bone Miner Res 2015;30:1709–16.
[84] Bailey CA, Brooke-Wavell K. Optimum frequency of exercise for bone health: randomised controlled trial of a high-impact unilateral intervention. Bone 2010;46:1043–9.
[85] Marques EA, Mota J, Carvalho J. Exercise effects on bone mineral density in older adults: a meta-analysis of randomized controlled trials. Age (Dordr) 2012;34:1493–515.
[86] Giangregorio LM, Papaioannou A, Macintyre NJ, Ashe MC, Heinonen A, Shipp K, et al. Too fit to fracture: exercise recommendations for individuals with osteoporosis or osteoporotic vertebral fracture. Osteoporos Int 2014;25:821–35.
[87] Robling AG, Burr DB, Turner CH. Recovery periods restore mechanosensitivity to dynamically loaded bone. J Exp Biol 2001;204(Pt 19):3389–99.
[88] Bolam KA, van Uffelen JG, Taaffe DR. The effect of physical exercise on bone density in middle-aged and older men: a systematic review. Osteoporos Int 2013;24:2749–62.
[89] Engelke K, Kemmler W, Lauber D, Beeskow C, Pintag R, Kalender WA. Exercise maintains bone density at spine and hip EFOPS: a 3-year longitudinal study in early postmenopausal women. Osteoporos Int 2006;17:133–42.
[90] Chen LR, Wen YT, Kuo CL, Chen KH. Calcium and vitamin D supplementation on bone health: current evidence and recommendations. Int J Gerontol 2014;8:183–8.
[91] Del Valle HB, Yaktine AL, Taylor CL, et al. Dietary reference intakes for calcium and vitamin D. Washington, DC: National Academies Press; 2011.
[92] Reid IR, Bolland MJ. Controversies in medicine: the role of calcium and vitamin D supplements in adults. Med J Aust 2019;211:468–73.
[93] Body JJ, Bergmann P, Boonen S, Boutsen Y, Bruyere O, Devogelaer JP, Goemaere S, Hollevoet N, Kaufman JM, Milisen K, et al. Non-pharmacological management of osteoporosis: a consensus of the belgian bone club. Osteoporos Int 2011;22:2769–88.
[94] Shapses SA, Sukumar D, Schneider SH, Schlussel Y, Brolin RE, Taich L. Hormonal and dietary influences on true fractional calcium absorption in women: role of obesity. Osteoporos Int 2012;23(11):2607–14. https://doi.org/10.1007/s00198-012-1901-5.
[95] Shapses SA, Sukumar D, Schneider SH, et al. Vitamin D supplementation and calcium absorption during caloric restriction: a randomized double-blind trial. Am J Clin Nutr 2013;97(3):637–45. https://doi.org/10.3945/ajcn.112.044909.
[96] Zhao JG, Zeng XT, Wang J, Liu L. Association between calcium or vitamin D supplementation and fracture incidence in community-dwelling older adults: a systematic review and meta-analysis. JAMA 2017;318:2466–82.
[97] Cano A, Chedraui P, Goulis DG, Lopes P, Mishra G, Mueck A, Senturk LM, Simoncini T, Stevenson JC, Stute P, et al. Calcium in the prevention of postmenopausal osteoporosis: EMAS clinical guide. Maturitas 2018;107:7–12.
[98] Bolland MJ, Leung W, Tai V, Bastin S, Gamble GD, Grey A, Reid IR. Calcium intake and risk of fracture: systematic review. BMJ 2015;351:4580.
[99] Bailey RL, Dodd KW, Goldman JA, Gahche JJ, Dwyer JT, Moshfegh AJ, Sempos CT, Picciano MF. Estimation of total usual calcium and vitamin D intakes in the United States. J Nutr 2010;140:817–22.
[100] Gorter EA, Krijnen P, Schipper IB. Vitamin D deficiency in adult fracture patients: prevalence and risk factors. Eur J Trauma Emerg Surg 2016;42:369–78.
[101] Bruyère O, Cavalier E, Reginster JY. Vitamin D and osteosarcopenia: an update from epidemiological studies. Curr Opin Clin Nutr Metab Care 2017;20:498.
[102] Duque G, Daly RM, Sanders K, et al. Vitamin D, bones and muscle: myth versus reality. Australas J Ageing 2017;36(Suppl 1):8–13.

[103] Holick MF. Vitamin D deficiency. N Engl J Med 2007;357:266–81.
[104] Karaguzel G, Holick MF. Diagnosis and treatment of osteopenia. Rev Endocr Metab Disord 2010;11:237–51.
[105] Houston DK, Nicklas BJ, Ding J, et al. Dietary protein intake is associated with lean mass change in older, community-dwelling adults: the health, aging, and body composition (health ABC) study. Am J Clin Nutr 2008;87:150–5.
[106] Coelho-Junior HJ, Milano-Teixeira L, Rodrigues B, et al. Relative protein intake and physical function in older adults: a systematic review and meta-analysis of observational studies. Nutrients 2018;10 [pii: E1330].
[107] Hannan MT, Tucker KL, Dawson-Hughes B, et al. Effect of dietary protein on bone loss in elderly men and women: the Framingham osteoporosis study. J Bone Miner Res 2000;15:2504–12.
[108] Koutsofta I, Mamais I, Chrysostomou S. The effect of protein diets in postmenopausal women with osteoporosis: systematic review of randomized controlled trials. J Women Aging 2019;31:117–39.
[109] Wallace TC, Frankenfeld CL. Dietary protein intake above the current RDA and bone health: a systematic review and meta-analysis. J Am Coll Nutr 2017;36:481–96.
[110] Joint WHO/FAO/UNU Expert Consultation. Protein and amino acid requirements in human nutrition. World Health Organ Tech Rep Ser 2007;(935):1–265.
[111] Rizzoli R, Stevenson JC, Bauer JM, et al. The role of dietary protein and vitamin D in maintaining musculoskeletal health in postmenopausal women: a consensus statement from the European society for clinical and economic aspects of osteoporosis and osteoarthritis (ESCEO). Maturitas 2014;79:122–32.
[112] Bauer J, Biolo G, Cederholm T, Cesari M, Cruz-Jentoft AJ, Morley JE, et al. Evidence based recommendations for optimal dietary protein intake in older people: a position paper from the PROT-AGE study group. J Am Med Dir Assoc 2013;14:542–59.
[113] Verlaan S, Maier AB, Bauer JM, Bautmans I, Brandt K, Donini LM, et al. Sufficient levels of 25-hydroxyvitamin D and protein intake required to increase muscle mass in sarcopenic older adults—the PROVIDE study. Clin Nutr 2016;37:1–7.
[114] Beavers KM, Beavers DP, Martin SB, et al. Change in bone mineral density during weight loss with resistance versus aerobic exercise training in older adults. J Gerontol A Biol Sci Med Sci 2017;72(11):1582–5. https://doi.org/10.1093/gerona/glx048. 28379325.
[115] Ensrud KE, Ewing SK, Stone KL, Cauley JA, Bowman PJ, Cummings SR. Intentional and unintentional weight loss increase bone loss and hip fracture risk in older women. J Am Geriatr Soc 2003;51(12):1740–7. 14687352.
[116] Chao D, Espeland MA, Farmer D, et al. Effect of voluntary weight loss on bone mineral density in older overweight women. J Am Geriatr Soc 2000;7(48):753–9.
[117] Kelleher JL, Beavers DP, Henderson RM, et al. Weighted vest use during dietary weight loss on bone health in older adults with obesity. J Osteoporos Phys Act 2017;5(4). https://doi.org/10.4172/2329-9509.1000210. pii: 210.
[118] Santanasto AJ, Glynn NW, Newman MA, et al. Impact of weight loss on physical function with changes in strength, muscle mass, and muscle fat infiltration in overweight to moderately older adults with obesity: a randomized clinical trial. J Obes 2011;2011. https://doi.org/10.1155/2011/516576. pii: 516576.
[119] Shah K, Armamento-Villareal R, Parimi N, et al. Exercise training in older adults with obesity prevents increase in bone turnover and attenuates decrease in hip BMD induced by weight loss despite decline in bone-active hormones. J Bone Miner Res 2011;26(12):2851–9. https://doi.org/10.1002/jbmr.475. 21786319.

[120] Villareal DT, Shah K, Banks MR, Sinacore DR, Klein S. Effect of weight loss and exercise therapy on bone metabolism and mass in older adults with obesity: a one-year randomized controlled trial. J Clin Endocrinol Metab 2008;93(6):2181–7. https://doi.org/10.1210/jc.2007-1473. 18364384.

[121] Zibellini J, Seimon RV, Lee CM, et al. Does diet-induced weight loss lead to bone loss in overweight or obese adults? A systematic review and meta-analysis of clinical trials. J Bone Miner Res 2015;30(12):2168–78. https://doi.org/10.1002/jbmr.2564. 26012544.

[122] Pines A. Weight loss, weight regain and bone health. Climacteric 2012;15(4):317–9. https://doi.org/10.3109/13697137.2012.667975. 22369637.

[123] Villalon KL, Gozansky WS, Van Pelt RE, et al. A losing battle: weight regain does not restore weight loss-induced bone loss in postmenopausal women. Obesity (Silver Spring) 2011;19(12):2345–50. https://doi.org/10.1038/oby.2011.263. 21852813.

[124] Von Thun NL, Sukumar D, Heymsfield SB, Shapses SA. Does bone loss begin after weight loss ends? Results 2 years after weight loss or regain in postmenopausal women. Menopause 2014;21(5):501–8. https://doi.org/10.1097/GME.0b013e3182a76fd5. 24149920.

[125] Waters DL, Vawter R, Qualls C, et al. Long-term maintenance of weight loss after lifestyle intervention in frail older adults with obesity. J Nutr Health Aging 2013;17(1):3–7. https://doi.org/10.1007/s12603-012-0421-5. 23299370.

[126] Jiang BC, Villareal DT. Weight loss-induced reduction of bone mineral density in older adults with obesity. J Nutr Gerontol Geriatr 2019;38(1):100–14. https://doi.org/10.1080/21551197.2018.1564721.

[127] Schibler U. The daily rhythms of genes, cells and organs. Biological clocks and circadian timing in cells. EMBO Rep 2005;6(Suppl 1):S9–13. https://doi.org/10.1038/sj.embor.7400424.

[128] Takahashi JS. Transcriptional architecture of the mammalian circadian clock. Nat Rev Genet 2017;18(3):164–79. https://doi.org/10.1038/nrg.2016.150.

[129] Schibler U, Naef F. Cellular oscillators: rhythmic gene expression and metabolism. Curr Opin Cell Biol 2005;17(2):223–9. https://doi.org/10.1016/j.ceb.2005.01.007.

[130] Schroder EA, Harfmann BD, Zhang X, Srikuea R, England JH, Hodge BA, et al. Intrinsic muscle clock is necessary for musculoskeletal health. J Physiol 2015;593(24):5387–404. https://doi.org/10.1113/JP271436.

[131] Hodge BA, Wen Y, Riley LA, Zhang X, England JH, Harfmann BD, et al. The endogenous molecular clock orchestrates the temporal separation of substrate metabolism in skeletal muscle. Skelet Muscle 2015;5:17. https://doi.org/10.1186/s13395-015-0039-5.

[132] Peek CB, Levine DC, Cedernaes J, Taguchi A, Kobayashi Y, Tsai SJ, et al. Circadian clock interaction with HIF1alpha mediates oxygenic metabolism and anaerobic glycolysis in skeletal muscle. Cell Metab 2017;25(1):86–92. https://doi.org/10.1016/j.cmet.2016.09.010.

[133] Riley LA, Esser KA. The role of the molecular clock in skeletal muscle and what it is teaching us about muscle-bone crosstalk. Curr Osteoporos Rep 2017;15(3):222–30 [PubMed: 28421465].

[134] Gorski JP, Huffman NT, Vallejo J, Brotto L, Chittur SV, Breggia A, et al. Deletion of Mbtps1 (Pcsk8, S1p, ski-1) gene in osteocytes stimulates soleus muscle regeneration and increased size and contractile force with age. J Biol Chem 2016;291(9):4308–22. https://doi.org/10.1074/jbc.M115.686626.

[135] Takarada T, Xu C, Ochi H, Nakazato R, Yamada D, Nakamura S, Kodama A, Shimba S, Mieda M, Fukasawa K, Ozaki K, Iezaki T, Fujikawa K, Yoneda Y, Numano R, Hida A, Tei H, Takeda S, Eiichi H. Bone resorption is regulated by circadian clock in osteoblasts. J Bone Miner Res 2017. https://doi.org/10.1002/jbmr.3053.

[136] van der Spoel E, Oei N, Cachucho R, Roelfsema F, Berbee JFP, Blauw GJ, Pijl H, Appelman-Dijkstra NM, van Heemst D. The 24-hour serum profiles of bone markers in healthy older men and women. Bone 2018;120:61–9. 30291970.

[137] Martinez-Nicolas A, Madrid JA, Garcia FJ, Campos M, Moreno-Casbas MT, Almaida-Pagan PF, Lucas-Sanchez A, Rol MA. Circadian monitoring as an aging predictor. Sci Rep 2018;8(1):15027. 30301951.

Chapter 16

Pharmacological management of osteosarcopenia

Jack Feehan[a,b] and Gustavo Duque[a,b]
[a]Australian Institute for Musculoskeletal Science (AIMSS), The University of Melbourne and Western Health, St. Albans, VIC, Australia, [b]Department of Medicine-Western Health, The University of Melbourne, St. Albans, VIC, Australia

Introduction

As the global population ages, the ongoing impact of osteosarcopenia is poised to strain or overwhelm healthcare systems around the world [1]. To combat this, effective treatment strategies are required beyond those that are already in place. The management of osteosarcopenia is an ongoing challenge in clinical practice. While the pharmacological strategies to manage osteoporosis are well defined, there are no approved compounds to treat sarcopenia, nor muscle and bone together. This necessitates an approach in which the clinician treats each component of the disease individually, i.e., osteoporosis medications, alongside adjunct therapies and nutritional approaches to improve muscle function and fall-related outcomes [2,3]. While this is not ineffective, there is growing interest in the identification of drug compounds that target both muscle and bone individually. While in its early days, there are a small number of agents in preclinical and clinical trials that may be able to improve function and outcomes across both muscle and bone simultaneously (Table 1). This chapter will discuss the current state of the evidence on compounds affecting both muscle and bone, as well as the challenges they face.

Targeting the endocrine system for muscle and bone anabolism

The central role the endocrine system plays in the development and maintenance of musculoskeletal tissues has driven interest in the exploitation of these factors for the treatment of muscle and bone disease. Hormones such as testosterone and growth hormone, as well as synthetic compounds that manipulate their physiologies have all been investigated as agents amenable to drug development. The pathways evaluated in research on pharmaceutical manipulation of osteosarcopenia are summarized in Fig. 1.

Osteosarcopenia. https://doi.org/10.1016/B978-0-12-820088-9.00003-2

TABLE 1 Summary of the evidence regarding the effect of pharmacological agents on osteoporosis and sarcopenia-related outcomes.

Pharmacological agent	Osteoporosis	Sarcopenia
Denosumab	Significant improvement in BMD at lumbar spine, hip, and radius. Reduces fracture risk.	Reduction in falls in the Denosumab treatment group of the FREEDOM study. No evidence of an effect on muscle function in that study. Improves muscle strength and insulin sensitivity and reduces falls and fear of falling in high-risk older persons.
Testosterone	Intramuscular testosterone increased lumbar spine bone density in men.	Testosterone in older men with decreased testosterone levels and muscle weakness can improve muscle mass, strength, and physical performance.
SARMs-Ostarine	Increases lean body mass and muscle power in elderly men and postmenopausal women.	Improves bone mass and architecture in ovariectomized rats.
Growth hormone	Metaanalysis of 7 RCTs and one extension trial concluded that growth hormone may not improve bone density but decrease fracture risk in women with age-related bone loss.	Low-growth hormone levels with age contribute to a decrease in lean body mass and increase adipose tissue.
Antimyostatin antibodies	Antimyostatin antibody in combination with resistance exercise improved bone health in rats.	Antimyostatin antibodies increased muscle mass and strength in mice. Antimyostatin antibodies increased lean mass and may improve functional measures of muscle power.

Abbreviations: *BMD*, bone mineral density; *RCTs*, randomized controlled trials; *SARMS*, selective androgen receptor modulators.
(Adapted from Fatima, M, Brennan-Olsen, SL, Duque, G. Therapeutic approaches to osteosarcopenia: insights for the clinician. Ther Adv Musculoskelet Dis 2019;11:1759720X19867009.)

Androgens

The gonadal hormones play a major role in the development of all musculoskeletal tissues and have been the focus of research into potential compounds that could be used to improve bone and muscle mass in older adults. Estrogen and other compounds that selectively interact with its receptor in different tissues,

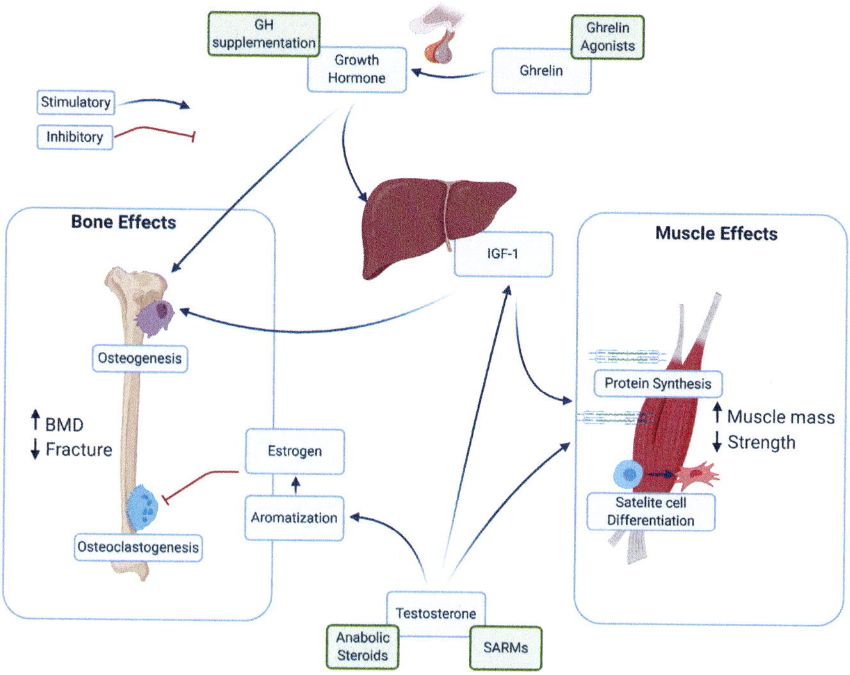

FIG. 1 Potential therapeutic targets for osteosarcopenia. *GH*, growth hormone; *SARMs*, Selective Androgen Receptor Modulators.

called selective estrogen receptor modulators (SERMs) were commonly used historically in the treatment of postmenopausal osteoporosis. However, from the perspective of osteosarcopenia, they are only a solution to half of the equation, with minimal effects on muscle [4]. As is well understood from a developmental perspective, androgens have a much stronger impact on the development of both bone and muscle mass, and this is reflected in their therapeutic use in osteoporosis and sarcopenia. Men with hypogonadism develop both osteoporosis and muscle wasting, and treatment with testosterone reverses these effects lending support to its use as an anabolic treatment for musculoskeletal disease [5].

The mechanisms by which testosterone imparts its anabolic effect vary based on the tissue. In bone, it undergoes aromatization and is converted to estrogen, where it inhibits osteoclast formation, while in muscle it acts directly to increase the synthesis of protein, leading to an overall increase in both muscle size and function. It also acts to increase the secretion of insulin-like growth factor-1 (IGF-1), which synergistically enhances the anabolic responses [5]. These actions are consistent in their magnitude throughout the lifespan, further supporting its use as a therapeutic strategy.

Testosterone has been shown to be effective in increasing both bone and muscle mass, particularly in men with hypogonadism. A systematic review of 8 trials, enrolling 365 men with the hypogonadal disease found an 8% increase in lumbar spine bone mineral density with intramuscular testosterone treatment [6]. However, it found no association with femoral neck BMD, and none of the studies examined fracture risk, leaving large questions unanswered [6]. These findings have been supported by other reviews, which also found no evidence to suggest that testosterone therapy could decrease the risk of fracture [7,8]. A more recent study of 211 men who received testosterone treatment for a year not only had similar findings showing increased spinal BMD but also demonstrating an improvement in femoral bone mass [9]. Another study of 100 obese men on very low-calorie diets who received intramuscular testosterone therapy for a year, found that it reduced serum c-telopeptide (CTX), a marker of bone resorption, suggesting it may aid in maintaining bone mineral density. However, they also found that while the testosterone treatment initially increased the bone formation marker N-terminal propeptide of type 1 procollagen (P1NP), it was marginally lower than baseline at the study end, painting a confusing picture of bone turnover with androgen treatment [10].

In muscle, testosterone is well known to cause increases in both muscle volume and strength [11,12]. Few studies have reported the effects of testosterone on both muscle and bone simultaneously, however. Two studies of transdermal testosterone injections in 67 [13] and 131 [14] men with low bioavailable testosterone found improvements in both bone mass and lean body mass, with an associated decrease in adipose tissue. One of these studies found an increase in lower limb muscle strength, though was confounded by simultaneous vitamin D supplementation [13], and the other found no change in functional measures [14]. A recent observational study had contrasting findings, showing that free testosterone and its precursor hormone dehydroepiandrosterone (DHEA) correlated to muscle strength and bone architecture in both older men and postmenopausal women [15]. While these studies lend support to testosterone as an anabolic agent in both bone and muscle, the lack of functional and fracture risk data leaves critical unanswered questions.

There is also little information available on the effects of testosterone on women, due to significant adverse effects related to its use, such as acne, male pattern baldness, cardiovascular disease, and potentially breast and gynecological malignancy [16]. At present, there are no widely approved indications for the use of testosterone in women [17]. As osteosarcopenia disproportionately affects women, this is a significant limitation in its use. Other androgenic compounds have been examined as potential candidates for a dual muscle-bone pharmacotherapeutic. The anabolic steroids are synthetic testosterone or androgen analogs that have classically been used in a sports context to enhance muscle strength, mass, and performance. Common anabolic steroids such as nandrolone decanoate have been shown to improve both bone [18,19] and muscle mass [19,20], as well as decrease fracture risk [19]. Unfortunately, due to their nonspecific action on androgen receptors, recipients of anabolic steroids suffer the same issues of widespread testosterone use, making their utilization for osteosarcopenia unlikely.

Selective androgen receptor modulators

In the face of these challenges, research has turned to selective androgen receptor modulators (SARMs) as a method to exploit the anabolic potential of testosterone in osteosarcopenia. The SARMs are ligand compounds that can activate androgen-mediated pathways in some tissues (i.e., bone and muscle) but have less or no impact on others such as the gonads [21]. This occurs by exploitation of the different androgen receptor isoforms expressed in different tissues showing preferential or specific action for the SARM ligands [22]. The perfect SARMs would provide the musculoskeletal anabolic effects of testosterone while having none of the off-target effects. There are a number of SARMs currently being evaluated, with some compounds currently being evaluated in clinical trials.

The SARMs andarine and the closely related ostarine have had the largest body of research behind them. Andarine is commonly described as an ideal SARM, due to its ready bioavailability and long half-life, as well as strong results with few side effects in preclinical studies [23,24], though it has principally been studied in the treatment of benign prostate hyperplasia [25]. However, it has more recently been replaced by ostarine as the compound leading the race to clinical utilization in musculoskeletal disease. Ostarine has been shown in a small number of studies to have anabolic effects in muscle and bone, both individually and together. Ostarine has been studied mostly in the treatment of secondary muscle wasting and sarcopenia. In phase II trials, ostarine (under the trade name Enobosarm) has been shown to increase lean body mass and muscle power in older men and postmenopausal women [26,27], as well as in cancer patients [28]. Interestingly, this effect appears to happen via multiple pathways, with androgen-independent impacts in satellite cells [29]. Unfortunately, Enobosarm failed to reach its primary endpoints in phase III trials in cancer patients, leading to delays in evaluation [30]. Ostarine has been shown to improve bone mass and architecture in ovariectomized rats, a common animal model of osteoporosis, after 5 weeks of administration [31]. It also improves bone healing after osteotomy in rats, alongside an increase in muscle mass, providing hope for a possible treatment for osteosarcopenia in the future, though currently, no studies have shown positive effects on bone in humans [32]. Though ostarine is the most well-studied compound, a number of other SARMs have also been shown to have benefits in muscle, or are currently being evaluated in trials [33], though none are currently investigating an effect on bone.

Growth hormone

Given the challenges facing the therapies utilizing androgen stimulation, interest has grown in other endocrine signaling pathways which may have the potential for therapeutic exploitation in osteosarcopenia. Principle among these is growth hormone for its well-defined role in the development of musculoskeletal tissues in puberty and young adulthood. Growth hormone is episodically released from the pituitary gland, with secretion peaking in the second decade. It has a large number of biological roles, but of particular import to osteosarcopenia is its direct stimulation of bone mineralization and muscle growth, via insulin-like growth factor 1 (IGF-1) secretion from the liver. A large protein molecule, growth hormone acts via cell surface membrane receptors in target tissues, with actions mediated by MAPK/ERK, JAK/STAT, and PI3K signaling resulting in specific actions in particular cell types.

Growth hormone is well correlated with musculoskeletal development. Deficiency of growth hormone leads to leads to short stature in children and osteoporosis and muscle wasting in older persons [34], while excess in early life leads to pituitary gigantism or acromegaly in adults. Growth hormone treatment has been evaluated with respect to effects in both muscle and bone with mixed results. Early studies found promising results, with increases in both bone and muscle mass after 6 months of treatment in older men [35]. However, the studies that followed had more inconsistent results. The evidence for growth hormone as an anabolic approach for muscle is relatively sound, generally finding that it increases muscle mass overall [36–38]. However, the improvements have tended to be small and have a limited impact on function [37,38]. In the treatment of bone, growth hormone does not appear to improve BMD, but it may reduce fracture risk in osteoporotic women [39]. Unfortunately, the use of growth hormone as treatment comes with an increased incidence of adverse events, limiting its utility, and diminishing research interest in recent years [36,40].

More recently, other agents in the physiological pathway of growth hormone have also been investigated. Ghrelin is a hormone produced by the gastrointestinal tract which stimulates the release of growth hormone. It is commonly referred to as the hunger hormone, as it strongly stimulates appetite in humans, with rising plasma levels rising before eating and falling after. It is presently being evaluated for use in cancer-associated anorexia and cachexia, due to its strong effect on appetite. However, as ghrelin stimulates a native pulsatile release of growth hormone, a hypothesis developed that it may be useful as a bone and muscle anabolic in osteosarcopenic patients. Studies have shown a small positive effect on muscle mass [41,42], but with inconsistent functional results. The ghrelin analog anamorelin was refused marketing approval by the European Medicines Agency in 2017, citing limited effectiveness, halting progress on its evaluation. There is a registered clinical trial evaluating the effect of anamorelin on osteosarcopenic patients (trial number: NCT04021706), which may shed light on the potential for its clinical use in the future.

Antifracture medications as muscle anabolics

Repurposing medications for osteoporosis for use in osteosarcopenia is an appealing strategy, however few of the approved medications have shown effect on muscle. At present, the only approved medication for osteoporosis with evidence suggesting an improvement in muscle is the monoclonal antibody treatment denosumab. Denosumab is a humanized monoclonal antibody targeting the receptor activator of nuclear factor κ-B ligand (RANKL), a key factor in the maturation of osteoclasts. It is marketed as Prolia for the treatment of postmenopausal osteoporosis, and as Xgexa for the treatment of malignant bone metastases. Inhibition of RANKL leads to a decrease in the number of active osteoclasts, with an associated decrease in bone resorption. Denosumab has been well-documented to be successful in preventing fractures [43], and is now in widespread use for the treatment of postmenopausal osteoporosis. New evidence has begun to identify a role for denosumab in the treatment of muscle loss, providing hope for treatment in osteosarcopenia. In the FREEDOM trial on osteoporotic fracture risk with denosumab treatment, it was found that in addition to the expected improvement in fracture rate and BMD, participants receiving denosumab also showed a significant decrease in falls—a hallmark of sarcopenia [44]. This prompted further research into the effect of denosumab on muscle function parameters, with studies finding that RANKL inhibition caused increased muscle strength, as well as insulin sensitivity [45]. Another study of community-dwelling adults taking either zoledronic acid or denosumab found improved gait velocity, balance and agility, and reduced fear of falling in those taking the RANKL inhibitor [46]. This provides some evidence for a role for RANKL inhibitors in the treatment of osteosarcopenia, however, more information is required to validate these findings. It is as yet unclear as to whether these muscle benefits are imparted through changes in lean mass, contractile force, or another unknown mechanism. Future studies on denosumab should include assessment of muscle function and volume in a larger clinical trial.

The crosstalk of muscle and bone as a therapeutic avenue

In recent times, a growing focus has been building on the crosstalk between muscle, bone, and fat [47]. With the discovery of agents that are secreted from one of these tissues that impact the others, a range of new targets for anabolic interventions were identified. One of the key agents in this area is myostatin, a myokine secreted by muscle tissue in response to decreased muscular loading such as inactivity, injury, or sarcopenia. Myostatin acts to diminish muscular differentiation and protein synthesis, in part through Akt signaling [48], and its exogenous administration causes muscle wasting in mice [49]. Considering these effects, myostatin inhibition has been evaluated as a therapeutic method to increase bone mass.

In animal models, myostatin inhibitors have been shown to cause improvements in muscle mass in models of aging [50], muscular dystrophy [51], and cancer-induced cachexia [52]. These compounds have also been evaluated in humans, with a study on older fallers finding improvements in both lean mass and muscle function [53]. Another study of muscular dystrophy found that a myostatin inhibitor improved contractile strength in humans [54]. Generally, the inhibitors have been well-tolerated, with few significant adverse events [55]. However, from the view of osteosarcopenia, their effect on bone is yet to be demonstrated. Myostatin is known to inhibit osteoblast differentiation and osteogenesis [56,57], as well as osteoclast formation through RANKL signaling [58]. In mice, inhibition of myostatin has been shown to have anabolic effects on bone. Myostatin deficient mice have been shown to have greater bone mineral content, particularly at sites of muscle attachment [59], a greater osteogenic response to exercise [60], and increased bone healing after fracture [61]. A myostatin inhibitor has also been shown to cause an increase in osteogenesis [62], though another compound tested in the same study improved muscle alone. While positive, effects of myostatin inhibition on bone are yet to be demonstrated, leaving this a hopeful, but an unproven candidate for the treatment of osteosarcopenia.

While myostatin has garnered the most attention as a therapeutic in muscle and bone, a range of other factors has been identified in recent years as having a dual role in both tissues. Compounds such as osteocalcin, irisin, and interleukin-6 have effects on both physiologies, however, no strong data has emerged yet to suggest a role for them as therapeutics [47].

Future directions and conclusions

Despite recent interest in dual anabolic therapies for muscle and bone in osteosarcopenia, potential therapeutics are still in their infancy. It is clear from recent developments that broad multisystem approaches are required to identify effective solutions. Crosstalk between muscle, bone, and fat is a key part of the pathogenesis of osteosarcopenia, and it stands to reason that consideration of the axes between these tissues will elucidate treatments for the disease [63]. Inhibitors of the lipotoxic effect of fat on muscle and bone, myokine stimulants or inhibitors of osteoclastogenesis, or completely external tissues which play a role in their development and maintenance could provide insight into efficacious methods of their treatment. Additionally, the approved or experimental treatments for osteoporosis or sarcopenia separately should be evaluated for an effect on their counterpart tissue. Their tightly interwoven physiologies of bone and muscle ensure that there is some likelihood of overlap in the therapeutic activity of these compounds, giving opportunity for fast progression in the area. For example, a study has found pamidronate, one of the first nitrogenous bisphosphonates was able to attenuate muscle loss after significant burns in children [64], however, this has not undergone further investigation to date. Finally, with the advent of cost-effective and efficient approaches for the assessment of genetics and the discovery of methods to manipulate genes safely, methods such as CRISPR may one day allow for targeting specific genetic pathways leading to disease. While still in the far future, as the exponential advance of medical sciences continues, these approaches will no doubt begin to be applied to the aging process in the musculoskeletal system.

While there have been some advances in finding dual muscle and bone pharmacotherapeutic approaches in recent years, there remains a long road ahead. As the focus on the androgen and endocrine pathways begins to recede, identification of new targets must become the priority, alongside evaluation of the promising molecules already identified. Understanding the interplay between the physiologies of bone, muscle and fat should be front and center of research efforts [63,65], as it will allow for the identification of the key factors and targets which co-regulate these tissues. These are likely to be the origin for the development of successful therapeutic approaches but will depend on the understanding of their role in health and disease.

References

[1] Kirk B, Zanker J, Duque G. Osteosarcopenia: epidemiology, diagnosis, and treatment—facts and numbers. J Cachexia Sarcopenia Muscle 2020.

[2] Fatima M, Brennan-Olsen SL, Duque G. Therapeutic approaches to osteosarcopenia: insights for the clinician. Ther Adv Musculoskelet Dis 2019;11, 1759720X19867009.

[3] Kirk B, et al. A clinical guide to the pathophysiology, diagnosis and treatment of osteosarcopenia. Maturitas 2020;140:27–33.

[4] Taaffe DR, et al. Estrogen replacement, muscle composition, and physical function: the Health ABC Study. Med Sci Sports Exerc 2005;37(10):1741–7.

[5] Herbst KL, Bhasin S. Testosterone action on skeletal muscle. Curr Opin Clin Nutr Metab Care 2004;7(3):271–7.

[6] Tracz MJ, et al. Testosterone use in men and its effects on bone health. A systematic review and meta-analysis of randomized placebo-controlled trials. J Clin Endocrinol Metabol 2006;91(6):2011–6.

[7] Chen J-F, et al. Androgens and androgen receptor actions on bone health and disease: from androgen deficiency to androgen therapy. Cell 2019;8(11):1318.

[8] Shigehara K, et al. Testosterone and bone health in men: a narrative review. J Clin Med 2021;10(3):530.

[9] Snyder PJ, et al. Effect of testosterone treatment on volumetric bone density and strength in older men with low testosterone: a controlled clinical trial. JAMA Intern Med 2017;177(4):471–9.

[10] Ng Tang Fui M, et al. Effect of testosterone treatment on bone remodelling markers and mineral density in obese dieting men in a randomized clinical trial. Sci Rep 2018;8(1):9099.

[11] Shin MJ, Jeon YK, Kim IJ. Testosterone and sarcopenia. World J Mens Health 2018;36(3):192–8.

[12] Griggs RC, et al. Effect of testosterone on muscle mass and muscle protein synthesis. J Appl Physiol 1989;66(1):498–503.

[13] Kenny AM, et al. Effects of transdermal testosterone on bone and muscle in older men with low bioavailable testosterone levels. J Gerontol A Biol Sci Med Sci 2001;56(5):M266–72.

[14] Kenny AM, et al. Effects of transdermal testosterone on bone and muscle in older men with low bioavailable testosterone levels, low bone mass, and physical frailty. J Am Geriatr Soc 2010;58(6):1134–43.

[15] Kong SH, et al. Dehydroepiandrosterone sulfate and free testosterone but not estradiol are related to muscle strength and bone microarchitecture in older adults. Calcif Tissue Int 2019;105(3):285–93.

[16] Shufelt CL, Braunstein GD. Safety of testosterone use in women. Maturitas 2009;63(1):63–6.

[17] Davis SR, et al. Global consensus position statement on the use of testosterone therapy for women. J Clin Endocrinol Metabol 2019;104(10):4660–6.

[18] Johansen JS, et al. Treatment of postmenopausal osteoporosis: is the anabolic steroid nandrolone decanoate a candidate? Bone Miner 1989;6(1):77–86.

[19] Frisoli Jr A, et al. The effect of nandrolone decanoate on bone mineral density, muscle mass, and hemoglobin levels in elderly women with osteoporosis: a double-blind, randomized, placebo-controlled clinical trial. J Gerontol A Biol Sci Med Sci 2005;60(5):648–53.

[20] Tsika R, Herrick R, Baldwin K. Effect of anabolic steroids on skeletal muscle mass during hindlimb suspension. J Appl Physiol 1987;63(5):2122–7.

[21] Narayanan R, Coss CC, Dalton JT. Development of selective androgen receptor modulators (SARMs). Mol Cell Endocrinol 2018;465:134–42.

[22] Bhasin S, et al. Drug insight: testosterone and selective androgen receptor modulators as anabolic therapies for chronic illness and aging. Nat Clin Pract Endocrinol Metab 2006;2(3):146–59.

[23] Mohler ML, et al. Nonsteroidal selective androgen receptor modulators (SARMs): dissociating the anabolic and androgenic activities of the androgen receptor for therapeutic benefit. J Med Chem 2009;52(12):3597–617.

[24] Gao W, et al. Comparison of the pharmacological effects of a novel selective androgen receptor modulator, the 5alpha-reductase inhibitor finasteride, and the antiandrogen hydroxyflutamide in intact rats: new approach for benign prostate hyperplasia. Endocrinology 2004;145(12):5420–8.

[25] Chen J, Kim J, Dalton JT. Discovery and therapeutic promise of selective androgen receptor modulators. Mol Interv 2005;5(3):173–88.

[26] Evans W, et al. Ostarine increases lean body mass and improves physical performance in healthy elderly subjects: implications for cancer cachexia patients. J Clin Oncol 2007;25(18_suppl):9119.

[27] Dalton JT, et al. The selective androgen receptor modulator GTx-024 (enobosarm) improves lean body mass and physical function in healthy elderly men and postmenopausal women: results of a double-blind, placebo-controlled phase II trial. J Cachexia Sarcopenia Muscle 2011;2(3):153.

[28] Dobs AS, et al. Effects of enobosarm on muscle wasting and physical function in patients with cancer: a double-blind, randomised controlled phase 2 trial. Lancet Oncol 2013;14(4):335–45.

[29] Dubois V, et al. Enobosarm (GTx-024) modulates adult skeletal muscle mass independently of the androgen receptor in the satellite cell lineage. Endocrinology 2015;156(12):4522–33.

[30] Le-Rademacher JG, et al. Overcoming obstacles in the design of cancer anorexia/weight loss trials. Crit Rev Oncol Hematol 2017;117:30–7.

[31] Hoffmann D, et al. Evaluation of ostarine as a selective androgen receptor modulator in a rat model of postmenopausal osteoporosis. J Bone Miner Metab 2019;37(2):243–55.

[32] Komrakova M, et al. The selective androgen receptor modulator ostarine improves bone healing in ovariectomized rats. Calcif Tissue Int 2020;106(2):147–57.

[33] Fonseca GWPD, et al. Selective androgen receptor modulators (SARMs) as pharmacological treatment for muscle wasting in ongoing clinical trials. Expert Opin Investig Drugs 2020;29(8):1–11.

[34] Zhao H-Y, et al. Relationships between insulin-like growth factor-I (IGF-I) and OPG, RANKL, bone mineral density in healthy Chinese women. Osteoporos Int 2008;19(2):221–6.

[35] Rudman D, et al. Effects of human growth hormone in men over 60 years old. N Engl J Med 1990;323(1):1–6.

[36] Liu H, et al. Systematic review: the safety and efficacy of growth hormone in the healthy elderly. Ann Intern Med 2007;146(2):104–15.
[37] Papadakis MA, et al. Growth hormone replacement in healthy older men improves body composition but not functional ability. Ann Intern Med 1996;124(8):708–16.
[38] De Spiegeleer A, et al. Pharmacological interventions to improve muscle mass, muscle strength and physical performance in older people: an umbrella review of systematic reviews and meta-analyses. Drugs Aging 2018;35(8):719–34.
[39] Barake M, et al. Effects of growth hormone therapy on bone density and fracture risk in age-related osteoporosis in the absence of growth hormone deficiency: a systematic review and meta-analysis. Endocrine 2018;59(1):39–49.
[40] Poidvin A, et al. Increased risk of bone tumors after growth hormone treatment in childhood: a population-based cohort study in France. Cancer Med 2018;7(7):3465–73.
[41] Nass R, et al. Effects of an oral ghrelin mimetic on body composition and clinical outcomes in healthy older adults: a randomized trial. Ann Intern Med 2008;149(9):601–11.
[42] White HK, et al. Effects of an oral growth hormone secretagogue in older adults. J Clin Endocrinol Metabol 2009;94(4):1198–206.
[43] Simpson E, et al. Clinical effectiveness of denosumab, raloxifene, romosozumab, and teriparatide for the prevention of osteoporotic fragility fractures: a systematic review and network meta-analysis. Bone 2020;130, 115081.
[44] Cummings SR, et al. Denosumab for prevention of fractures in postmenopausal women with osteoporosis. N Engl J Med 2009;361(8):756–65.
[45] Bonnet N, et al. RANKL inhibition improves muscle strength and insulin sensitivity and restores bone mass. J Clin Invest 2019;129(8):3214–23.
[46] Phu S, et al. Effect of denosumab on falls, muscle strength, and function in community-dwelling older adults. J Am Geriatr Soc 2019;67(12):2660–1.
[47] Kirk B, et al. Muscle, bone, and fat crosstalk: the biological role of myokines, osteokines, and adipokines. Curr Osteoporos Rep 2020;18(4):388–400.
[48] Trendelenburg AU, et al. Myostatin reduces Akt/TORC1/p70S6K signaling, inhibiting myoblast differentiation and myotube size. Am J Physiol Cell Physiol 2009;296(6):C1258–70.
[49] Zimmers TA, et al. Induction of cachexia in mice by systemically administered myostatin. Science 2002;296(5572):1486–8.
[50] Camporez J-PG, et al. Anti-myostatin antibody increases muscle mass and strength and improves insulin sensitivity in old mice. Proc Natl Acad Sci U S A 2016;113(8):2212–7.
[51] Nakatani M, et al. Transgenic expression of a myostatin inhibitor derived from follistatin increases skeletal muscle mass and ameliorates dystrophic pathology in mdx mice. FASEB J 2008;22(2):477–87.
[52] Klimek MEB, et al. Acute inhibition of myostatin-family proteins preserves skeletal muscle in mouse models of cancer cachexia. Biochem Biophys Res Commun 2010;391(3):1548–54.
[53] Becker C, et al. Myostatin antibody (LY2495655) in older weak fallers: a proof-of-concept, randomised, phase 2 trial. Lancet Diabetes Endocrinol 2015;3(12):948–57.
[54] Krivickas LS, Walsh R, Amato AA. Single muscle fiber contractile properties in adults with muscular dystrophy treated with MYO-029. Muscle Nerve 2009;39(1):3–9.
[55] Wagner KR, et al. A phase I/IItrial of MYO-029 in adult subjects with muscular dystrophy. Ann Neurol 2008;63(5):561–71.
[56] Qin Y, et al. Myostatin inhibits osteoblastic differentiation by suppressing osteocyte-derived exosomal microRNA-218: a novel mechanism in muscle-bone communication. J Biol Chem 2017;292(26):11021–33.

[57] Hamrick MW, et al. Loss of myostatin (GDF8) function increases osteogenic differentiation of bone marrow-derived mesenchymal stem cells but the osteogenic effect is ablated with unloading. Bone 2007;40(6):1544–53.
[58] Dankbar B, et al. Myostatin is a direct regulator of osteoclast differentiation and its inhibition reduces inflammatory joint destruction in mice. Nat Med 2015;21(9):1085–90.
[59] Hamrick MW, McPherron AC, Lovejoy CO. Bone mineral content and density in the humerus of adult myostatin-deficient mice. Calcif Tissue Int 2002;71(1).
[60] Hamrick MW, et al. Increased muscle mass with myostatin deficiency improves gains in bone strength with exercise. J Bone Miner Res 2006;21(3):477–83.
[61] Kellum E, et al. Myostatin (GDF-8) deficiency increases fracture callus size, Sox-5 expression, and callus bone volume. Bone 2009;44(1):17–23.
[62] Bialek P, et al. A myostatin and activin decoy receptor enhances bone formation in mice. Bone 2014;60:162–71.
[63] Colón-Emeric C, et al. AGS and NIA bench-to bedside conference summary: osteoporosis and soft tissue (muscle and fat) disorders. J Am Geriatr Soc 2020;68(1):31–8.
[64] Børsheim E, et al. Pamidronate attenuates muscle loss after pediatric burn injury. J Bone Miner Res 2014;29(6):1369–72.
[65] Zanker J, Duque G. Osteoporosis in Older Persons: Old and New Players. J Am Geriatr Soc 2019;67(4):831–40. https://doi.org/10.1111/jgs.15716.

Chapter 17

The social context of osteosarcopenia: Risk factors and social impact

Sharon L. Brennan-Olsen[a,b,c,d], Kate Anderson[a,d], Alison Beauchamp[b,c,e], Jordan O'Connor[g], and Rachel L. Duckham[b,c,f]

[a]*Deakin University, School of Health and Social Development, Geelong, VIC, Australia,* [b]*Department of Medicine-Western Health, University of Melbourne, St Albans, VIC, Australia,* [c]*Australian Institute for Musculoskeletal Science (AIMSS), University of Melbourne and Western Health, St Albans, VIC, Australia,* [d]*Institute for Health Transformation, Deakin University, Geelong, VIC, Australia,* [e]*School of Rural Health, Monash University, Warragul, VIC, Australia,* [f]*Institute for Physical Activity and Nutrition (IPAN), Deakin University, Geelong, VIC, Australia,* [g]*Federation University, School of Health and Life Science, Ballarat, VIC, Australia*

It is well-documented that "...the conditions in which people are born, grow, work, live, and age..." [1] can negatively, or positively, influence our health. With few exceptions, an inverse association is reported between social advantage and chronic disease [2,3]: this has been also observed across the lifecourse whereby childhood exposures negatively influence health outcomes in later life [4–6]. One of the earlier, now superseded, models to introduce the notion of how social factors and structures at the micro, meso, and macro levels influence health was posited by Dahlgren and Whitehead; known colloquially as the "rainbow model" [7] (Fig. 1). Subsequent models acknowledge multidirectional influences of social determinants, and the role of accumulated disadvantage over the lifecourse. Some are even inclusive of financial and social support on which one can draw in times of need, health policy, "norms," health literacy, and access to quality and/or preventive healthcare. What is consistent across the models is the imperative role of social and environmental factors in determining risk for chronic disease [2,3], indeed a large range of evidence suggests that the lifestyle-related risk factors for musculoskeletal conditions, and the conditions themselves, are no exception to this paradigm [2,3,8–14].

Osteosarcopenia. https://doi.org/10.1016/B978-0-12-820088-9.00016-0

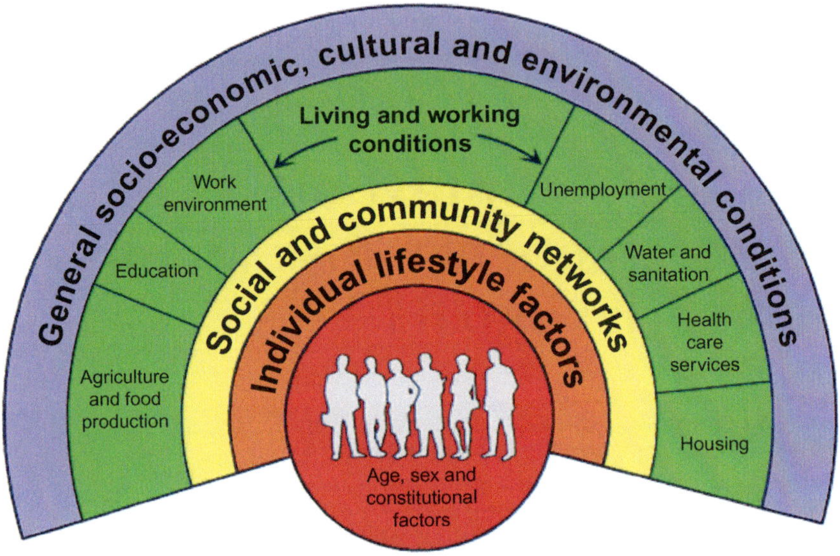

FIG. 1 Dahlgren and Whitehead "rainbow model" of social determinants of health outcomes [7]. *(Reprinted with permission from Dahlgren G, Whitehead M, World Health Organization Regional Office for Europe. Levelling up (part 2): a discussion paper on European strategies for tackling social inequities in health. Copenhagen: WHO Regional Office for Europe; 2008. https://apps.who.int/iris/handle/10665/107791, with permission from the World Health Organization.)*

Socially patterned risk factors for osteosarcopenia

The evidence of crosstalk between muscle and bone is increasing [15–17], in addition to evidence regarding muscle and bone being interconnected biochemically [18–20]. Furthermore, lifestyle-related factors that influence one tissue are likely to also influence the other. Not only are there many commonalities in lifestyle risk factors for sarcopenia and osteoporosis, and thus osteosarcopenia, these factors are also influenced by social determinants. For sarcopenia, three of the key modifiable risk factors are sedentary lifestyles, inadequate dietary protein intake, and vitamin D deficiency [21,22]. For osteoporosis, common modifiable risk factors are low body weight, alcohol intake of ≥ 30 g/day, current smoking, low dietary calcium intake, low serum vitamin D, and a range of chronic conditions [23]. The majority of these modifiable risk factors for osteoporosis and sarcopenia (and thus osteosarcopenia) all relate to economic and geographical access, and indeed affordable, available and accessible opportunities for education, housing, access to fresh foods, and social security policies, among many other social determinants. Other modifiable risk factors for osteosarcopenia include smoking and alcohol consumption, for which the association with education and income have been well-documented [24].

Childhood precursors to osteosarcopenia in later life?

Environmental factors and the interplay between social and biological factors during childhood are integral to the musculoskeletal system. These may not only dictate risk for osteosarcopenia in later life, but the accumulation of disadvantages over the lifecourse may increase the trajectory of bone and muscle loss. Here, we discuss the biological plausibility for such a suggestion, taking a focus on physical activity and dietary calcium intake.

The accrual of bone mass begins in utero and continues until reaching peak bone mass around the third decade of life [25] (Fig. 2). After a consolidation period, age-related bone loss involves a gradual and progressive decline [25,26] which is a result of a predominance of bone resorption over the bone formation [27]. Although a significant reduction in bone formation is associated with increasing age for both sexes [25], a steeper decline in bone loss is observed for women compared to men [26]: a factor primarily associated with low levels of estrogens across the menopausal years (Fig. 2). Interestingly, muscle mass also begins to decline with advancing age, with a decline of between 1% and 2% being observed every year after the age of 40 years [28], and an acceleration of this loss after the age of 65 years.

Bone

In a study of 729 participants in the Midlife in the United States Biomarker project, both childhood socioeconomic advantage and adult educational attainment, but not adult financial status, were associated with higher adult lumbar spine bone mineral density [29]. Another study from the same cohort investigated childhood social adversity and bone strength in adults, including the ability of the femoral neck to withstand axial compressive loading (compression strength

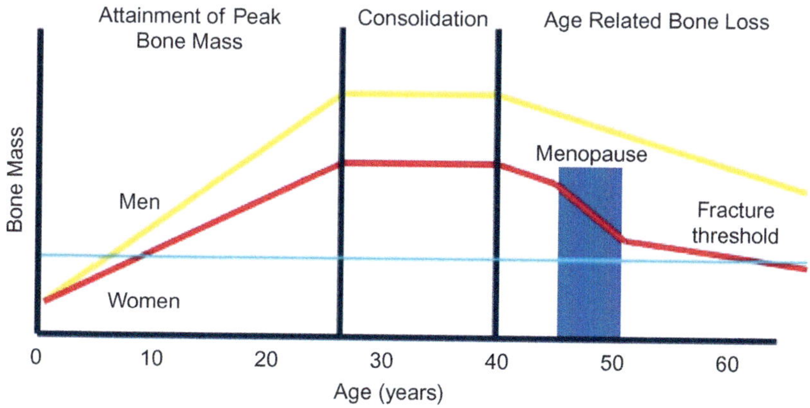

FIG. 2 Age-related changes in bone mass across the lifecourse. *(Modified from Compston JE. Review: osteoporosis. Clin Endocrinol (Oxf) 1990;33:653–82, and reprinted with permission from John Wiley and Sons, Inc.)*

index), the ability to withstand bending (bending strength index), and the ability to absorb the energy of an impact associated with a fall from standing height (impact strength index) [30]. The authors of that study reported that for every standard deviation (SD) increment of childhood advantage score, femoral neck indices increased by between 0.18 SD and 0.26 SD: those associations remained unchanged after adjustment for adult socioeconomic status [30]. Interestingly, only bending strength remained significant after adjustment was made for lifestyle behaviors [30]. Those data suggest an influential role in childhood social circumstances in bone acquisition. Furthermore, it is important to note that in older, community-dwelling women, each SD increment in femoral neck strength indices is associated with 57%–66% relative reduction in hip fracture risk over 10 years [30]. Given this, if strength indices had comparable fracture risk associations in older white men, we would expect 36% lower hip fracture risk in those with an advantaged childhood compared to those with the most disadvantaged childhood [30].

Muscle

Global estimates suggest that young people and older adults are among the most sedentary groups spending ~60% of their waking hours engaged in sedentary behaviors [31,32]. While it is well established that sedentary behavior increases the risk of pediatric obesity [33–35], and potentially results in early-onset cardio-metabolic diseases such as type II diabetes and cardiovascular disease [36], there is less consensus, however, about the potential detrimental impacts childhood, sedentary behavior may have on the musculoskeletal system, despite biological plausibility. Too much time spent sedentary, such as during extreme bed rest, can negatively affect muscle health and indeed increase muscle wasting [37]. Data suggest that increased sedentary behavior may result in skeletal muscle fiber replacement by noncontractile (fat) components potentially resulting in a deterioration of muscle quality from a younger age, which may be linked to muscle weakness and poor muscle function across the lifecourse [38]. In growing girls (age 9–12 years), Farr et al. [39] showed a negative association between low physical activity and skeletal muscle, fat, bone density, and strength parameters. Furthermore, that study showed low levels of physical activity were associated with lower muscle density [39]. Combined, these data suggest that reduced muscle density and lower physical activity may put children at risk of suboptimal skeletal loading. It is plausible that these findings may be heightened in children and adolescents with long-term sedentary behavior, resulting in a greater associated risk for early-onset osteosarcopenia later in life. However, in healthy growing children whether long-term sedentary behavior acts to undermine these effects of physical activity in a similar way remains unclear. Data hints at this issue, however, as in a study of 1403 UK-based men and women, low birth weight at birth and 1 year was significantly associated with poor adult grip strength even after adjustment for adult size [40,41].

Synergistic role of bone and muscle

To argue for biological plausibility, we highlight that muscle and bone both adapt mass and strength in response to mechanical load [42,43]. Therefore, mechanical loading, particularly in early life, plays essential role in the health of bone and muscle development [44,45]. Currently, there exists a paucity of data regarding the simultaneous contribution of muscle mass and strength to bone health during childhood. However, observational studies are suggestive of an indirect pathway between muscle power and bone strength [46,47]. It is plausible that these findings may be heightened in children and adolescents with long-term sedentary behavior, resulting in a greater associated risk for early-onset osteosarcopenia later in life.

Contemporary studies of children show unprecedented higher proportions of inactive and obese Australian children and adolescents. These measures of disproportionately increasing body habitus in children will have much potential to negatively influence the accrual of bone and muscle, plausibly increasing the risk of early-onset osteosarcopenia later in life.

Both muscle contraction and gravitational loading must be of sufficient magnitude and rate, and be sufficiently dynamic and multidirectional in their application, to provide the necessary stimuli to drive bone adaptation during growth [48]. This optimal loading stimulus may not be obtained in children who are spending a large proportion of their time in sedentary activities.

Conceptual model: The social-biological nexus

Based on a large evidence-base of research in the field of social disadvantage and osteoporosis [8–12], we have posited that socially patterned risk factors impact osteoporosis risk across the lifecourse, thus influencing the likelihood of osteoporotic fracture [49]. Here, we argue that the conceptual model for osteoporosis (Fig. 3) could be refocused to encompass the geriatric condition of osteosarcopenia. Indeed, it is not just the direct biological effect of risk factors, but the biological mechanisms at different life-stages [50], and what that may mean for the onset of osteosarcopenia.

In utero

While poor bone health is more commonly the domain of gerontologists, it has been postulated that osteoporosis is, in fact, a "pediatric disease with geriatric consequences" [51]. The "Barker hypothesis," which was initially about coronary heart disease, suggested that "...adverse environmental influences in utero and during infancy, associated with poor living standards, directly increased susceptibility to the disease" [4,5]. From this came the Developmental Origins of Health and Disease (DOHaD) theory, which suggested biological "programming" occurring in utero. Combined, the environmental, nutritional, and genetic influences in utero have the potential for long-term impact upon a broad range

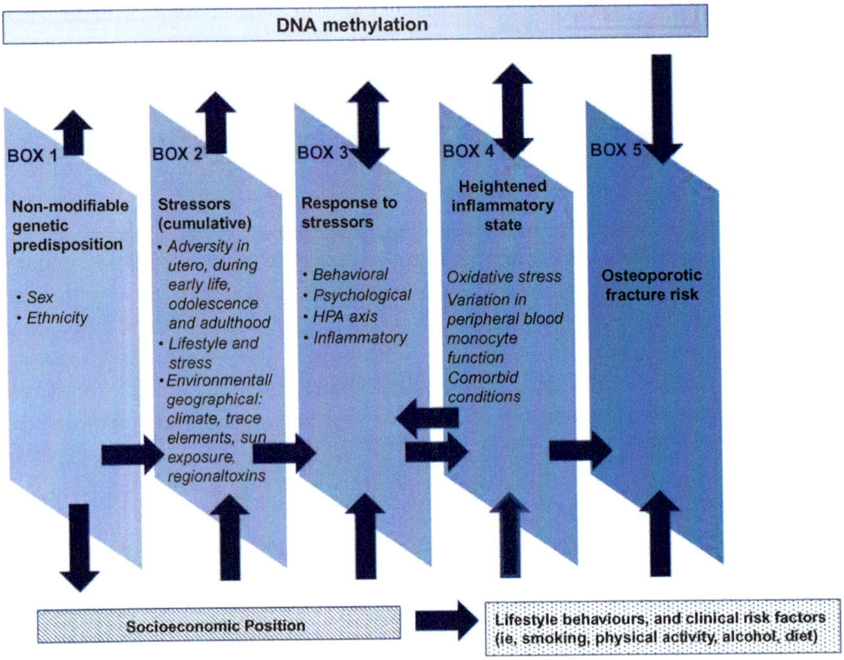

FIG. 3 A conceptual model of the relationship between socioeconomic factors and osteoporosis risk. *(Revised from Bone with permission Brennan-Olsen SL, Page RS, Berk M, Riancho JA, Leslie WD, Wilson SG, et al. DNA methylation and the social gradient of osteoporotic fracture: a conceptual model. Bone 2016;84:204–12.)*

of offspring health outcomes [6]: given this has been argued for osteoporosis [24,49,50] and sarcopenia [22], we must consider plausibility for including osteosarcopenia in this argument.

Various maternal conditions influence conditions in utero; the most common include stress, nutrition, and vitamin D [52]. These conditions can alter metabolism, influence placental calcium transporters, influence alterations to neuroendocrine-immune network set-points, upregulate immune function and inflammatory responses (via the HPA axis and/or sympathetic nervous system), increase the expression of glucocorticoid receptors, influence the methylation of the RXRA promoter, and alter the eNOS promoter [49]. In human growth muscle development first occurs in the formation of fibers approximately 6 weeks gestation [53]. The development of primary muscle fibers is controlled by genetic influences, whereas the development of secondary fibers (during week 8 and 21 gestations) are more sensitive to maternal and prenatal environmental factors such as nutrition and hormonal release [54]. That environmental sensitivity extends further into the postnatal period [22,55]. This notion can further be supported through the relationship of birth weight and adult grip strength suggesting the prenatal and postnatal period may have long-term importance for muscle function. The reports that the relationship of birth weight and grip strength remains following adjustment for adult size further supports the influence of early life on later muscle function. Although the mechanism remains unknown it is postulated that it reflects altered fiber type, proportion, and quality which may have consequences not only on the attenuation of peak muscle but also on the subsequent muscle decline [40].

Early childhood

It is argued that genetics and environment both significantly impact growth [49]; however, there are periods across the lifecourse in which one or the other factor appears dominant. For instance, at birth, we obtain a particular genetic blueprint that indicates our specific potential for growth and development without the influence of our environment [56]. However, our ability to meet that potential is often influenced by our environment, particularly during the first 1000 days of life [56]. Importantly, the timing, duration, frequency, and strength at which these environmental triggers occur in addition to the age and gender of the child will impact our potential to develop [56]. The primary control mechanism affected by environmental insults is the endocrine system (responsible not only for the control of specific hormones but also for complex associations with key tissue responses). It is important to note, that at some point in our life we will all experience environmental insult [56]. This is evident right from intrauterine in which growth would have been restrained by the size of our mother's uterus. Similarly, during childhood, many would have experienced childhood illness or disease negatively impacting growth and in particular that of bone and muscle tissue. These naturally occurring insults have previously been likened by Waddington to the movement of a boulder rolling down the groove of a valley [57]: whereby, if an insult occurs, the boulder is pushed out of its groove and forced up onto the walls of the valley. The magnitude of the deviation from the natural pathway will depend on the timing, duration, and strength of the insult. A greater more severe insult will result in greater long-lasting effects on growth and thus an associated affected to the development of bone and muscle [56].

A specific example during infancy and childhood is that in which environment insult results in the increased secretion of stress hormones and altered levels of cortisol, altering the HPA axis response, increasing proinflammatory cytokines, and heightening the inflammatory response resulting in differences in gene expression patterns [49]. A link between chronic stress and impaired bone growth and development in children has been documented [58]. The growth plate is targeted by stress through different mechanisms, including increased serum concentrations of proinflammatory cytokines and cortisol [58]. The impaired actions of the growth hormone-insulin-like growth factor-1 (IGF-1) axis have direct effects on the growth plate [59–61] and disrupt growth plate vasculature [58,60]. Proinflammatory cytokines and cortisol adversely affect several aspects of chondrogenesis in the growth plate [58,60]. Indeed, high levels of stress experienced in early life may reset the neurological and hormonal systems, thus permanently affecting children's epigenetic processes and phenotypic expression of disease risk [62–64].

Lower health literacy

We argue that there is a growing body of evidence to suggest that the relationship between social disadvantage and poorer bone health may be, in part, mediated by health literacy [24,65–68]. Health literacy is a multidimensional concept that encapsulates the capacity to access, understand, appraise, and apply health information to make decisions about health care, disease prevention, and health promotion [24,69]. Lower health literacy is a concern in both developed and developing countries including Australia and Europe where up to 60% of the population has less than adequate health literacy [70–72]. Health literacy is strongly associated with adverse health outcomes including a higher prevalence of chronic conditions, increased risk of mortality, delayed treatment, and increased hospitalizations [73–77].

Health literacy and risk factors

Suboptimal health literacy is most common in older populations, and those with a lived experience of social disadvantage [75,78–81]. Low health literacy is also associated with a higher prevalence of some risk factors for osteosarcopenia including nutrition, smoking, physical inactivity, and vitamin D knowledge [82–84], and has been associated with prefrailty and frailty [83,85]. Finally, risk factors for osteosarcopenia are greater among groups with lower socioeconomic status [86]. The combination of low health literacy and social disadvantage will thus disproportionately increase the likelihood that risk factors for osteosarcopenia are present.

Health literacy and prevention and treatment

Use of health services

Health care systems are increasingly difficult to navigate and evidence strongly indicates that low health literacy contributes to adverse health outcomes in these systems [73,74], including delayed care or access to providers [87]. Among older people, particularly those from CALD backgrounds there are difficulties accessing transport to health services, long waiting times for appointments, gender sensitivity, and feelings of shame when receiving care from a nonfamily member [88]. Socioeconomic disadvantage is also shown to be associated with increased length of hospital stay, fewer visits to specialists, and shorter waiting times [89–91]. For culturally and linguistically diverse (CALD) populations, access and uptake of services are also limited [92]. People with disabilities, particularly intellectual or developmental disabilities, are also subjected to health service exclusion as they age [93–96].

Ability to self-manage

Inadequate health literacy may also limit a person's ability to participate in decision-making, follow self-care recommendations, and implement self-management behaviors [97,98]. This is also the case for older adults, although one study identified that simple self-management tasks such as taking medication were achievable in adults aged over 75 years, even among those with lower health literacy [99]. Low health literacy may also be a risk factor for the physical decline in older adults [100], thus further impacting their ability to self-manage.

Adherence to treatment recommendations

The ability to adhere to treatment recommendations is compromised by age-related changes in health literacy, which may be partly explained by cognitive ability [101–104]. Mild cognitive impairment is associated with lower health literacy, with a stronger association seen in those with lower education [103]. Low health literacy and declining cognitive functioning may thus be barriers to adherence to treatment recommendations, more so among lower socioeconomic groups [81].

The combination of multimorbidity and lower health literacy also increase difficulty in adhering to treatment regimes. Multimorbid patients often have a high treatment burden and poorer quality of life and this has been associated with lower levels of health literacy in several studies [105–107]. Mechanisms may include difficulties with understanding and applying complex health information and instructions [107], particularly in relation to polypharmacy [108]. Limited affordability related to multimorbidity and associated high health care use may also be an issue for older people [88].

Given that low health literacy may be likely to contribute to premature bone deterioration, and thus disability and dependency with subsequent greater reliance on acute care, this prompts a shift toward addressing disparities in health outcomes by ensuring the delivery of health information and services in ways that address health literacy needs [108,109], particularly of older adults.

Social impact of osteosarcopenia

Quality of life

Older adults with osteosarcopenia are at higher risk of falls, fractures, and entry into a nursing home, thus exacerbating the trajectory of poorer quality of life [15]. Data shows that quality of life and health utility reduce significantly with the number of fractures experienced [110,111]. In older women aged 65 years and over, data suggest a greater likelihood of depression after experiencing a fracture compared to their counterparts of the same age that had not experienced a fracture [112]. For sarcopenia, a systematic review and metaanalyses reported an independently associated almost twofold increased likelihood of reporting depression [113]; while these findings were based on the observational studies alone, and thus causality cannot be determined, such a relationship is plausible due to the significant loss of muscle strength and functionality that accompanies sarcopenia [110,111]. The reduced aspirations of/and attainment of quality of life that accompanies depression, therefore, indicate the imperative of considering depression for those with osteosarcopenia.

Identity

Identity for older people bears a close relationship to concepts such as independence, autonomy, and a sense of belonging [114]. A person's self-concept is likely to play a significant role in their experience of osteosarcopenia; identity can be profoundly affected by physical and psychosocial consequences of osteosarcopenia, yet can also act as a powerful mechanism for coping and thriving with the condition [114]. Older community-dwelling adults recovering from recent hip fracture surgery [114,115] have described the importance of identity factors (including their dignity and independence, the ability to express personality traits, such as creativity, persistence, and positivity, and being reunited with familiar rituals and environments), as key facilitators in their self-confidence and overall recovery. Data from a qualitative study of men (age range 52″86 years) suggests that some men still consider osteoporosis, and thus plausibly osteosarcopenia, as being a "woman's" disease' [116]. Consider the impact of medical terminology on identity and empowerment: Taylor [117] reveals the concept of "frailty" as a double-edged sword for older people, on the one hand soliciting care and support for elders, yet at the same time risking the dignity and empowerment of this already marginalized population. Indeed, very recent qualitative data suggest that older adults' perspectives on the concept of frailty are highly negative-some have indicated that frailty is perceived as an unmodifiable state strongly associated with fragility, lowered self-worth, loss of control, and the end of life [118]. Further, being labeled as frail has been associated with "...a loss of interest in participating in social and physical activities, poor physical health and increased stigmatisation" for older adults [119]. Given this, and the self-reported value for older people with osteoporosis in identifying as "capable" and "resilient" [114,115], we might consider whether applying a label of "frail" to all older patients with musculoskeletal decline maybe, in fact, counterproductive [119].

Older people reported actively resist accepting a medical determination of frailty by using a range of strategies including maintaining meaningful task regimes (e.g., gardening, cooking, etc.), positively comparing their own situation to others', and compartmentalizing health conditions to avoid acknowledging an overall state of illness or physical weakness. Particularly for men, qualitative data has suggested that older men may apply more importance to the physical functionality of their body-a construct of masculinity-than women of the same generation [116,120,121]. Yet, despite drawing on their identity as a source of strength, older fracture survivors have also described experiences of fracture and vulnerability in the face of lost capabilities, or from their increased dependency and perceived burden on others [114].

People diagnosed with osteosarcopenia or its constituent conditions can struggle to accept their new diagnosis as part of their identity, especially when the conditions are not visibly manifest [122]. From a systematic review of qualitative studies concerning the lived experience of osteoporosis [122], it is observed that a lack of noticeable symptoms at the time of diagnosis can obscure patients' appreciation of fracture risk or disease severity. Without perceptible evidence to the contrary, people with low bone density may continue to identify as strong and at low-risk, or may see themselves as being the wrong "type" of person to develop osteoporosis [122–124]. Conversely, others may become unnecessarily anxious or risk-averse based on the medical or media hyperbole [125]. Meanwhile, the presence of visible or apparent disease markers (such as pain, fracture loss of height, or spinal deformity) often results in compromised biographical integrity, where once-healthy identities are threatened by struggles with isolation, vulnerability, and dependence on others [114,122]. Older adults with chronic physical conditions including osteoporosis report struggling with the appearance and increasing unreliability of their bodies, at times expressing feelings of shame, embarrassment, and reduced self-worth [126,127]. Regression analyses have similarly confirmed an association between frail/prefrail status and low self-esteem [128]. Traumatic events such as a fracture can result in a rapid and radical disruption to personal identity [114,115,122], leaving older fracture survivors especially vulnerable. Coping with a diagnosis is further complicated by ambiguous medical advice and media reporting around fracture risk, prognosis, and treatment options [123,124]. At the same time, some older people with osteoporosis [126] or hip fracture [114,115] seem to have accepted physical suffering and functional restrictions as a reality of "becoming old," and have described a gradual and successful adaptation to a new way of life, achieved through the use of adaptive aids, new supports, or the vicarious enjoyment of inaccessible activities.

Osteoporosis is often positioned as a "female disease" [116] and qualitative studies have reported descriptives such as "... the crumbly status of old age" (p. 32). These framings of osteoporosis can give rise to additional identity conflict for men and individuals who did not previously view themselves as elderly or frail [122]. There is also some evidence of the influence of belief systems and cultural variation in the way that osteoporosis is conceptualized and managed [129], which can, and perhaps should be, extrapolated to understanding osteosarcopenia. For example, "ageism" is a notion that refers to the stereotyped and discriminatory view of older persons based on their age; importantly, it is a contemporary paradigm of the Western world [129–131], and, while taking care not to apply a different stereotype to Asian-Pacific cultures, there exists an obvious east-west variation in filial piety. Negative stereotypes of older persons differ between countries and indeed between lower income vs moderate-higher income countries, thus indicative of not sharing a "western" value regarding advancing age [129], nor the potential for independence continuing through older age. Aligned with this issue is that aged care homes are predominantly a western phenomenon [129]. Although sarcopenia is still a relatively new disease and thus has little awareness in the public domain and is suboptimal in the clinical domain, it too is likely to develop these associations and corresponding identity challenges in time.

Social exclusion

Loneliness and social isolation among older adults can lead to adverse mental and physical health outcomes [132–134] including frailty [135] and increased risk of nursing home admission [136]. In turn, poor health and limited mobility can lead to social exclusion [137], further exacerbating the risk of social isolation. There is also evidence that the combination of social isolation, loneliness, and low socioeconomic status significantly increases the risk of poor health behaviors [138]. Both loneliness and social isolation are more prevalent among older adults with lower health literacy [99]. This may be due to less effective communication skills among older adults with low health literacy, limiting their ability to maintain a large social network [99]. Also, social isolation has been reported to increase the more times a fracture occurs [110]. Social participation has, however, been observed to facilitate both the maintenance of functional skills and recovery from serious fractures [114]. Older adults with osteoporosis or recent fracture report physical environments to be a major participation barrier [114,122]; it, therefore, follows that the provision of safe, accessible, and dignified transport and other spaces may enhance participation and wellbeing outcomes for older populations including those with osteosarcopenia. Additionally, older individuals whose social isolation is compounded by cognitive or communication disability should be referred for speech-language pathology or other allied health support, to ensure better participation in healthcare decision-making and wellbeing outcomes.

Entry into a nursing home

Having osteosarcopenia significantly increases the risk of entry into a nursing home [15]. As discussed earlier, while data are sparse it is likely that osteosarcopenia risk is associated with lower health literacy, and the condition itself has been well-documented as associated with poorer quality of life, we argue that older adults with osteosarcopenia are disproportionately disadvantaged. Considering the combination of lower health literacy, poor quality of life, having a little-understood geriatric condition, an increased risk of entry into an aged care facility, and an attributable increased risk of depression and lowered self-esteem or self-worth, it is vital in the clinical and research domains to consider the social context of osteosarcopenia. In terms of entry into an aged care facility, given this is determined by access to financial resources, the choice of a nursing home may be limited. Also, once residing in an aged care facility, personal visits may be fewer from their social circle and/or family. In one study, up to 40% of the nursing home, residents reported being lonely, with family relationships and level of mobility determining the degree of the loneliness felt by residents [139]. Nursing home residents report that this lack of meaningful relationships, in turn, leads to more loneliness and loss of self-determination [140], introducing a downward spiral toward a loss of purpose for living.

Conclusion

In this chapter, we posited a conceptual lifecourse model: the utility of which includes targeting those most at risk of developing osteosarcopenia by addressing causative environmental pathways that are greater for socially disadvantaged persons. We suggest that if we are to positively influence the process of healthy aging and reduce the plausibility for inequitable disparities in osteosarcopenia risk seen across social groups, we may need to focus on younger ages and address the modifiable lifestyle factors that are socially patterned. In older adults, clinical attention could be focused on identifying those most-at-risk and affording extra time to ensure effective health communications, thus ameliorating the negative effect of low health literacy on the likelihood of this condition. Although there exists a plethora of community-based health promotion programs that encompass an array of lifestyle modification options to enhance bone and muscle health, national health-related and multisectoral policies and strategies must prioritize health inequities and overall inclusion for this population [2,3,24,141].

References

[1] World Health Organization, https://www.who.int/social_determinants/en/.

[2] Marmot M. Achieving health equity; from root causes to fair outcomes. Lancet 2007;370:1153–63.

[3] Marmot M. Addressing the causes of the causes. Lancet 2018;391(10117):186–8.

[4] Barker D. The origins of the developmental origins theory. J Intern Med 2007;261(5):421–7.

[5] Barker D. Fetal origins of coronary heart disease. BMJ 1995;311(6998):171–4.

[6] Gluckman PD, Hanson MA, Cooper C, Thornburg KL. Effect of in utero and early-life conditions on adult health and disease. N Engl J Med 2008;359:61–73.

[7] Dahlgren G, Whitehead M. Policies and strategies to promote social equity and health. Copenhagen: World Health Organisation; 1992.

[8] Brennan SL, Holloway KL, Williams LJ, Kotowica MA, Bucki-Smith G, Moloney DJ, et al. The social gradient of fractures at any skeletal site in men and women: data from the Geelong osteoporosis study fracture grid. Osteoporos Int 2015;26:1351–9.

[9] Brennan SL, Yan L, Lix LM, Morin SN, Majumdar SR, Leslie WD. Sex and age-specific associaitons between income and incident major osteoporotic fracgtures in Canadian men and women: a population-based analysis. Osteoporos Int 2015;26:59–65.

[10] Brennan SL, Leslie WD, Lix LM. Associations between adverse social position and bone mineral density in women aged 50 years or older: data from the Manitoba Bone Density Program. Osteoporos Int 2013;24(9):2405–12.

[11] Leslie WD, Brennan SL, Prior HJ, Lix LM, Metge C, Elias B. The contributions of first nations ethnicity and income on post-fracture mortality; a population-based analysis. Osteoporos Int 2013;24(4):1247–56.

[12] Brennan SL, Winzenberg T, Pasco JA, Wluka AE, Dobbins AG, Jones G. Social disadvantage, bone mineral density and vertebral wedge deformities in the Tasmanian Older Adult Cohort. Osteoporos Int 2013;24(6):1909–16.

[13] Brennan SL, Henry MJ, Kotowicz MA, Nicholson GC, Zhang Y, Pasco JA. Incident hip fracture and social disadvantage in an Australian population aged 50 years or greater. Bone 2011;48(3):607–10.

[14] Brennan SL, Pasco JA, Urquhart DM, Oldenburg B, Wang Y, Wluka AE. Association between socioeconomic status and bone mineral density in adults: a systematic review. Osteoporos Int 2011;22(2):517–27.

[15] Hassan EB, Duque G. Osteosarcopenia: a new geriatric syndrome. Aust Fam Physician 2017;46(11):849–53.

[16] Sepulveda WA, Phu S, Bani Hassan E, Brennan-Olsen SL, Zanker J, Vogrin S, et al. The joint occurrence of osteoporosis and sarcopenia (osteosarcopenia): definitions and characteristics. J Am Med Dir Assoc 2020;21(2):220–5.

[17] Fatima M, Brennan-Olsen SL, Duque G. Therapeutic approaches to osteosarcopenia: insights for the clinician. Ther Adv Musculoskelet Dis 2019;11:1–15.

[18] Kirk B, Al Saedi A, Duque G. Osteosarcopenia: a case of geroscience. Aging Med (Milton) 2019;1–10.

[19] Kirk B, Phu S, Brennan-Olsen SL, Bani Hassan E, Duque G. Associations between osteoporosis, the severity of sarcopenia and fragility fractures in community-dwelling older adults. Eur Geriatr Med 2020;11:443–50 [online 11 March 2020].

[20] Laurent MR, Dedeyne L, Dupon TJ, Mellaerts B, Dejaeger M, Gielen E. Age-related bone loss and sarcopenia in men. Maturitas 2019;122:51–6.

[21] Brennan-Olsen SL, Hayes A, Duque G. Musculoskeletal health and healthy aging. In: Coll PP, editor. Healthy aging: a complete guide to clinical management. Springer; 2019.

[22] Shaw SC, Dennison EM, Cooper C. Epidemiology of sarcopenia; determinants throughout the lifecourse. Calcif Tissue Int 2017;101:229–47.

[23] Royal Australian College of General Practioners. Clinical guidelines for the prevention and treatment of osteoporosis in postmenopausal women and men [Internet]; 2010.

[24] Brennan-Olsen SL, Hyde NK, Duckham RL, Zengin A, Talevski J, Green D, et al. Bone quality in socially and ethnically diverse groups: downstream and upstream determinants across the lifecourse. In: Miszkiewicz JJ, Brennan-Olsen SL, Riancho JA, editors. Bone health: a reflection of the social mosaic. Springer; 2019.

[25] Demontiero O, Vidal C, Duque G. Aging and bone loss: new insights for the clinician. Ther Adv Musculoskelet Dis 2012;4(2):61–76.

[26] Compston JE. Review: osteoporosis. Clin Endocrinol (Oxf) 1990;33:653–82.

[27] Raisz L, Seeman E. Causes of age related bone loss and bone fragility: an alternate view. J Bone Miner Res 2001;16(11):1948–52.

[28] McLean RR, Kiel DP. Developing consensus criteria for sarcopenia: an update. J Bone Miner Res 2015;30(4):588–92.

[29] Crandall CJ, Merkin SS, Seeman TE, Greendale GA, Binkley N, Karlamangla AS. Socioeconomic status over the life-course and adult bone mineral density: the Midlife in the US Study. Bone 2012;5(1):107–13.

[30] Karlamangla AS, Mori T, Merkin SS, Seeman TE, Greendale GA, Binkley N, et al. Childhood socioeconomic status and adult femoral neck bone strength: findings from the Midlife in the United States Study. Bone 2013;56(2):320–6.

[31] Colley RC, Garriguet D, Janssen I, Creaig CL, Clarke J, Tremblay MS. Physical activity of Canadian children and youth: accelerometer results from the 2007 to 2009 Canadian Health Measures Survey. Health Rep 2011;22(1):15–23.

[32] Matthews CE, Chen KY, Freedson PS, Buchowski MS, Beech BM, Pate RR, et al. Amount of time spent in sedentary behaviors in the United States, 2003–2004. Am J Epidemiol 2008;167(7):875–81.

[33] Rey-Lopez JP, Vicente-Rodriguez G, Biosca M, Moreno LA. Sedentary behavior and obesity development in children and adolescents. Nutr Metab Cardiovasc Dis 2008;18(3):242–51.

[34] Hughes AR, Henderson A, Orti-z-Rodriguez V, Artinou ML, Reilly JJ. Habitual physical activity and sedentary behavior in a clinical sample of obese children. Int J Obes (Lond) 2006;30:1494–500.

[35] Mihrshahi S, Gow ML, Baur LA. Contemporary approaches to the prevention and management of paediatric obesity: an Australian focus. Med J Aust 2018;209(6):267–74.

[36] Healy GN, Mathrews CE, Dunstan DW, Winkler EA, Owen N. Sedentary time and cardio metabolic biomarkers in US adults NHANES 2003-06. Eur Heart J 2011;32(5):590–7.

[37] Koedijk JB, van Rijswijk J, Oranje WA, van den Bergh JP, Bours SP, Savelberg HH, et al. Sedentary behaviour and bone health in children, adolescents and young adults: a systematic review-supplementary presentation. Osteoporos Int 2017;28(10):3075–6.

[38] Farr JN, Laddu DR, Blew RM, Lee VR, Going SB. Effects of physical activity and muscle quality on bone development in girls. Med Sci Sports Exerc 2013;45(12):2332–40.

[39] Farr JN, Funk JL, Chen Z. Skeletal muscle content is inversely associated with bone strength in young girls. J Bone Miner Res 2011;26(9):2217–25.

[40] Sayer AA, Syddall HE, Martin HJ, Dennison EM, Anderson FH, Cooper C. Falls, sarcopenia, and growth in early life: findings from the hertfordshire cohort study. Am J Epidemiol 2006;164(7):665–71.

[41] Dodds RM, Roberts HC, Cooper C, Sayer AA. The epidemiology of sarcopenia. J Clin Densitom 2015;18(4):461–6.

[42] Robling AG. Is bone's response to mechanical signals dominated by muscle forces? Med Sci Sports Exerc 2009;41(11):2044–9.

[43] Hart NH, Nimphius S, Rantalainen T, Ireland A, Siafarikas A, Newton RU. Mechanical basis of bone strength: influence of bone material, bone structure and muscle action. J Musculoskelet Neuronal Interact 2017;17(3):114–39.

[44] Turner CH. Site-specific skeletal effects of exercise: importance of interstitial fluid pressure. Bone 1999;24(3):161–2.

[45] Anderson JJ. The important role of physical activity in skeletal development: how exercise may counter low calcium intake. Am J Clin Nutr 2000;71(6):1384–6.

[46] Hyde NK, Duckham RL, Wark JD, Brennan-Olsen SL, Hosking SM, Holloway-Kew KL, et al. The association between muscle mass and strength in relation to bone measures in a paediatric population: sex-specific effects. Calcif Tissue Int 2020;107:121–5.

[47] Janz KF, Letuchy EM, Burns TL, Francis SL, Levy SM. Muscle power predicts adolescent bone strength: Iowa bone development study. Med Sci Sports Exerc 2015;47(10):2201–6.

[48] Robling AG. Is bones response to mechanical signal domimated by muscle forces? Med Sci Sports Exerc 2009;41(11):2044–9.

[49] Brennan-Olsen SL, Page RS, Berk M, Riancho JA, Leslie WD, Wilson SG, et al. DNA methylation and the social gradient of osteoporotic fracture: a conceptual model. Bone 2016;84:204–12.

[50] Santurtun A, Riancho J, Riancho JA. The influence of maternal and social factors duirng intrauterine life. In: Miszkiewicz JJ, Brennan-Olsen SL, Riancho JA, editors. Bone health: a reflection of the social mosaic. Springer; 2019 [chapter 8].

[51] Hightower I. The origins of the developmental origins theory. J Intern Med 2007;261(5):412–7.
[52] Brennan-Olsen SL, Riancho J, Miszkiewicz JJ. The social context of bone health: conclusions and future directions. In: Miszkiewicz JJ, Brennan-Olsen SL, Riancho J, editors. Bone health: a reflection of the social mosaic. Springer; 2019.
[53] Phillips DI. Relation of fetal growth to adult muscle mass and glucose tolerance. Diabet Med 1995;12(8):686–90.
[54] Syddall HE, Aihie Sayer A, Dennison EM, Martin HJ, Barker DJ, Cooper C. Cohort profile: the Hertfordshire cohort study. Int J Epidemiol 2005;34(6):1234–42.
[55] Lohman TG, Roche AF, Martorell R. Anthropometric standardization reference manual. Champaign, IL: Human Kinetics Books; 1988.
[56] Cameron N. The human growth curve, canalization and catch-up growth. In: Cameron N, Bogin B, editors. Human growth and development. 2nd ed. Boston: Academic Press; 2012. p. 1–22 [chapter 1].
[57] Waddington CH. The strategy of the genes. London: Allen and Unwin; 1957.
[58] Sävendahl L. The effect of acute and chronic stress on growth. Sci Signal 2012;5(247):pt9.
[59] De Luca F. Impaired growth plate chondrogensis in children with chronic illnesses. Pediatr Res 2006;59(5):625–9.
[60] Wu S, Yang W, De Luca F. Insulin-like growth factor-independent effects of growth hormone on growth plate chondrogenesis and longitudinal bone growth. Endocrinology 2015;156(7):2541–51.
[61] Wong SC, Dobie R, Altowati MA, Werther GA, Farquharson C, Ahmed SF. Growth and the growth hormon-insulin like growth factor 1 axis in children with chronic inflammation current evidence, gaps in knowledge, and future directions. Endocr Rev 2016;37(1):62–110.
[62] Hunter RG. Epigenetic effects of stress and corticosteroids in the brain. Front Cell Neurosci 2012;6(18):1–18.
[63] Gudsnuk K, Champagne FA. Epigenetic influence of stress and the social environment. ILAR J 2012;53(3–4):279–88.
[64] Champagne FA. Epigenetic influence of social experiences across the lifespan. Dev Psychobiol 2010;52(4):299–311.
[65] Howard DH, Sentell T, Gazmararian JA. Impact of health literacy on socioeconomic and racial differences in health iin an elderly population. J Gen Intern Med 2006;21(8):857–61.
[66] Mantwill S, Monestel-Umana S, Schulz PJ. The relationship between health literacy and health disparities: a systematic review. PLoS One 2015;10(12):e0145455.
[67] van der Heide I, Wang J, Droomers M, Spreeuwenberg P, Rademakers J, Uiters E. The relationship between health, education, and health literacy: results from the Dutch Adult Literacy and Life Skills Survey. J Health Commun 2013;18:172–84.
[68] Friis K, Lasgaard M, Rowlands G, Osborne RH, Maindal HT. Health literacy mediates the relationship between educational attainment and health behaviour: a Damish population-based study. J Health Commun 2016;21(Suppl. 2):54–60.
[69] WHO Health Evidence Network synthesis report 65. In: WHO, editor. What is the evidence on the methods, frameworks and indicators used to evaluate health literacy policies, programmes and interventions at the regional, national and organizational levels? Copenhagen: WHO Regional Office for Europe; 2019.
[70] Health Literacy, Australia. In: ABo, editor. Statistics. Australian Bureau of Statistics: Canberra; 2008.
[71] World Health Organization. Health literacy: the solid facts. In: Healthy cities 21st century. Regional Office for Europe; 2013.
[72] Sørensen K, Pelikan JM, Röthlin F, Ganahl K, Slonska Z, Doyle G, et al. Health literacy in Europe: comparative results of the European health literacy survey (HLS-EU). Eur J Public Health 2015;25(6):1053–8.

[73] Berkman ND, Sheridan SL, Donahue KE, Halpern DJ, Viera A, Crotty K, et al. Health literacy interventions and outcomes: an updated systematic review. Evid Rep Technol Assess 2011;199(1):1–941.
[74] Ioka G. The relationship between health literacy and health outcomes in Australian, Canadian and New Zealand adults: a scoping review of interventions within the literature. An unpublished thesis submitted in partial fulfilment of the requirements for the degree of Master of Osteopathy, Auckland, New Zealand: Unitec Institute of Technology; 2018.
[75] MacLeod S, Musich S, Gulyas S, Cheng Y, Tkatch R, Cempellin D, et al. The impact of inadequate health literacy on patient satisfaction, healthcare utilization, and expenditures among older adults. Geriatr Nurs 2017;38(4):334–41.
[76] McNaughton CD, Cawthon C, Kripalani S, Liu D, Storrow AB, Roumie CL. Health literacy and mortality: a cohort study of patients hospitalized for acute heart failure. J Am Heart Assoc 2015;4(5):e001799.
[77] Bostock S, Steptoe A. Association between low functional health literacy and mortality in older adults: longitudinal cohort study. BMJ 2012;344:e1602.
[78] Beauchamp A, Buchbinder R, Dodson S, Batterham RW, Elsworth GR, McPhee C, et al. Distribution of health literacy strengths and weaknesses across socio-demographic groups: a cross-sectional survey using the Health Literacy Questionnaire (HLQ). BMC Public Health 2015;15:678.
[79] Hosking SM, Brennan-Olsen SL, Beauchamp A, Buchbinder R, Williams LJ, Pasco JA. Health literacy in a population-based sample of Australian women: a cross-sectional profile of the Geelong Osteoporosis Study. BMC Public Health 2018;18(1):876.
[80] Rikard RV, Thompson MS, McKinney J, Beauchamp AJ. Examining health literacy disparities in the United States: a third look at the National Assessment of Adult Literacy (NAAL). BMC Public Health 2016;16(1):975.
[81] Geboers B, Uiters E, Reijneveld SA, Jansen CJM, Almansa J, Nooyens ACJ, et al. Health literacy among older adults is associated with their 10-years' cognitive functioning and decline—the Doetinchem cohort study. BMC Geriatr 2018;18(1):77.
[82] Jayasinghe UW, Harris MF, Parker SM, Litt J, van Driel M, Mazza D, et al. The impact of health literacy and life style risk factors on health-related quality of life of Australian patients. Health Qual Life Outcomes 2016;14(1):68.
[83] Shirooka H, Nishiguchi S, Fukutani N, Adachi D, Tashiro Y, Hotta T, et al. Association between comprehensive health literacy and frailty level in community-dwelling older adults: a cross-sectional study in Japan. Geriatr Gerontol Int 2017;17(5):804–9.
[84] Christides T. Older adults' beliefs, knowledge and preferences for achieving healthy vitamin D status: a narrative review. Geriatrics (Basel) 2018;3(2):26.
[85] Huang CH, Lai Y-C, Lee YC, Teong XT, Kuzuya M, Kuo K-M. Impact of health literacy on frailty among community-dwelling seniors. J Clin Med 2018;7(12):481.
[86] Mackenbach JP, Valverde JR, Bopp M, Brønnum-Hansen H, Deboosere P, Kalediene R, et al. Determinants of inequalities in life expectancy: an international comparative study of eight risk factors. Lancet Public Health 2019;4(10):e529–37.
[87] Levy H, Janke A. Health literacy and access to care. J Health Commun 2016;21(Suppl):43–50.
[88] van Gaans D, Dent E. Issues of accessibility to health services by older Australians: a review. Public Health Rev 2018;39:20.
[89] Filc D, Davidovich N, Novack L, Balicer RD. Is socioeconomic status associated with utilization of health care services in a single-payer universal health care system? Int J Equity Health 2014;13(1):115.
[90] Moscelli G, Siciliani L, Gutacker N, Cookson R. Socioeconomic inequality of access to healthcare: does choice explain the gradient? J Health Econ 2018;57:290–314.

[91] Cookson R, Propper C, Asaria M, Raine R. Socio-economic inequalities in health care in England. Fisc Stud 2016;37(3–4).
[92] Page J, Comino E, Burgess M, Cullen J, Harris E. Participation in hospital in the home for patients in inner metropolitan Sydney: implications for access and equity. Aust Health Rev 2018;42(5):557–62.
[93] VicHealth. Enabling Health: Taking action to improve the health of people with a disability. Victorian Health Promotion Foundation: VicHealth, Melbourne; 2014. p. 2014.
[94] Krahn G, Hammond L, Turner A. A cascade of disparities: health and health care access for people with intellectual disabilities. Ment Retard Dev Disabil Res Rev 2006;12:70–82.
[95] Michael J, Richardons A. Healthcare for all: the independent inquiry into access to healthcare for people with learning disabilities. Tizard Learn Disabil Rev 2008;13(4):28–34.
[96] Ziviani J, Lennox N, Allison H, Lyons M, DelMar C. Meeting in the middle: improving communication in primary healthcare consultations with people with an intellectual disability. J Intellect Dev Disabil 2004;29(3):211–25.
[97] Ishikawa H, Yano E. Patient health literacy and participation in the health-care process. Health Expect 2008;11(2):113–22.
[98] van der Heide I, Uiters E, Rademakers J, Struijs JN, Schuit AJ, Baan CA. Associations among health literacy, diabetes knowledge, and self-management behavior in adults with diabetes: results of a dutch cross-sectional study. J Health Commun 2014;19(Suppl. 2):115–31.
[99] Geboers B, de Winter AF, Spoorenberg SLW, Wynia K, Reijneveld SA. The association between health literacy and self-management abilities in adults aged 75 and older, and its moderators. Qual Life Res 2016;25(11):2869–77.
[100] Smith SG, O'Conor R, Curtis LM, Waite K, Deary IJ, Paasche-Orlow M, et al. Low health literacy predicts decline in physical function among older adults: findings from the LitCog cohort study. J Epidemiol Community Health 2015;69(5):474–80.
[101] Kobayashi LC, Smith SG, O'Conor R, Curtis LM, Park D, von Wagner C, et al. The role of cognitive function in the relationship between age and health literacy: a cross-sectional analysis of older adults in Chicago, USA. BMJ Open 2015;5(4):e007222.
[102] Wilson RS, Yu L, James BD, Bennett DA, Boyle PA. Association of financial and health literacy with cognitive health in old age. Aging Neuropsychol Cognit 2017;24(2):186–97.
[103] Han SD, Boyle PA, James BD, Yu L, Bennett DA. Poorer financial and health literacy among community-dwelling older adults with mild cognitive impairment. J Aging Health 2015;27(6):1105–17.
[104] Fawns-Ritchie C, Starr JM, Deary IJ. Role of cognitive ability in the association between functional health literacy and mortality in the Lothian Birth Cohort 1936: a prospective cohort study. BMJ Open 2018;8(9):e022502.
[105] N'Goran AA, Pasquier J, Deruaz-Luyet A, Burnand B, Haller DM, Neuner-Jehle S, et al. Factors associated with health literacy in multimorbid patients in primary care: a cross-sectional study in Switzerland. BMJ Open 2018;8(2):e18281.
[106] Herzig L, Zeller A, Pasquier J, Streit S, Neuner-Jehle S, Excoffier S, et al. Factors associated with patients' and GPs' assessment of the burden of treatment in multimorbid patients: a cross-sectional study in primary care. BMC Fam Pract 2019;20(1):88.
[107] Friis K, Lasgaard M, Pedersen MH, Duncan P, Maindal HT. Health literacy, multimorbidity, and patient-perceived treatment burden in individuals with cardiovascular disease. A Danish population-based study. Patient Educ Couns 2019;102(10):1932–8.
[108] Parekh N, Ali K, Davies K, Rajkumar C. Can supporting health literacy reduce medication-related harm in older adults? Ther Adv Drug Saf 2018;9(3):167–70.

[109] Remshardt MA. The impact of patient literacy on healthcare practices. Nurs Manage 2011;42(11):24–9.

[110] Oleksik A, Lips P, Dawson A, Minshall ME, Shen W, Cooper C, et al. Health-related quality of life in postmenopausal women with low BMD with or without prevalent vertebral fractures. J Bone Miner Res 2000;15(7):1384–92.

[111] Palacios S, Neyro JL, Fernandez de Cabo S, Chaves J, Rejas J. Impact of osteoporosis and bone fracture on health-related quality of life in postmenopausal women. Climacteric 2014;1(17):1384–92.

[112] Williams LJ, Berk M, Henry MJ, Stuart AL, Brennan SL, Jacka FN, et al. Depression following fracture in women: a study of age-matched cohorts. BMJ Open 2014;4(2):e004226.

[113] Chang KV, Hsu TH, Wu WT, Huang KC, DS H. Is sarcopenia associated with depression? A systematic review and meta-analysis of observational studies. Age Aging 2017;46(5):738–46.

[114] Rasmussen B, Nielsen C, Uhrenfeldt L. Being active after hip fracture; older people's lived experiences of facilitators and barriers. Int J Qual Stud Health Well Being 2018;13(1):1554024. https://doi.org/10.1080/17482631.2018.1554024.

[115] Pol M, Peek S, van Nes F, van Hartingsveldt M, Buurman B, Kröse B. Everyday life after a hip fracture: what community-living older adults perceive as most beneficial for their recovery. Age Aging 2019;48(3):440–7.

[116] Solimeo SL. Living with a 'women's disease': risk appraisal and management among men with osteoporosis. J Men's Health 2011;8(3):185–91.

[117] Taylor BC. Elderly identity in conversation: producing frailty. J Appl Commun Res 1992;19(4):493–515.

[118] Archibald M, Lawless M, Ambagtsheer RC, Kitson A. Older adults' understandings and perspectives on frailty in community and residential aged care: an interpretive description. BMJ Open 2020;10(3):e035339. https://doi.org/10.1136/bmjopen-2019-035339.

[119] Warmoth K, Lang IA, Phoenix C, Abraham C, Andrew MK, Hubbard RE, et al. Thinking you're old and frail: a qualitative study of frailty in older adults. Ageing Soc 2016;7:1483.

[120] Nielsen DS, Brixen K, Huniche L. Men's experiences of living with osteoporosis: focus group interviews. Am J Mens Health 2011;5(2):166–76.

[121] Compton M, Mortenson WB, Sale J, Crossman A, Ashe MC. Men's perceptions of living with osteoporosis: a systematic review of qualitative studies. Int J Orthop Trauma Nurs 2019;1(33):11–7.

[122] Barker KL, Toye F, Lowe CJ. A qualitative systematic review of patients' experience of osteoporosis using meta-ethnography. Arch Osteoporos 2016;11(1):33.

[123] Otmar R, Reventlow SD, Morrow M, Nicholson GC, Kotowicz MA, Pasco JA. A cultural models approach to osteoporosis prevention and treatment. SAGE Open 2012;2(4):1–16.

[124] Reventlow S, Bang H. Brittle bones: ageing or threat of disease exploring women's cultural models of osteoporosis. Scand J Public Health 2006;320–6.

[125] Erol M. Melting bones: the social construction of postmenopausal osteoporosis in Turkey. Soc Sci Med 2011;73(10):1490–7.

[126] Cott CA, Gignac MAM. Independence and dependence for older adults with osteoarthritis or osteoporosis. Can J Aging 1999;18(1):1–25.

[127] Clarke LH, Griffin M, PACC Research Team. Failing bodies: body image and multiple chronic conditions in later life. Qual Health Res 2008;18:1084–95.

[128] Guerrero-Escobedo P, Tamez-Rivera O, Amieva H, Avila-Funes JA. Frailty is associated with low self-esteem in elderly adults. J Am Geriatr Soc 2014;6(2):396–8.

[129] Brennan-Olsen SL, Quirk SE, Hosking SM, Hyde NK, Duckham R, Millar L. Cultural and socioeconomic determinants of health aging'. In: Healthy aging. Springer Nature; 2019 [chapter 31].

[130] Palmore E. Ageism comes of age. J Gerontol 2015;706(6):873–5.

[131] Kite ME, Stockdale GD, Whitley BE, Johnson BT. Attitudes toward young and older adults: an updated meta-analytic review. J Soc Issues 2005;61(2):241–66.

[132] Courtin E, Knapp M. Social isolation, loneliness and health in old age: a scoping review. Health Soc Care Community 2017;25(3):799–812.

[133] Cantarero-Prieto D, Pascual-Sáez M, Fernández CB. Social isolation and multiple chronic diseases after age 50: a European macro-regional analysis. PLoS One 2018;13(10):392–7.

[134] Gardiner C, Geldenhuys G, Gott M. Interventions to reduce social isolation and loneliness among older people: an integrative review. Health Soc Care Community 2018;26(2):147–57.

[135] Gale CR, Westbury L, Cooper C. Social isolation and loneliness as risk factors for the progression of frailty: the English Longitudinal Study of Ageing. Age Ageing 2018;47(3):392–7.

[136] Hanratty B, Stow D, Collingridge Moore D, Valtorta NK, Matthews F. Loneliness as a risk factor for care home admission in the English Longitudinal Study of Ageing. Age Ageing 2018;47(6):896–900.

[137] Sacker A, Ross A, MacLeod CA, Netuveli G, Windle G. Health and social exclusion in older age: evidence from Understanding Society, the UK household longitudinal study. J Epidemiol Community Health 2017;71(7):681–90.

[138] Algren MH, Ekholm O, Nielsen L, Ersbøll AK, Bak CK, Andersen PT. Social isolation, loneliness, socioeconomic status, and health-risk behaviour in deprived neighbourhoods in Denmark: a cross-sectional study. SSM Popul Health 2020;10:100546.

[139] Trybusińska D, Saracen A. Loneliness in the context of quality of life of nursing home residents. Open Med (Wars) 2019;14:354–61.

[140] Paque K, Bastiaens H, Van Bogaert P, Dilles T. Living in a nursing home: a phenomenological study exploring residents' loneliness and other feelings. Scand J Caring Sci 2018;32(4):1477–84.

[141] Brennan-Olsen SL, Friel S. Australia's health divide: time to address the underlying causes. Med J Aust 2018;208(10):461–2.

Chapter 18

Models of care for falls and fracture prevention: A historical perspective

Naaz Parmar[a,b,c] and Larry Dian[a,b,d]
[a]*Division of Geriatrics, Faculty of Medicine, University of British Columbia, Vancouver, BC, Canada,* [b]*Faculty of Medicine, University of British Columbia, Vancouver, BC, Canada,* [c]*Pacific Geriatricians Group, Vancouver, BC, Canada,* [d]*Center for Hip Health and Mobility, Faculty of Medicine, University of British Columbia, Vancouver, BC, Canada*

Models of care for falls and fracture prevention

The authors of this chapter work at Vancouver General Hospital, a quaternary care center in British Columbia, Canada. As a major medical and surgical center, a large number of patients admitted following a fall require surgical interventions and often a prolonged hospitalization. A decline in functional status often follows this. In 2008, the local Centre for Hip Health, Vancouver Coastal Health Research Institute, and the University of British Columbia collaborated to form the Falls Prevention Clinic. This clinic accepted patients referred from acute care and the community who fulfilled their research criteria. All those who did not fulfill research criteria were referred for assessment and treatment in a General Geriatric Medicine Clinic as a Comprehensive Geriatric Assessment (CGA) was accepted as standard care. Patients at the Falls Prevention Clinic initially complete the Physiological Profile Assessment (PPA), which is then combined with a CGA to provide a treatment plan.

A CGA is a tool that has been shown in multiple metaanalyses to better identify, treat and prognosticate outcomes in older adults than standard medical assessment alone. In Struck et al.'s 1993 metaanalysis, a CGA was shown to decrease mortality by 14%–35%, have an odds ratio (OR) of 1.80 of living at home at 6 months, and reduce total readmission rates by 12% [2]. A metaanalysis by Ellis et al. in 2011 showed a CGA increased likelihood in patients being alive and living in their own home with a number needed to treat (NNT) of 17 for mortality benefit and an OR of 0.78 of needing to move to long-term care [3].

A CGA follows a multidomain model that is implemented in care settings spanning acute, outpatient, and long-term care. The CGA begins with the usual

Osteosarcopenia. https://doi.org/10.1016/B978-0-12-820088-9.00015-9

medical assessment domains of history of presenting illness and past medical and surgical history. Additional information recorded includes a functional review of Activities of Daily Living (ADLs) and Independent Activities of Daily Living (IADLs). A Review of Systems of the so-called "Geriatric Giants" including cognition, mobility (including falls), mood and mental health, sleep, pain, nutrition, continence, and polypharmacy is completed as an overlap with a basic functional review. A social history is then obtained with attention to the patient's support network and their personal history of educational status, work history, smoking, alcohol, and drug use. A review of their current living situation is also completed with questions regarding housing accessibility and knowledge of community supports. A physical examination as per a usual medical exam is then conducted with the addition of special tests for cognition, mobility, and mood. Standard investigations are reviewed, and additional ones are requested based upon a patient's presenting complaint (Fig. 1).

The PPA was developed in 2003 by the Falls and Balance Research Group of the Prince of Wales Medical Research Institute, Sydney, Australia [4]. The PPA consists of five parts: contrast sensitivity, position sense, muscle strength, reaction time, and postural sway. This information is collected and collated versus normative data, and deficits are identified. A printout of the information is created for the patient. Nonphysical risk factors for falls risk, including cognition and mood, are also assessed as the first stage of the Falls Prevention Clinic visit as part of a CGA. The information is then provided to a specialist in Geriatric Medicine (Geriatrician) who completes a CGA along with the PPA and can offer a targeted treatment plan for the patient. Of particular help is the printout of the PPA to illustrate the deficits and the goals for improvement. Patients are then followed in the 6-month interval to complete three visits (0, 6, 12 months). At each visit, the patient undergoes the same testing. The PPA is repeated, and the information is provided in a printout to the patient. The cognitive and mood screens of the CGA are also repeated. With the objective information, physicians and patients are able to track progress (Figs. 2 and 3).

The combined CGA and PPA identified several subtypes of patients concerning the etiology of the falls. The biggest group of our Falls patient population is generally frail with diffuse muscle weakness clinically labeled as sarcopenia. This is clearly seen when using the PPA with the predominance of patients falling below -2SD, and often -3SD, on postural sway. In about 20%–25% of patients, we identify polypharmacy or adverse drug reactions as a primary or major cause of falls. Medications that affect cognition and alertness are particularly important risk factors. Classes include major tranquilizers, neuroleptics, sedative-hypnotics, anticonvulsants, and antidepressants. Antihypertensives causing postural hypotension are also a concern. Medications that have high anticholinergic properties are particularly troublesome. The commonly used polypharmacy tools such as the Beers' Criteria [7] and STOPP/START [8] are helpful to identify particular culprit medications for a fall risk. Patients with a known neurodegenerative disorder are typically not seen in this clinic as it is felt these patients are best served in a clinic targeted to their movement disorder. However, we have found that falls can often be the first sign of these disease processes and

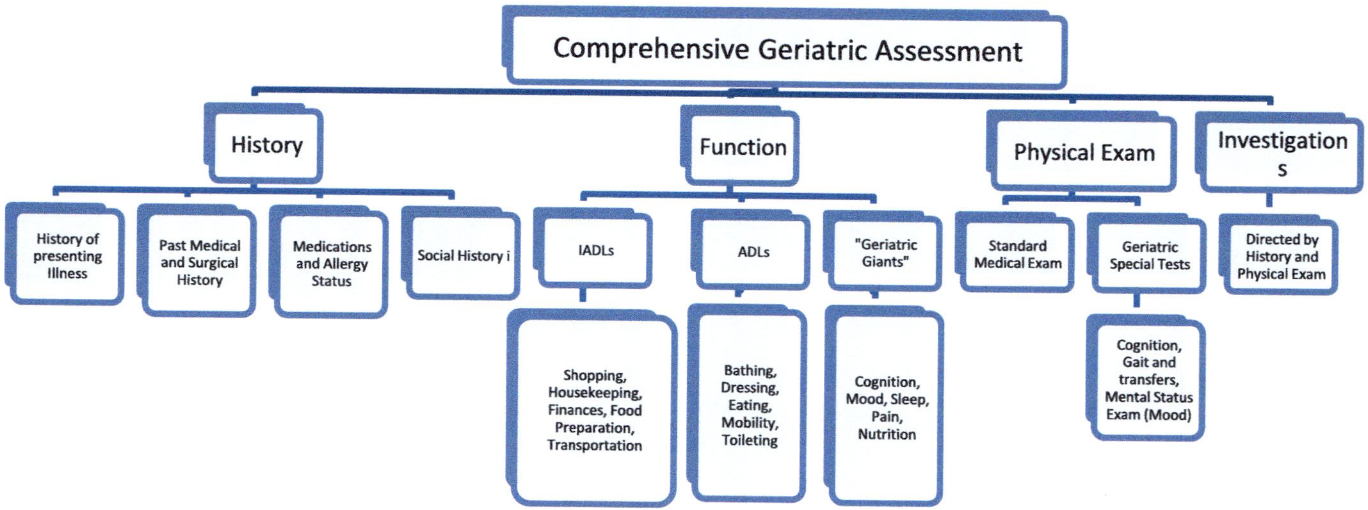

FIG. 1 Comprehensive geriatric assessment.

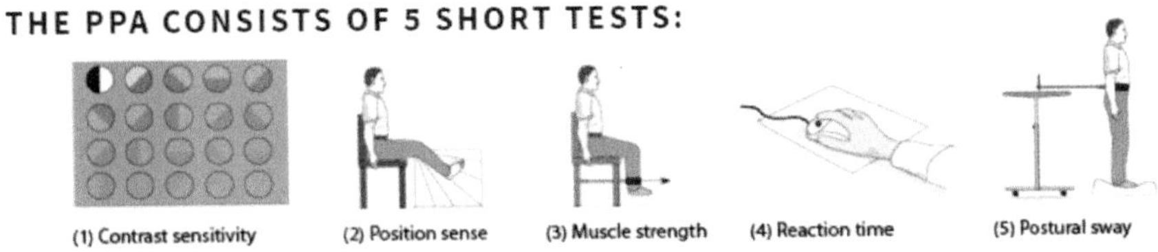

FIG. 2 From NeuRA the components of a PPA [5].

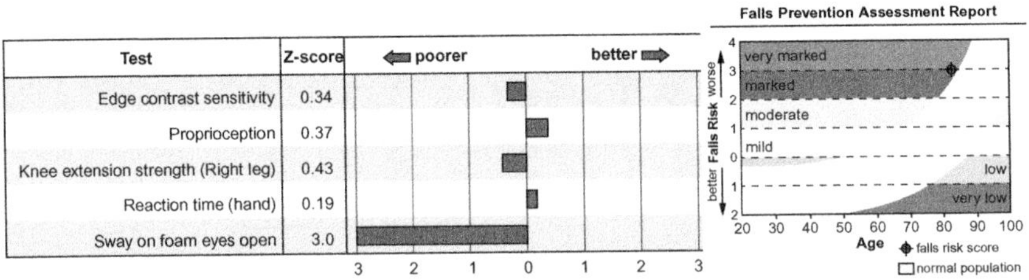

FIG. 3 Example of presentation of information for physician interpretation and patient education [6].

go unrecognized until a CGA and PPA unmask them. Approximately 10%–15% of our Falls Clinic population receive new diagnoses such as Parkinson's disease or Parkinson's plus syndrome, cervical myelopathy, or proximal muscle myopathy due to a primary neurological disorder. In about 10% of the population, no single major cause can be identified. In the setting, we have found it helpful to address all the potential risk factors. In doing this, the small incremental benefit that occurs is often sufficient to raise people out of the high-risk zone.

At the inception of the Falls Prevention Clinic, the first research question was "Does a home-based exercise program reduce falls among community-dwelling older adults who present to a fall prevention clinic after a fall?" [9]. This study was carried out from 2009 to 2018. This was a randomized control trial with a primary outcome of self-reported falls. The control arm received standard care from a Geriatrician. The intervention arm received usual care plus visits, and telephone follow-up with a physical therapist providing a strength and balance training exercise program. Both the control and intervention were carried out for 12 months. The absolute difference in fall incidence was 0.74, and there were no adverse events related to the intervention. From this research experience, the authors learned that the usual care of a CGA and treatment plan could be further optimized with a formalized exercise program. This could be through a direct connection with the clinic or a referral to community services offering similar programs.

The Falls Clinic requires more manpower than a standard clinic with support staff to complete the PPA and a Geriatrician to interpret and provide treatment plans. As such, a feasibility and acceptability study was conducted [10]. A 12-month prospective cohort study was conducted. This focused on >70-year-old community-dwelling adults attending the Falls Prevention Clinic. Clinic attendance was used as an assessment for feasibility. Acceptability was measured by compliance with recommendations, completion of monthly fall reporting calendars, and patient experience. The most common clinical recommendations were referrals to other healthcare workers, medication changes, exercise prescriptions, and lifestyle modifications. Feasibility was demonstrated by 65% attendance. Acceptability was demonstrated with 69% compliance. Referrals to other healthcare professionals and medication changes had a 78% compliance rate. Exercise prescription from the Geriatrician had a 58% compliance and lifestyle modifications 35%. Based upon this outcome, the team at the clinic was encouraged by the positive benefit to patients. It also highlighted that there is more to be done to improve the outcomes for patients and grow the clinic in scope and efficacy.

Osteoporosis care in our region was scattered across many different clinics. The largest of these was located at the local Women's Hospital, but the clinic was closed due to restructuring. Left without a hospital-based program and patients pending follow-up, a new Osteoporosis clinic was created and temporarily housed in the exact location as the Falls Prevention Clinic. Due to the overlap of Geriatricians involved in Falls and Osteoporosis, this worked well. Over time the strong relationship between Osteoporosis and Falls care became apparent. The history and physical exams required by both groups of patients are very similar. Treatment plans for both are parallel. The co-location of these clinics also sparked discussion among the clinicians and researchers involved. Many patients presented with both falls and fractures but those with only falls appeared to carry a higher fracture risk, and those with only fractures were worrisome for their falls risk (Fig. 4).

Patients were often referred from one clinic to the other to complete a workup when the Geriatrician discovered falls or fracture history during a CGA. The majority of the falls patients were over the age of 65 years and required an age-appropriate screening Bone Mineral Density or had other risk factors for osteoporosis. At the Osteoporosis clinic, a patient presenting with a fracture may not have a history of falls documented by emergency or primary care but, during the CGA reports worsening balance or falls in the last 12 months were identified. To optimize their care, they were then referred to the Falls Prevention Clinic to complete a PPA. From this experience, the idea of providing a combined Falls and Fracture Clinic rather than separate entities was born. The same collaborators from the initial Falls Clinic came together again to review potential research topics. With the added collaboration of Orthopedics a research proposal focused on hip fractures and a formal exercise program was begun. The next step will be to recruit these patients through the Fracture Liaison Service (FLS). FLS is a well-validated clinical pathway whereby patients who suffer a fragility fracture are identified, investigated, and treated (Fig. 5).

The creation of the Falls Prevention Clinic in 2008 demonstrated the benefit of exercise. The relocation of an Osteoporosis Clinic a decade later exposed the overlap and the need for a clinic covering the continuum of these diseases known as osteosarcopenia. Moving forward, we plan a Fracture Liaison Service to improve the scope of osteoporosis patients screened for osteosarcopenia. Falls frequently lead to fragility fractures, with over 95% of hip surgeries being due to a fall. Vertebral, radial, and humeral fractures are also an increasing concern

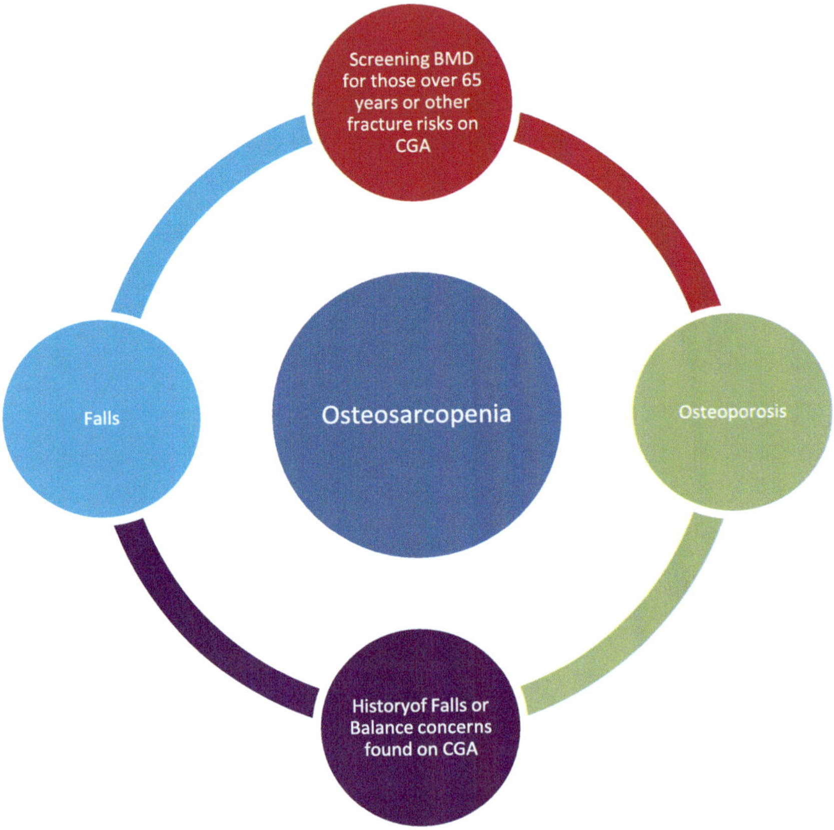

FIG. 4 Continuum of osteosarcopenia identified by individual falls and osteoporosis clinics leading to the falls and fracture prevention clinic.

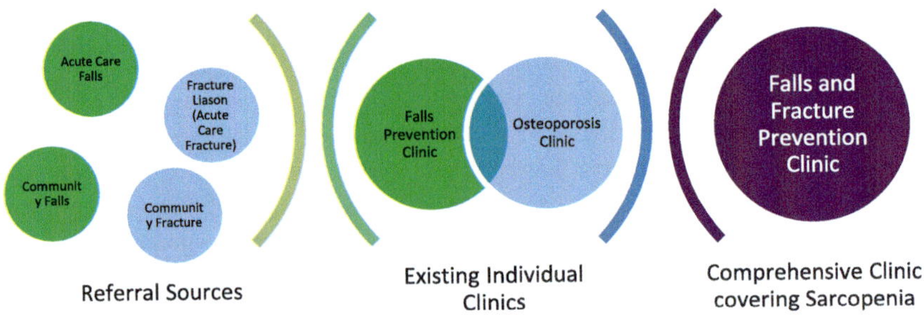

FIG. 5 Evolution of clinical care to a combined service.

with higher morbidity and mortality. The subsequent development would be to identify patients admitted to the hospital having sustained a fragility fracture. To this end, we are planning to initiate a randomized study to determine whether the standardized approach shown to work in community-based populations would be equally effective for a frail hospitalized patient population.

Summary

The presentations and health outcomes of sarcopenia [11] and osteoporosis often overlap. Increased mobility concerns, morbidity, and mortality are documented in both. A CGA is standard care for both. A history of the presenting complaint, past history, geriatric review of systems, medication reconciliation, and physical exam are crucial elements. A PPA is a tool for targeted physical exams and aids in information dissemination. Thus, we suggest the model of a single clinic receiving referrals for falls from the acute care setting and community, osteoporosis from the community, and the FLS from acute care. A single clinic allows these patients recognized at a high risk of osteosarcopenia to be screened by a PPA and a CGA. A comprehensive treatment plan outlining lifestyle, medication, and exercise modifications can then be presented, and the patient provided objective measures to follow from the PPA. Follow-up over the 6 and 12-month interval tracks progress and allows for clinical adjustments and reinforcement of suggestions to improve outcomes (Fig. 6).

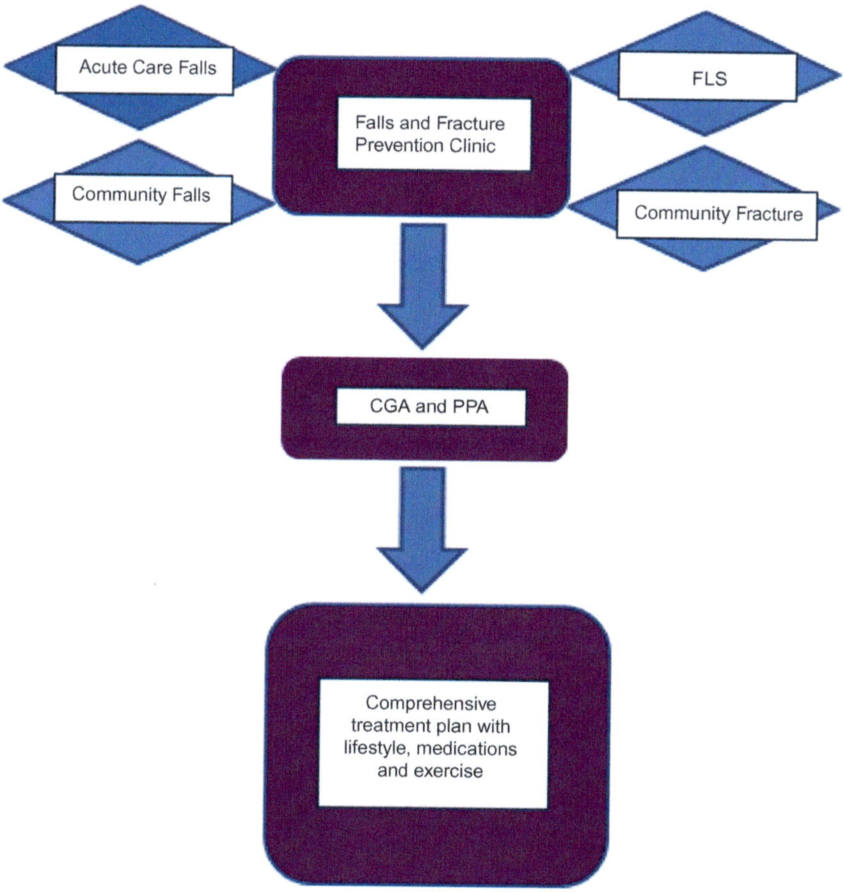

FIG. 6 Model of care for osteosarcopenia.

References

[1] Centers for Disease Control and Prevention., 2017, https://www.cdc.gov/features/older-adult-falls/index.html. [accessed 27.05.21].

[2] Stuck AE, Siu AL, Wieland GD, Rubenstein LZ, Adams J. Comprehensive geriatric assessment: a meta-analysis of controlled trials. Lancet 1993;342(8878):1032–6.

[3] Ellis G, Whitehead MA, Robinson D, O'Neill D, Langhorne P. Comprehensive geriatric assessment for older adults admitted to hospital: meta-analysis of randomized controlled trials. BMJ 2011;343. https://doi.org/10.1136/bmj.d6553, d6553.

[4] Lord SR, Menz HB, Tiedemann A. A physiological profile approach to falls risk assessment and prevention. Phys Ther Rehabil Sci 2003;83(3):237–52.

[5] Fallscreen The Falls Risk Calculator., 2021, https://www.neura.edu.au/wp-content/uploads/2016/05/Short-Form-Test-quads.png. [accessed 27.05.21].

[6] Fall Screen Clinic Information., 2021, https://www.neura.edu.au/research-clinic/fbrg/. [accessed 27.05.21].

[7] By the 2019 American Geriatrics Society Beers Criteria® Update Expert Panel. American Geriatrics Society 2019 updated AGS Beers Criteria® for potentially inappropriate medication use in older adults. J Am Geriatr Soc 2019;67(4):674–94. https://doi.org/10.1111/jgs.15767. Epub 2019 Jan 29 30693946.

[8] O'Mahony D. STOPP/START criteria for potentially inappropriate medications/potential prescribing omissions in older people: origin and progress. Expert Rev Clin Pharmacol 2019;13(1):15–22. https://doi.org/10.1080/17512433.2020.1697676. Epub 2019 Nov 30 31790317.

[9] Liu-Ambrose T, Davis JC, Best JR, Dian L, Madden K, Cook W, Hsu CL, Khan KM. Effect of a home-based exercise program on subsequent falls among community-dwelling high-risk older adults after a fall: a randomized clinical trial. JAMA 2019;321(21):2092–100. Erratum in: JAMA. 2019 Jul 9;322(2)174 31162569. PMC6549299.

[10] Davis JC, Dian L, Parmar N, Madden K, Khan KM, Chan W, Cheung W, Rogers J, Liu-Ambrose T. lGeriatrician-led evidence-based Falls Prevention Clinic: a prospective 12-month feasibility and acceptability cohort study among older adults. BMJ Open 2018;8. https://doi.org/10.1136/bmjopen-2017-020576, e020576. 30518579. PMC6286621.

[11] Beaudart C, Zaaria M, Pasleau F, Reginster J-Y, Bruyere O. Health outcomes of sarcopenia: a systematic review and meta-analysis. PLoS One 2017;12(1). https://doi.org/10.1371/journal.pone.0169548, e0169548. 28095426. PMC5240970.

Index

Note: Page numbers followed by *f* indicate figures and *t* indicate tables.

T

U

V

W

X

CPI Antony Rowe
Eastbourne, UK
January 24, 2024